COLORECTAL CANCER

BOERHAAVE SERIES FOR POSTGRADUATE MEDICAL EDUCATION
Vol. 18

PROCEEDINGS OF BOERHAAVE COURSES
ORGANIZED BY
THE FACULTY OF MEDICINE, UNIVERSITY OF LEIDEN
THE NETHERLANDS

COLORECTAL CANCER

edited by

K. WELVAART
Leiden University Hospital, Leiden

L.H. BLUMGART
Royal Postgraduate Medical School, Hammersmith Hospital, London

J. KREUNING
Leiden University Hospital, Leiden

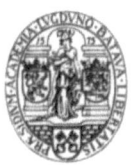

1980

LEIDEN UNIVERSITY PRESS
THE HAGUE / BOSTON / LONDON

Distributors:

for the United States and Canada

Kluwer Boston, Inc.
190 Old Derby Street
Hingham, MA 02043
USA

for all other countries

Kluwer Academic Publishers Group
Distribution Center
P.O. Box 322
3300 AH Dordrecht
The Netherlands

Library of Congress Cataloging in Publication Data   CIP

Main entry under title:

Colorectal cancer.
    (Boerhaave series for postgraduate medical education; v. 18)
    Includes index.
    1. Colon (Anatomy) – Cancer. 2. Rectum – Cancer. I. Welvaart, K. II. Blumgart, L.H. III. Kreuning, J. IV. Series. [DNLM: 1. Colonic neoplasms – Congresses.
2. Rectal neoplasms – Congresses. W3 B0672 v. 18 / W1520 C7193]
RC280.C6C66   616.99'4347   80-18688

ISBN-13: 978-94-009-9160-6   e-ISBN-13: 978-94-009-9158-3
DOI: 10.1007/978-94-009-9158-3

Cover design: Paul Burg

PREFACE

This book is based on the proceedings of a successful Boerhaave International Symposium on colorectal cancer held at the University of Leiden, 6-9 June, 1979. I would like to offer grateful thanks to the eminent clinicians and scientists who contributed both to the Symposium and to this book.

Colorectal cancer is a very common form of malignancy, particularly in the Western world, and there have been a number of recent developments in the management of this condition. This book has attempted to collate information on the current methods of investigation and treatment and I believe that it will prove valuable to all those interested in oncology.

The contents range widely, covering the entire field from epidemiology through screening methods, diagnostic approaches and therapy of both primary and secondary disease.

Perhaps the most outstanding new areas discussed and reflected in the proceedings are the possible range and scope of screening techniques, the new possibilities both in treatment and in endoscopic surgery now available as a result of developments in fibre-optic endoscopy, and new approaches and important parameters in staging of the disease.

Significant contributions were presented in relation to therapy and especially with approaches to the low rectal cancer and the use of newly developed stapling instruments in approaches to treatment. Adjuvant chemotherapy and radiotherapy were also discussed and in addition to treatment of primary disease there was a major section of the programme devoted to the management of disseminated malignancy. The possibility of surgical cure for secondary disease in the liver was reviewed and encouraging results reported.

L. H. BLUMGART

CONTENTS

PART VI. POSTOPERATIVE MANAGEMENT

CONTRIBUTORS

L.H. Blumgart, M.D., Royal Postgraduate Medical School, Hammersmith Hospital, Ducane Road, London W12 0HS, United Kingdom

D.M. van den Boomgaard, M.D., Department of Gastroenterology, Leiden University Hospital, Rijnsburgerweg 10, 2333 AA Leiden, The Netherlands

D.W. Day, M.D., Department of Pathology, University of Liverpool, P.O. Box 147, Liverpool L69 3BX, United Kingdom

A. Eardley, M.D., Department of Epidemiology and Social Research, University Hospital of South Manchester, Manchester M20 9QL, United Kingdom

V.W. Fazio, M.D., Department of Colon and Rectal Surgery, Cleveland Clinic, 9500 Euclid Avenue, Cleveland Ohio 44106, USA

G. Feifel, M.D., Department of Surgery, University Clinics Grosshadern, Marchioninistrasse 15, 8000 München, West Germany

P. Frühmorgen, M.D., Department of Medicine, University Clinic, Krankenhausstrasse 12, D 8520 Erlangen, West Germany

A.J.Ch. Haex, M.D., Department of Gastroenterology, Leiden University Hospital, Rijnsburgerweg 10, 2333 AA Leiden, The Netherlands

M.G. Herben, M.D., Department of Medical Oncology, Leiden University Hospital, Rijnsburgerweg 10, 2333 AA Leiden, The Netherlands

M.J. Hill, M.D., Bacterial Metabolism Research Laboratory, Central Public Health Laboratory, Colindale Avenue, London NW9 5HT, United Kingdom

O.M. Jensen, M.D., Centre International de Recherche sur le Cancer, 150 Cours Albert-Thomas, 69372 Lyon, France

J. Kreuning, M.D., Department of Gastroenterology, Leiden University Medical Hospital, Wassenaarseweg 62, 2333 AL Leiden, The Netherlands

M. Lipkin, M.D., Memorial Sloan-Kettering Cancer Center, 1300 York Avenue, New York NY 10021, USA

P. Lopes Cardozo, M.D., Department of Hematomorphology and Clinical Cytology, Leiden University Hospital, Wassenaarseweg 62, 2333 AL Leiden, The Netherlands

A. York Mason, M.D., St. Mark's Hospital, City Road, London EC1V 2PS, United Kingdom

P. de Ruiter, M.D., Department of Surgery, St. Elizabeth Hospital, Alkmaar

D.J. Ruiter, M.D., Department of Pathology, Leiden University Medical Hospital, Wassenaarseweg 62, 2333 AL Leiden, The Netherlands

W. Schellerer, M.D., Surgical Clinic, University of Erlangen-Nürnberg, Maximiliansplatz, D 8520 Erlangen, West Germany

E.A. van Slooten, M.D., Antoni van Leeuwenhoek Hospital, Plesmanlaan 121, 1066 CX Amsterdam, The Netherlands

J. Spierdijk, M.D., Department of Anaesthesiology, Leiden University Hospital, Rijnsburgerweg 10, 2333 AA Leiden, The Netherlands

M.W. Stearns, Jr., M.D., Memorial Sloan-Kettering Cancer Center, 1300 York Avenue, New York NY 10021, USA

P. Thomas, M.D., Department of Radiotherapy, Leiden University Hospital, Rijnsburgerweg 10, 2333 AA Leiden, The Netherlands

R.B. Turnbull, M.D., Department of Surgery, Santa Barbara Medical Foundation Clinic, Calle Real at San Marcos Pass Road, Santa Barbara CA 93102, USA

K. Welvaart, M.D., Department of Surgical Oncology, Leiden University Hospital, Rijnsburgerweg 10, 2333 AA Leiden, The Netherlands

R.C.J. Verschueren, M.D., Department of Surgery, Groningen University Hospital, Oostersingel 59, 9700 RB Groningen, The Netherlands

C.B. Williams, M.D., St. Mark's Hospital, City Road, London ECIV 2PS, United Kingdom

C.B. Wood, M.D., Department of Surgery, Royal Postgraduate Medical School, Hammersmith Hospital, London W12 0HS, United Kingdom

PART I

GENERAL ASPECTS

1. EPIDEMIOLOGY OF COLORECTAL CANCER

OLE M. JENSEN

Cancer of the large bowel, colon and rectum is among the most frequent cancers in Western Europe and its associated cultures of North America, Australia and New Zealand. In the United States, 2.7% of all deaths are caused by colorectal cancer, and, according to the Connecticut Cancer Registry, about 17.2% and 17.4% of all cancers in males and females, respectively, are located in the large bowel. Similar figures prevail in Northern Europe (e.g. proportion of all cancers in the United Kingdom: males 11.9%, females 14.8%; Denmark: males 15.9%, females 14.4%). In contrast these tumours are less frequent in Africa and Asia, e.g. 1.9% of all deaths are caused by colorectal cancer in Japan, where about 6.7% and 8.1% of all tumours in males and females, respectively, are located in the large bowel (1).

The life-time risk of developing colonic and rectal cancer may be approximated by the cumulative incidence from age 0 to 74 (2), which in Northwestern Europe and the United States is about 5%, e.g. Connecticut, U.S.A.: colonic cancer: males 3.5%, females 3.1%; rectal cancer: males 2.2%, females 1.3% (3).

Valid comparisons of the frequency of large bowel cancer in different populations and between various time periods can, however, only be made on the basis of mortality or incidence rates, i.e. when expressed as the number of deaths or new cases per 100,000 inhabitants per year. Due to the relatively favourable prognosis of large bowel cancer after treatment, comparisons of the occurrence of large bowel cancer are best based on incidence data and population differences in age distribution are taken into account by adjustment according to age of the 'World' standard population (1).

Such comparisons of routinely collected data, often denoted as descriptive epidemiology, have formed the basis for hypotheses concerning the determinants of colo-rectal cancer. Such hypotheses need testing by *ad hoc* designed studies of the case-control or cohort type. The following outlines briefly variations in the occurrence of colorectal cancer and the various aetiological hypotheses which have been suggested on this basis.

4

VARIATIONS WITH AGE AND SEX

Like most other malignant neoplasms of epithelial origin, the incidence of cancer of the colon and rectum increase with increasing age, Fig. 1. This is true for both males and females; but whereas the colonic cancer age incidence curves for the two sexes are approximately the same, the slope for cancer of the rectum is steeper for males than for females.

These characteristics of the age incidence curves translate themselves into different male/female ratios for cancer of the colon and cancer of the rectum, Table 1. In most countries, cancer of the colon is equally frequent among men and women, i.e. sex ratio around 1. In contrast, cancer of the rectum is almost invariably more frequent among men than among women. This feature has been taken to indicate that the aetiological factors of cancer of the colon and cancer of the rectum may in part be different. It should, nevertheless, be mentioned that there is a highly positive correlation between the occurrence of cancer of the colon and cancer of the rectum (4, 5).

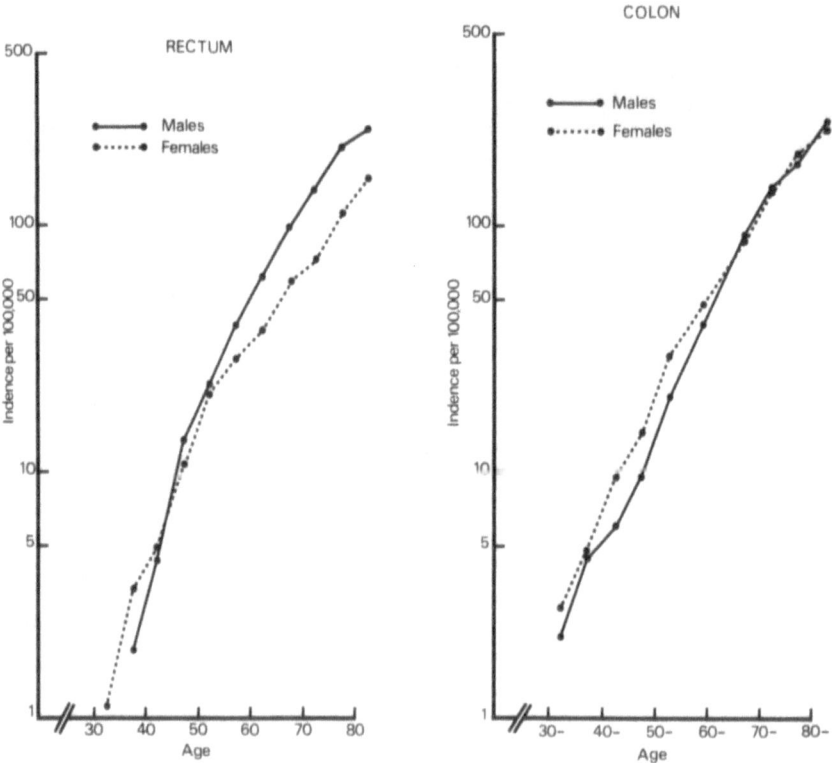

Fig. 1. Age-specific incidence of cancer of the colon and rectum among males and females. Denmark 1963-1968.

Table 1. World-wide distribution of colonic and rectal cancer and male/female ratio. Age-standardized incidence[a] per 100,000.

Registry	Colon (ICD 153)			Rectum (ICD 154)		
	Male	Female	M/F	Male	Female	M/F
Africa						
Nigeria, Ibadan	1.3	1.2	1.1	1.2	2.0	0.6
Bulawayo, African	7.0	5.8	1.2	1.3	0.0	—
America						
Brazil, Recife	2.8	4.1	0.7	2.7	7.7	0.4
Brazil, Sao Paulo	8.7	10.8	0.8	6.9	7.0	1.0
Canada, Alberta	17.1	18.5	0.9	10.6	6.9	1.5
Canada, Brit. Colombia	23.5	24.1	1.0	15.9	10.5	1.5
Canada, Manitoba	20.7	20.4	1.0	13.7	9.0	1.5
Canada, Mar. Prov.	19.3	23.4	0.8	13.5	9.9	1.4
Canada, Newfoundland	24.7	24.2	1.0	13.1	6.0	2.2
Canada, Quebec	16.2	18.1	0.9	12.7	8.5	1.5
Canada, Saskatchewan	17.8	18.9	0.9	13.8	9.4	1.5
Colombia, Cali	3.2	3.4	0.9	3.1	3.3	0.9
Cuba	6.9	8.7	0.8	4.2	4.2	1.0
Jamaica, Kingston	9.1	7.9	1.2	4.9	4.0	1.2
Alameda: White	25.3	22.2	1.1	15.0	10.2	1.5
Alameda: Black	23.0	19.4	1.2	10.7	6.1	1.8
Bay Area: White	28.3	24.0	1.2	15.2	10.4	1.5
Bay Area: Black	24.0	21.2	1.1	10.8	7.8	1.4
Bay Area: Chinese	23.5	13.8	1.7	19.5	9.4	2.1
Connecticut	30.1	26.1	1.2	18.2	11.1	1.6
Iowa	24.8	25.0	1.0	13.4	8.6	1.6
Detroit: White	26.2	21.8	1.2	16.0	8.9	1.8
Detroit: Black	24.5	22.7	1.1	13.8	8.2	1.7
New Mexico: Spanish	8.7	11.0	0.8	6.7	4.7	1.4
New Mexico: Other White	23.3	22.6	1.0	12.1	8.9	1.4
New Mexico: Amer. Indian	1.7	5.2	0.3	4.9	3.6	1.4
New York State	24.6	22.6	1.1	13.7	8.7	1.6
El Paso: Spanish	9.3	10.4	0.9	5.5	4.4	1.3
El Paso: Other White	15.4	17.1	0.9	6.8	6.2	1.1
Puerto Rico	6.0	6.7	0.9	4.2	5.0	0.8
Utah	16.3	16.9	1.0	9.2	6.9	1.3
Asia						
India, Bombay	4.6	3.3	1.4	4.4	2.6	1.7
Israel: all Jews	11.6	11.7	1.0	10.6	9.9	1.1
Israel: born Israel	8.7	5.4	1.6	5.1	8.3	0.6
Israel: born Eur. Amer.	12.9	13.4	1.0	11.9	11.2	1.1
Israel: born Africa, Asia	5.1	5.3	1.0	4.2	4.1	1.0
Israel: non Jews	2.3	1.6	1.4	3.8	1.2	3.2
Japan: Miyagi	5.6	5.4	1.0	6.8	5.0	1.4
Japan: Okayama	5.0	4.7	1.1	7.0	5.5	1.3
Japan: Osaka	6.3	5.0	1.3	6.9	4.7	1.5
Singapore: Chinese	11.9	9.5	1.3	10.0	7.0	1.4
Singapore: Malay	3.4	3.6	1.0	4.7	2.2	2.1
Singapore: Indian	5.0	13.0	0.4	6.4	5.3	1.2

Table 1 (continued).

Registry	Colon (ICD 153)			Rectum (ICD 154)		
	Male	Female	M/F	Male	Female	M/F
Europe						
Denmark	16.2	17.5	0:9	16.7	10.8	1.6
Finland	7.9	8.0	1.0	7.7	6.1	1.3
East Germany	9.6	9.6	1.0	11.3	8.4	1.4
West Germany: Hamburg	13.6	13.6	1.0	12.0	9.3	1.3
West Germany: Saarland	15.5	14.7	1.1	16.9	11.1	1.5
Hungary: Szabolcs	3.1	2.8	1.1	5.2	3.7	1.4
Hungary: Vas	9.1	7.7	1.2	11.0	7.0	1.6
Iceland	12.3	13.8	0.9	7.9	5.4	1.5
Malta	7.0	5.3	1.3	5.8	3.4	1.7
Norway	12.7	13.0	1.0	10.1	7.1	1.4
Poland: Cieszyn etc.	4.9	5.7	0.9	8.7	5.3	1.6
Poland: Cracow	6.0	5.3	1.1	6.0	4.0	1.5
Poland: Katowice	6.8	5.3	1.3	6.6	5.3	1.3
Poland: Warsaw City	10.9	8.6	1.3	7.7	5.4	1.4
Poland: Warsaw Rural	4.2	4.0	1.1	3.8	2.6	1.5
Romania, Timis	3.0	3.6	0.8	8.1	7.1	1.1
Spain, Zaragoza	6.5	5.5	1.2	6.9	4.4	1.6
Sweden	15.8	14.7	1.1	10.5	6.9	1.5
Switzerland, Geneva	18.9	13.5	1.4	13.8	8.0	1.7
UK: Birmingham	16.5	15.0	1.1	16.1	8.7	1.9
UK: Oxford	15.7	15.4	1.0	13.1	7.7	1.7
UK: Sheffield	13.8	13.0	1.1	13.3	7.2	1.9
UK: SMCR	13.9	13.7	1.0	11.2	7.1	1.6
UK: South West	14.7	15.3	1.0	12.7	8.3	1.5
UK: Liverpool	17.1	16.1	1.1	15.1	10.1	1.5
UK: Ayrshire	16.6	18.9	0.9	14.0	7.2	1.9
Yugoslavia, Slovenia	6.0	6.0	1.0	11.4	6.6	1.7
Hawaii: Hawaiian	14.1	16.9	0.8	9.4	2.9	3.2
Hawaii: Caucasian	23.9	22.9	1.0	13.5	12.0	1.1
Hawaii: Chinese	28.7	20.9	1.4	20.4	5.9	3.5
Hawaii: Filipino	16.8	15.3	1.1	14.5	0.0	—
Hawaii: Japanese	22.4	18.8	1.2	16.3	10.1	1.6
New Zealand: Maori	7.4	14.2	0.3	4.6	1.8	2.6
New Zealand: non-Maori	23.0	23.2	1.0	15.4	10.1	1.5

[a] World standard population (1)
Source: (1)

TIME TRENDS

Figs. 2 and 3 show the recent trends for cancer of the colon and cancer of the rectum, respectively.

For both sexes colonic cancer increases gradually in almost all of the countries or regions shown. The average annual increase in incidence is most

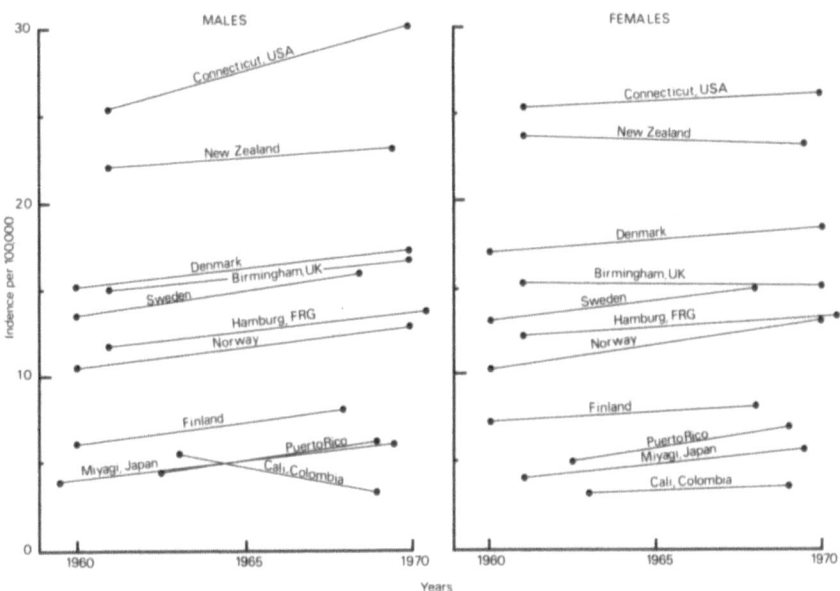

Fig. 2. Trends in incidence of cancer of the colon, 1960-1979, in selected cancer registry areas.

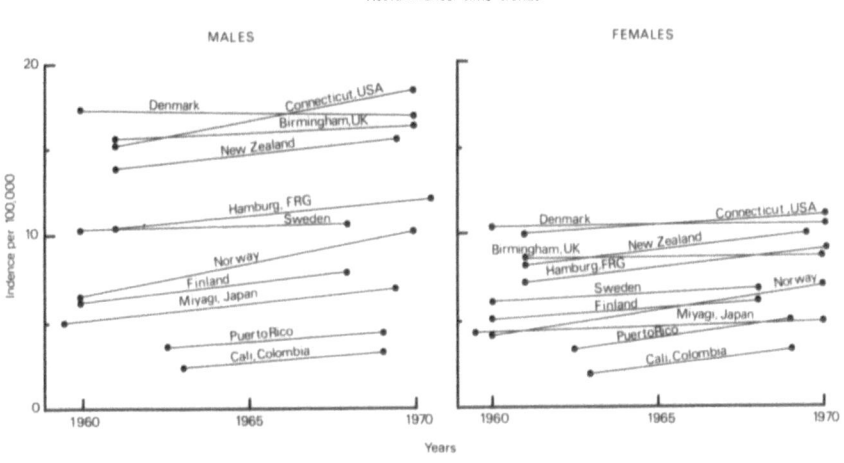

Fig. 3. Trends in incidence of cancer of the rectum, 1960-1970, in selected cancer registry areas.

marked in the medium and low incidence areas (e.g. Miyagi, Japan: 4.4%; Finland: 3.7%), and less so in high incidence areas (e.g. Denmark and Birmingham, U.K.: 1.5%; New Zealand 0.6%; Connecticut 2.1%).

The pattern observed for rectal cancer is less uniform, with increases like those observed for colon cancer prevailing in some countries; in others, like Birmingham, U.K., Denmark and Sweden, rectal cancer is stable or has even dropped slightly. Examining the time trends in areas with long-standing cancer registration, like Connecticut, U.S.A. (since 1935) and Denmark (since 1943), it appears that these trends in colorectal cancer have prevailed throughout a period covering 3 to 4 decades.

The validity of these upward trends has been questioned (6), in view of the simultaneous fall in gastric cancer, implying that part of the increase (and fall, respectively) may be due to the improved accuracy of the diagnosis of intra-abdominal tumours. It is not possible to evaluate the extent to which the increase was influenced by such artefacts, but it seems unlikely that improved diagnostic facilities provide the full explanation and the incidence of colonic cancer is undoubtedly increasing slowly in many parts of the world.

Such changes in disease frequency with time are generally held to indicate that environmental factors play a role in the aetiology, but recent attempts to relate such trends to dietary factors have not always been satisfactory (7).

GEOGRAPHICAL DIFFERENCES

International Variations

The main features of the international variations in large bowel cancer appear in Table 1, which shows an approximately 20-fold variation between selected countries or regions; this table is based on information taken from 'Cancer Incidence in Five Continents' (1). The highest incidences of both colonic and rectal cancer are seen in Western Europe and North America, whereas intermediate rates prevail in Eastern Europe. The lowest rates are seen in Asia, Africa and South America with the exception of high rates in Argentina, possibly related to a high consumption of meat.

Some of these differences may be due to underreporting in the low incidence areas, cancer of the large bowel being a disease which requires the availability of sophisticated technical equipment, surgical services or pathology services to be diagnosed. Inaccuracy in diagnosis and incomplete recording in such areas are, however, thought to account for only a small part of the international variation, as testified by the low rates in highly developed Japan. Comparisons between Denmark and Finland show that the differences encountered between the two countries seem to be real (8).

It appears from Table 1 that the incidence of cancer of the rectum varies somewhat less internationally than cancer of the colon. This is in accordance with the suggestion that in low incidence countries cancer of the rectum occurs relatively more frequently than cancer of the colon (9).

Within-Country Variations

International variations are generally much larger for cancer of the colon and rectum than the variations within any given country. Large bowel cancer occurs, however, in general more frequently in urban than in rural areas, e.g., Denmark, Poland (1, 6). In the United States an increase in the incidence of colonic cancer in blacks has followed the internal migration of blacks from rural to urban areas (10).

No marked differences in the incidence of colonic cancer are associated with socio-economic status in Western Europe or the United States. Some studies have, however, indicated that cancers of the sigmoid occur slightly more often in upper socio-economic classes, whereas rectal cancers show the opposite trend with higher risks for the lower socio-economic classes (11). In low incidence areas, like Hong Kong, a higher risk of colonic cancer has been demonstrated for the highest socio-economic class (12).

The risk of colorectal cancer among religious groups with special dietary habits has been studied within the United States. Seventh-Day Adventists, largely ovo-lacto-vegetarians who abstain from meat, have been shown to have a reduced risk of large bowel cancer (13).

The between and within-country distributions of colorectal cancer thus show that these tumours are associated with Western European culture and affluency. The low rates in Japan do not corroborate a risk associated with industrialization as such, and hypotheses have been centered around the dietary patterns of Europe and North America (10), supported by identification of the above-mentioned low-risk religious groups.

MIGRANTS

A decisive indicator of the role of environmental rather than genetic factors in the aetiology of large bowel cancer is provided by studies of migrants. The risk of colonic cancer increases among Japanese as they move from low incidence Japan to high incidence United States – Table 1 – and the finding of a higher risk of colonic cancer both among Japanese-born (Issei) and US-born (Nisei) Japanese in the United States than among Japanese in Japan (14) has been taken to suggest the importance of environmental factors during adult life in the aetiology of colorectal cancer. Recent comparative studies of Japanese in Hawaii and Japanese in Japan show that the migrants adopt the dietary habits of the American host population, thus adding further evidence for the aetiological role of Western food habits in colonic cancer (15).

Similar evidence for the role of the environment is provided by the higher rates of colonic cancer among European-born than among Asian-African-born Jews in Israel (16) and the fact that the incidence rates among American blacks are 10-20 times higher than those prevalent in West Africa, where many of these people come from (1).

DISTRIBUTION OF CANCER WITHIN THE LARGE BOWEL

Most tumours of the large bowel in Western European cultures are located in the sigmoid colon and upper rectum including the rectosigmoid junction. The distribution of malignant neoplasms within the large bowel follows the same pattern in both high and low incidence areas, Fig. 4, with decreasing frequencies from the ascending to the transverse and descending colon, followed by higher frequencies in the sigmoid and rectum. Various investigators (4, 17) have pointed out the relative lack of cancers of the sigmoid in low incidence areas, and it has been suggested that the aetiological factors responsible for

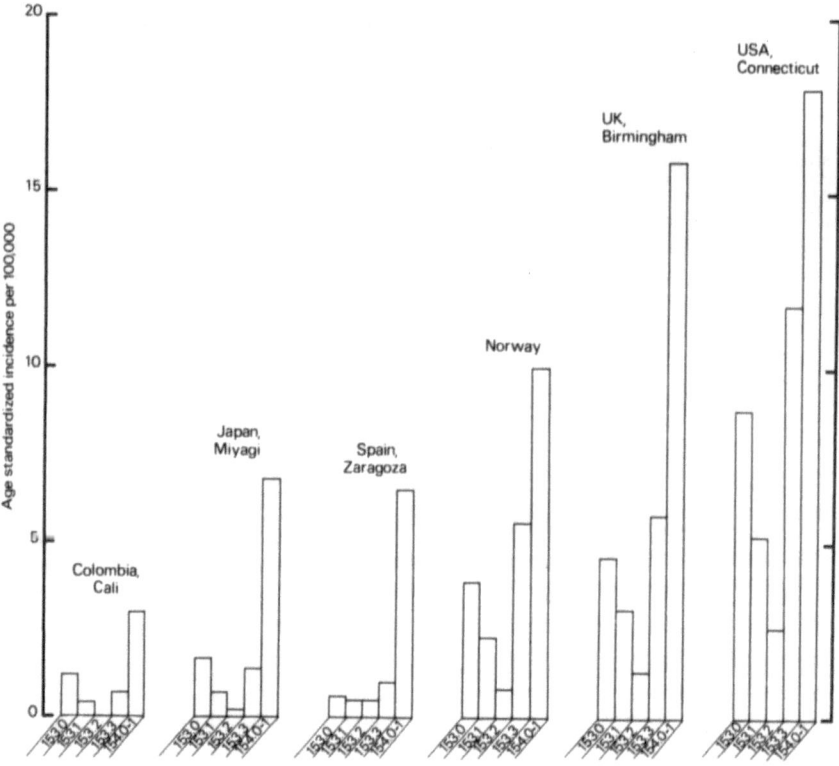

Fig. 4. Distribution of cancer within the large bowel among males in selected cancer registry areas. (153.0 = Appendix, cecum, ascending colon; 153.1 = Transverse colon; 153.2 = Descending colon; 153.3 = Sigmoid colon; 154.0, 1 = Rectosigmoid and rectum).

the high incidence in Western Europe and North America first lead to an increase in the frequency of cancers of the sigmoid, which is later followed by an increase in cancers of the right colon (17). Although these suggestions need to be substantiated, the implication would be that more than one aetiological factor determines the incidence of colonic cancer.

Cancers of the upper rectum seem epidemiologically to behave like cancers of the sigmoid; as a result it has been suggested that the two are aetiologically related in contrast to cancers of the lower rectum (5).

Due to well-known uncertainties in determining the boundary between the colon and the rectum, it is difficult to classify cancers of the most cancer-prone part of the large bowel as belonging to either of these sites. Specific comparative studies of the distribution of tumours in the rectum, the recto-sigmoid junction and the sigmoid colon are needed to tell us more about the variation among populations in the frequency of tumours of this area; only then can firm conclusions be drawn concerning the aetiological differences between cancers of the lower rectum and the remainder of the large bowel.

CLUES TO AETIOLOGY

Descriptive epidemiology thus points to factors associated with westernized societies as being of aetiological importance in large bowel cancer. Although family studies have provided evidence for a genetically determined suscepti-bility in some cases (18), the studies of migrants and religious groups referred to above show that environmental factors are of overwhelming importance.

When considering the possible environmental factors of importance in cancer of the large bowel, it is natural to concentrate on food or components thereof. Energy-rich, highly refined food is characteristically eaten in high incidence areas. A high fat intake has been proposed as a risk factor since, by stimulating bile acid production and modifying the bacterial flora of the gut in an anaerobic direction, it may lead to an increase in the faecal concentra-tion of the co-carcinogenic steroid degradation products of bile acids (19, 20). National statistics on fat and meat consumption correlate positively with the incidence of colonic cancer (21, 22), and recent case-control studies have provided support for the role of these dietary items as risk factors in colonic cancer (23, 24).

On the basis of the international distribution of colonic cancer, it has also been suggested that the low amounts of fibre in western diets are responsible for the high incidence of colonic cancer by diminishing the faecal bulk and the mouth-anus transit time (25). Although crude fibre consumption does not correlate internationally with colonic cancer (22), recent comparative studies of Scandinavians (26) and Japanese (15) have shown that factors other than fat and bile acids may determine the risk of colonic cancer; one study provided support for the role of dietary fibre as a possible protective food component with an as yet unknown mode of action (26).

There are few aetiological studies of rectal cancer available, although the slight differences in the distribution of colonic and rectal cancer (e.g. sex ratio, socio-economic trends, time trends) suggest partly different aetiologies. Beer consumption has been advanced as a possible risk factor for cancer of the rectum (27) but a recent cohort study contrasting a group of heavy beer consumers with the general population in Denmark provides no support for a causal association between beer and rectal cancer (28).

CONCLUSION

The epidemiology of large bowel cancer points to environmental factors as determinants of the disease. Aetiological differences may exist for various segments of the bowel, in particular for the rectum and the colon. There is evidence that the aetiology is associated with the western life style, in particular the consumption of a high fat - low fibre diet. Further substantiation of the individual role of these food items as well as their interaction is needed before preventive dietary measures should be attempted.

REFERENCES

1. Waterhouse JAH, Muir CS, Correa P and Powell J (eds): *Cancer Incidence in Five Continents, Volume III,* Lyon, International Agency for Research on Cancer (IARC Scientific Publications No. 15), 1976.
2. Day N: A new measure of age standardized incidence, the cumulative rate. In: *Cancer Incidence in Five Continents, Volume III,* Waterhouse JAH, Muir CS, Correa P and Powell J (eds), Lyon, International Agency for Research on Cancer (IARC Scientific Publications No. 15), 1976, p 443-445.
3. Stukonis MK: Cancer Incidence Cumulative Rates – International comparison based on data from 'Cancer Incidence in Five Continents'. IARC Internal Technical Report No. 78/002, International Agency for Research on Cancer, Lyon, 1978.
4. de Jong U, Day NE, Muir CS, Barclay THC, Bras G, Foster FH, Jussawalla DJ, Kurihara M, Linden G, Martinez I, Payne PM, Pedersen E, Ringertz N and Shanmugaratnam T: The distribution of cancer within the large bowel. *Int J Cancer* 10: 463-477, 1972.
5. Berg JW and Howell MA: The geographic pathology of bowel cancer. *Cancer* 34: 807-814, 1974.
6. Clemmesen J: *Statistical Studies in the Aetiology of Malignant Neoplasms, Volume V, Trends and Risks, Denmark 1943-72.* Supplementum 261, *Acta path microbiol Scand,* Munksgaard, Copenhagen, 1977.
7. Enstrom J: Colorectal cancer and beer drinking. *Br J Cancer* 35: 674-683, 1977.
8. Jensen OM, Mosbech J, Salaspuro M and Ihamäki T: A comparative study of the diagnostic basis for cancer of the colon and cancer of the rectum in Denmark and Finland. *Int J Epid* 3: 183-186, 1974.

9. Hutt MSR: Epidemiology of chronic intestinal disease in Middle Africa. *Israel J Med Sci* 15: 314-317, 1979.

10. UICC. *Colo-rectal cancer*. UICC Technical Report Series, Volume 19. International Union Against Cancer, Geneva, 1975.

11. Office of Population Censuses and Surveys: Occupational Mortality. The Registrar General's decennial supplement for England and Wales, 1970-1972, series DS No 1. London, Her Majesty's Stationery Office, 1978.

12. Crowther JS, Drasar BS, Hill MJ, MacLennan R, Magning D, Peach S and Teoh-Chan CH: Faecal steroids and bacteria and large bowel cancer in Hong Kong by socio-economic groups. *Br J Cancer* 34: 191-197, 1976.

13. Phillips RL: Role of lifestyle and dietary habits in risk of cancer among Seventh-Day Adventists. *Cancer Res* 35: 3513-3522, 1975.

14. Haenszel W: Cancer mortality among the foreign born in the United States. *J Natl Cancer Inst* 26: 37-132, 1961.

15. Mower HF, Ray RM, Shoff R, Stemmermann GN, Nomura A, Glober GA, Kamiyama S, Shimada A and Yamakawa H: Fecal bile acids in two Japanese populations with different colon cancer risks. *Cancer Res* 39: 328-331, 1979.

16. Modan B: Patterns of gastrointestinal neoplasms in Israel. *Israel J Med Sci* 15: 301-304, 1979.

17. Haenszel W and Correa P: Cancer of the colon and rectum and adenomatous polyps. *Cancer* 28: 14-24, 1971.

18. Anderson DE: Familial susceptibility. In: *Persons at high risk of cancer. An approach to cancer etiology and control*. Fraumeni Jr. JF (ed), Academic Press Inc., New York, 1975.

19. Aries V, Crowther JS, Drasar BS, Hill MJ and Williams REO: Bacteria and the aetiology of cancer of the large bowel *Gut* 10: 334-335, 1969.

20. Hill MJ, Drasar BS, Meade TW, Cox AG, Simpson JEP and Morson BC: Faecal bile-acids and clostridia in patients with cancer of the large bowel. *Lancet* i: 535-539, 1975.

21. Armstrong B and Doll R: Environmental factors and cancer incidence and mortality in different countries, with special reference to dietary practices. *Int J Cancer* 15: 617-631, 1975.

22. Drasar BS and Irving D: Environmental factors and cancer of the colon and breast. *Br J Cancer* 27: 167-172, 1973.

23. Haenszel W, Berg JW, Segi M, Kurihara M and Locke FB: Large-bowel cancer in Hawaiian Japanese. *J Natl Cancer Inst* 51: 1765-1779, 1973.

24. Dales LG, Friedman GD, Ury HK, Grossman S and Williams S: A case-control study of relationships of diet and other traits to colorectal cancer in American Blacks. *Am J Epidemiol* 109 (2): 132-144, 1978.

25. Burkitt DP: Epidemiology of cancer of the colon and rectum. *Cancer* 28: 3-13, 1971.

26. IARC Microecology Group: Dietary fibre, transit-time, fecal bacteria, steroids and colon cancer in two Scandinavian populations. *Lancet* ii: 207-211, 1977.

27. Breslow NE and Enstrom JE: Geographic correlations between cancer mortality rates and alcohol-tobacco consumption in the United States. *J Natl Cancer Inst* 53: 631-639, 1974.

28. Jensen OM: Cancer morbidity and causes of death among Danish brewery workers. *Int J Cancer* 23: 454-463, 1979.

2. BACTERIAL FACTORS IN THE AETIOLOGY OF LARGE BOWEL CANCER

M.J. HILL

INTRODUCTION

The incidence of large bowel cancer shows a geographical variation, being high in North-West Europe, North America and Australasia and low in much of Africa, South-East Asia and the Andean regions of South America. Initially this distribution appears to favour a major link between the disease and genetic racial factors, since the populations with a high incidence of the disease include all of the Anglo-Saxon countries together with the North and West European peoples and very few others. However, studies of migrants have led to the rejection of this possibility since first generation Japanese migrants to California experience greatly increased incidence of the disease, as do migrants from Eastern Europe to the United States and to Australia. Thus the disease appears to have an environmental rather than a genetic aetiology.

Environmental factors can be divided into two classes; the physical and the cultural environment. The physical environment includes, for example, altitude, climate, lattitude and air pollution whilst the cultural environment includes the more personal factors such as diet, smoking habits, personal hygiene etc. Studies have been made of the various religious groups in Bombay, of the various racial groups in Johannesburg and of the various subgroups of Chinese living in Singapore; in all three studies the populations compared had a shared physical environment but distinct cultural habits and a range of incidences of bowel cancer (table 1). This, together with much other evidence, has convinced most epidemiologists that bowel cancer is caused by some factor in the cultural environment probably dietary. The epidemiology of large bowel cancer has been reviewed extensively elsewhere (1, 2).

Although there is a near consensus on a role for dietary factors in large bowel carcinogenesis there is no agreement on the actual dietary component involved and most items of the diet have been implicated by somebody at some time (table 2). It is inevitable that the picutre will be confused since the diet is so closely interrelated (a person eating much more meat will be eating much less of some other item). The search for a single dietary item causing large bowel is therefore likely to fail, and argument about whether, for example, fat or fibre is more important in the aetiology of the disease is more

Table 1. Types of study indicating that large bowel cancer is due to cultural factors rather than the physical environment.

Populations compared	Location of populations	Reference

Religious groups
  Hindus
  Moslems
  Parsees
  Christians
	Bombay	16

Racial groups
  Black
  White
  Coloured
  Indian
	South Africa	17

Racial groups
  Caucasian
  Japanese
  Hawaiian
	Hawaii	17

Chinese groups
  Hokkien
  Teachow
  Canton
	Singapore	18

Table 2. Dietary items implicated in the causation of colorectal cancer.

Dietary item	Direction of correlation	Reference
Meat	positive	Armstrong and Doll (1975)[a]
– fat	positive	Drasar and Irving (1975)[a]
– protein	positive	Gregor et al. (1969)[a]
Fibre	negative	Burkitt (1971)[a]
	positive	Crowther et al. (19)
Refined carbohydrate	positive	Cleave (1974)[a]
Vitamins A and C	negative	Bjelke (1974)[a]
Alcohol	positive	Enstrom (20)
Ammonia	positive	Tjopping and Visek (21)

[a] For detailed references see Hill (11).

likely to divert us from the real problem than it is to reveal the correct answer. I propose, therefore, to leave the discussion of dietary relationships, as such, and move on to mechanisms by which diet might be related to colorectal carcinogenesis.

MECHANISM OF COLORECTAL CARCINOGENESIS

In order to study further the relationship between diet and colorectal carcinogenesis a postulated mechanism was needed and the simplest was that the diet contained carcinogens directly responsible for the disease. Analyses of a wide range of dietary items have revealed a wide range of dietary carcinogens including the aflatoxins and other mycotoxins, N-nitroso compounds, polycyclic aromatic hydrocarbons, products of the cooking process (such as harman and nor-harman) and carcinogenic glycosides such as cycasin. These are present in greater amounts in the diets of peoples with a low incidence of bowel cancer and in hindsight this is not unsurprising; most of them are lipophilic and so would be readily absorbed from the upper small intestine and would not reach the large bowel to cause a carcinoma unless they were organ-specific. Consequently we put forward the postulate that the carcinogen or co-carcinogen was produced *in situ* in the colon from some benign substrate, and that the concentration of this substrate in the colon was determined by the diet (3, 4).

If this is so, then clues to the nature of the substrate should be found in the epidemiological results relating diet to large bowel carcinogenesis. Of the items implicated, fibre is claimed to exert its protective effect by modifying the physiology of the gut; vitamins A and C might inhibit carcinogen formation or action and alcohol could aid the absorption of a carcinogen. All of these are modifying the effect of a carcinogen or its mode of action but are not acting as substrates for carcinogen formation. Meat, on the other hand, might provide a wide range of carcinogens or promoters and so in the search for a substrate for bacterial carcinogen formation meat is the obvious starting point. A range of the possible substrates derived from meat is listed in table 3

Table 3. Possible substrates for bacterial production of carcinogens or promoters (for details and references see Hill (1)).

Meat component	Possible substrate	Suggested product
Protein → amino acids		
	methionine	ethionine
	tyrosine	phenol, p-cresol
	tryptophan	3-hydroxykynurenine
		3-hydroxyanthranilic acid
		indoleacetic acid
		8-hydroxyquinaldic acid
		xanthenuric acid
		quinaldic acid
	basic amino acids	secondary amines → N-nitroso compounds
Fat	cholesterol	various products (inactive)
	bile acids	deoxycholic acid
		lithocholic acid
		unsaturated bile acids

and these will be discussed in turn. They have been reported more fully by Hill (5) and references can be obtained from these.

Methionine

Methionine can be converted to its S-ethyl analogue ethionine by bacteria in the presence of sulphate ions *in vitro*. The reaction has still to be demonstrated *in vivo*, and so its possible significance cannot be assessed, but ethionine has been shown to be carcinogenic in rodents.

Tyrosine

Tyrosine is metabolised by gut bacteria to the volatile phenols: phenol, 4-methylphenol (p-cresol) and 4-ethylphenol; these are absorbed from the gut and are excreted in the urine. In normal western persons about 10-20 mg phenol, 50-100 mg p-cresol and less than 1 mg 4-ethyl phenol are excreted in the urine each day; as shown in table 4 the amounts are increased with increased dietary protein and with increased bowel transit time (6). They have been shown to be promotors of carcinogenesis in the rodent skin.

In a small case-control study the amounts of urinary volatile phenols were no greater in patients with large bowel cancer than in persons with other intestinal diseases. From this, it would appear that these compounds are unlikely to be of major importance in colorectal carcinogenesis.

Tryptophan

Tryptophan is metabolised by bacteria to a wide range of metabolites some of which have been shown to be co-carcinogenic in the rodent bladder. The faecal tryptophan concentration is related to the amount of dietary protein (table 4) and so is a suitable candidate for the bacterial production of co-carcinogens implicated in colorectal carcinogenesis.

Our results to date are equivocal with respect to this substrate; we find a weak correlation in six populations between the colon cancer incidence and their mean faecal tryptophan level, but since the correlation is less good than those between colon cancer incidence and either animal protein or meat intake the correlation with tryptophan could easily be coincidental. We also found higher faecal tryptophan levels in persons with colorectal cancer than in control persons, but this might be the result of the blood in the stools of the colorectal cancer patients. Thus, although we cannot rule out a role for

Table 4. The relation between dietary protein and (a) urinary volatile phenol secretion, or (b) faecal tryptophan (data from Cummings et al. (6)).

Dietary protein (g/day)	Dietary fibre (g/day)	Urinary volatile phenols (mg/day)	Faecal tryptophan (mg/day)
62.7	23 g	74±14	2.40±.13
136	22 g	108±15	2.98±.34
136	53 g	81± 5	5.40±.89

tryptophan metabolites there is, as yet, not good evidence in their favour.

N-Nitroso Compounds

N-nitroso compounds are formed by the action of nitrite on a suitable nitrogen compound and this reaction can be catalysed by the presence of bacteria. Nitrite is formed by the bacterial reduction of nitrate which, although entirely of dietary origin, is secreted in saliva, sweat, tears, gastric juice, vaginal secretion and colonic secretions. In the sites of all of these secretions bacteria and nitrosatable amine are also present and the production of N-nitroso compounds has been demonstrated in all these sites except the skin following tears or sweat secretion. N-nitrosamines are organotropic and give rise to tumours often at a site distant from that of their formation or introduction, but nitrosamides and N-nitrosoureas are locally acting carcinogens; whichever is formed, the amount should be related to the dietary nitrate concentration and so there should be a relation between the amount of dietary nitrate and the incidence of cancer of the target organ (in the case of N-nitrosamines) or the principal site of formation (in the case of N-nitrosamides and N-nitrosoureas). The small number of studies carried out to date indicate a relation between nitrate intake and gastric cancer incidence (7) but none with colorectal cancer.

It is unlikely, therefore, that N-nitroso compounds are important in determining the incidence of large bowel cancer.

Cholesterol Metabolites

It has been suggested by Cruse et al. (8) that cholesterol is a potent colon carcinogen promoter and that it is important in colon carcinogenesis; support for this would come from the studies of Wilkins and Hackman (9) which indicate that about 30% of normal Americans carry an intestinal bacterial flora which fails to reduce colonic cholesterol (and consequently would be at greater risk of colorectal carcinogenesis). In our case control study (10) we found no difference between cases and controls in the amount of faecal neutral steroid, and only a tiny proportion of either group carried an intestinal flora which failed to reduce cholesterol to coprostanol. In my opinion cholesterol is very unlikely to be important in colorectal carcinogenesis.

Bile Acid Metabolites

Of the possible substrates for carcinogen production by gut bacteria, the strongest evidence is in favour of the bile acids. The evidence in humans has all come from metabolic epidemiology and has been reviewed by Hill (11). In summary:

(i)   In 9 populations from various countries, some with a high incidence and some with a very low incidence of bowel cancer, the incidence of colorectal cancer was roughly proportional to the faecal bile acid (FBA) concentration;

(ii)   Populations within a country and who belong to the same race and live in the same physical environment but who belong to different socioeconomic classes have a bowel cancer incidence proportional to their mean FBA concentration;

(iii)   In comparisons of large bowel cancer cases with patients with other gastrointestinal diseases, the mean FBA concentration was higher in the colorectal cancer cases than in the controls;

(iv)   Patients with diseases that carry a high risk of colorectal cancer have a high mean FBA concentration.

Studies of animal models provide very convincing evidence of a role for bile acid metabolites (12) but suffer from the defect that the model itself is a highly artifical one.

POSSIBLE BACTERIAL PRODUCTS

If we assume that the bile acids are the most likely substrates, then there is evidence in favour of two types of bacterial metabolite (reviewed by Hill (13)). These are the products of 7α-dehydroxylation and the products of nuclear dehydrogenation.

The evidence in favour of the products of 7α-dehydroxylation is that the two major products, deoxycholic acid (from cholic acid) and lithocholic acid (from chenodeoxycholic acid), are the only two saturated bile acids which are co-carcinogenic in animal studies (14); further, in the study of 9 populations from 4 continents the colorectal cancer incidence correlated much more strongly with the faecal deoxycholic acid concentration than with the total FBA concentration.

The evidence in favour of nuclear dehydrogenation, which appears to be carried out only be certain clostridia (referred to as NDC, or *nuclear-dehydrogenating-clostridia*), is that in our case-control study (10) the combination of high FBA concentration with carriage of NDC provided a very good discriminant between colorectal cancer cases and controls (table 5). This was mainly because whereas only about 40% of control patients carried NDC more than 80% of the colorectal cancer cases carried these organisms. The high rate of carriage of NDC in colorectal cancer has been confirmed by Calman et al. (15). The combination of high FBA /NDC is a good discriminant in colorectal cancer of the left-side and of Dukes A and B. It is much less good for right-sided colon carcinomas and poor for carcinomas which have metastasised to the liver (unpublished results).

These two enzymic activities are, of course, not incompatible and a postulated co-carcinogen involving both enzymic activities has been described by Hill (11). The value of the NDC/FBA discriminant is currently being tested in a large prospective study of 8000 normal healthy persons aged 45-75, and in prospective studies of high risk patient groups (such as those with ulcerative colitis with total involvement of the colon for more than 10 years, patients who have had a colorectal carcinoma resected and are therefore at higher risk than normal of developing a second primary colorectal cancer). These studies have been summarized by Hill (11).

FUTURE STUDIES

If the FBA/NDC discriminant proves to be of value prospectively then it offers a real prospect of cancer prevention. Approximately 3-4% of the population will develop colorectal cancer during their lifetime, and almost all of these occur in persons over 50 years old. If we can identify, by faecal analysis, a sub-group of the population with, for example, a 20-30% risk of developing the disease then we could hope to be able to persuade those persons to adopt a diet which would substantially reduce their risk of car-

Table 5. The value of the combination of high faecal bile acid (FBA) concentration and the carriage of the relevent clostridia (NDC) in characterising patients with large bowel cancer.

Group of patients	Number studied	% with high FBA* and carrying NDC
Control persons	100	8
All colorectal cancers	116	74%
sigmoid and rectum	96	78%
caecum and asc. colon	20	40%
Dukes A and B	90	80%
Dukes C	8	0

cinogenesis. The FBA concentration can be reduced substantially by reducing the amount of dietary fat or by increasing faecal bulk (Hill, 1975); a pilot study of the effect of this diet (or the 'prudent diet' recommended for prevention of coronary heart disease) on the incidence of large bowel cancer would clearly be of great value.

ACKNOWLEDGEMENTS

The studies on colon carcinogenesis carried out in this laboratory are entirely financially supported by the Cancer Research Campaign, to whom I would like to express my gratitude.

REFERENCES

1. Hill MJ: *Crit Rev Toxicol* 4: 31-82, 1975.
2. Wynder EL and Reddy BS: *Cancer* 34: 801-806, 1974.
3. Aries VC, Crowther JS, Drasar BS, Hill MJ and Williams REO: *Gut* 10: 334-335, 1969.
4. Hill MJ, Drasar BS, Aries VC, Crowther JS, Hawksworth GM and Williams REP: *Lancet* i: 95-100, 1971.
5. Hill MJ: In: *Topics in gastroenterology* Vol 5, Truelove S and Lee E (eds), Blackwell, Oxford, 1977a, p 45-64.
6. Cummings J, Hill MJ, Bone ES, Branch WJ and Jenkins DJ: *Am J Clin Nutr* 32: 2094-2101, 1979.
7. Hill MJ: In: *The 9th International Symposium of the Princess Takamatsu Research Fund*, Miller, EC et al. (eds), Univ Park Press, Baltimore, 1979, p 229-240.
8. Cruse P, Lewin M and Clark CG: *Lancet* i: 752-755, 1979.
9. Wilkins TD and Hackman AS: *Cancer Res* 34: 2250-2254, 1974.
10. Hill MJ, Drasar BS, Williams REO, Meade TW, Cox AG, Simpson JEP and Morson BC: *Lancet* i: 535-538, 1975.
11. Hill MJ: In: *Origins of human cancer*, Hiatt H, Watson J and Winster J (eds), Cold Spring Harbour Lab, New York, 1977b, p 1627.
12. Hill MJ: *Br Med Bull* 36: 89-94, 1980.
13. Hill MJ: *Front Gastrointest Res* 4: 1-16, 1979b.
14. Narisawa T, Magadia N, Weisburger J and Wynder EL: *J Natl Cancer Inst* 53: 1093-1097, 1974.
15. Blackwood A, Murray W, Mackay C and Calman K: *Br J Cancer* 38: 175, 1978.
16. Paymaster JC, Sanghvi LD and Gangadharan P: *Cancer* 21: 279-288, 1968.
17. Doll R, Muir C and Waterhouse J (eds): *Cancer in five continents*, Vol. II, Springer-Verlag, Berlin, 1970.
18. Shanmuguratnam K and Wee A: *Host environment interactions and the etiology of cancer in man*, IARC, Lyon, 1974.
19. Crowther JC, Drasar BS, Hill MJ, MacLennan R, Magnin D, Peach S and Teoh-Chan CH: *Br J Cancer* 34: 191-198, 1976.
20. Enstrom JE: *Br J Cancer* 35: 674, 1977.
21. Topping DC and Visek WJ: *J Nutr* 106: 1583-1590, 1976.

3. CLINICAL DIAGNOSIS OF COLORECTAL CANCER

A.J.CH. HAEX

This course on colorectal cancer is very useful, not only because the incidence of colorectal cancer is increasing in the West, but also to emphasise that our profession (especially those in the first echelon) should be alert for early diagnosis as there is a chance to help these cases adequately.

Of course it is impossible and unnecessary to be extensive in considering the symptoms which can be found in colorectal cancer. Therefore, I shall confine myself to accentuating some problems relevant to this subject.

THE NON-SPECIFICITY OF EACH SEPARATE SYMPTOM

In general it is the combination of symptoms and other signs and facts which is essential in the diagnosis and treatment. It is up to the experienced clinician to translate these symptoms, signs and facts into a probable diagnosis.

It has definitely been established that in almost all asymptomatic patients in whom colon cancer is detected, the disease is localised and therefore potentially curable at surgery. Miller (1) stated that less than 4% have distant metastases and that the 5-year survival approaches 90%. These percentages are by far not as favourable in patients with symptoms.

To discover those 'silent' cases, preventive medicine of some kind is needed. Preventive medicine is good medicine. I was recently shocked by an instructor of doctor's-training for the first echelon, who gave his opinion that preventive medicine was not of any importance. To this I can only say that if all that squabbling in the diagnostic sector of our profession about social matters is taking the place of true medicine, the doctor is not executing his profession in accordance with his medical duties. We are not social workers!

We have to pay special attention to the people at risk. We must not forget that although the chances of patients with colon cancer and symptoms are not zero, the prognosis in these cases is very bad. Extensive surgery, aggressive chemo- and advanced radio-therapy have not improved the cure-rate at all. Thus, earlier diagnosis is a must! A screening procedure is an absolute necessity. The validity of a screening approach was already illustrated in 1960 in the Memorial Sloan-Kettering Cancer Center. In this course other speakers will inform us about their experiences in this field. In my opinion exfoliative

K. Welvaart et al. (eds.), Colorectal Cancer, 23-27. All rights reserved.
Copyright © 1980 by Martinus Nijhoff Publishers, The Hague/Boston/London.

cytology in expert hands is a good method, provided that the specimens are collected and prepared with the greatest care and under optimal conditions.

THE SIGNIFICANCE OF SOME IMPORTANT COMPLAINTS

The sharp cramping abdominal pain with a history of vague abdominal discomfort for several months prior to the onset is important.

The symptoms characterised as a dyspeptic syndrome, in which the complaints do not seem to be of colonic origin, but rather suggest a chronic gallbladder disease, are also important. The danger here is: *the delay.*

The sharp cramping abdominal pain, in older age, with acute onset and sometimes connected with the bowel movement may be of very great importance in diagnosing a colon tumor.

I am not so sure about the significance of the so-called change in bowel movement habits. In my opinion the significance is often exaggerated. The question remains to what extend this symptom should be considered to be an important warning. How many patients and normal individuals do have periodic changes in their bowel movement habits? It seems most likely that these alterations are physiologic or due to motility disorders in most cases. Still, it is better to pay attention to these complaints, especially again in older age, than to dismiss them as primarily functional.

> Once I saw a patient with acute abdominal pain for some days and the clinical picture of an obstruction (subileus). The patient reported as a possible cause the swallowing of a drumstick. At operation the surgeon found this object which got stuck in a stenosing circular carcinoma of the sigmoid.

Sometimes the symptoms of a carcinoma of the coecum are similar to those of appendicitis. In other cases the symptoms are weight loss and anemia only.

Blood Loss, Macro- or Microscopic

This symptom needs attention. In cases of coecum carcinoma, anemia is very often the only symptom.

Even blood loss during medication with anticoagulants calls for special attention and does not cancel the suspicion of a malignant lesion.

It seems to be recommendable to develop a system for Hemoccult test, enabling doctors in the first echelon to detect microscopic or occult blood loss.

Low Back Pain

In general, the practitioner is inclined to disregard the prevalent symptom of low back pain. This is often the main reason for a considerable delay. The responsibility for this delay, generally speaking, in 25% of the cases is attributed to the patient and in another 25% to the doctor.

DIGITAL EXAMINATION

I want to stress that the value of digital examination is more often than not underestimated. Yet in not a few cases this examination, when properly applied, may lead us to the diagnosis straight away. It should be applied routinely and with the utmost care, especially in patients over 45 years of age and in patients with blood loss and/or local anal symptoms.

RADIOLOGY

The barium enema is a diagnostic method which requires technical expertness and thoroughness. Sometimes the value is suboptimal. This is not a negative appreciation of this discipline, but a normal limitation. We all have observed a remarkable improvement in the quality of radiology during the last 10 to 15 years. It goes without saying that the clinician is bound to give adequate information to the radiologist.

In this connection I would like to describe briefly to you the following four cases.

a. A woman of about 75 years of age with a long history of functional colon complaints presented these complaints for the hundredth time to the doctor. For safety another X-ray examination of the colon was performed, the third one in 20 years. As before the radiologist's report was reassuring: no abnormalities. The complaints, however, continued to a high degree and in the end the clinical picture of a subileus developed. Surgical intervention was necessary and a carcinoma of the colon at the level of the hepatic flexure was found. Re-evaluation of the last X-ray (one and a half years before the operation) showed that the lesion was already visible at that time.

b. A man of about 60 years of age had some abdominal complaints and anemia. A barium enema showed a carcinoma in the coecum. The patient was operated upon and the tumor was removed; there were no metastases. Ten years later the patient payed another visit to the doctor, who found a palpable mass in the sigmoid region. The X-ray of the colon showed again a carcinoma; the surgeon, however, did not find a malignant tumor, but a diverticulitis.

c. A patient of Dr. Kuenen had a mobile mass in the abdomen. The X-ray was suspicious, and the report of the radiologist did not settle the matter. Operation showed a malignant tumor (adeno-carcinoma).

The phenomenon of the mobile mass – insufficiently recognized now – does not exclude a malignant tumor. G. Dieulafoy (2) already described this symptom 75 years ago: 'L'induration cancéreuse n'est pas toujours accessible à la palpation abdominale; si le sujet est amaigri, si le ventre est retracté on aperçoit la tumeur, et on constate généralement qu'elle est mobile; mais si le ventre est ballonné la recherche de la tumeur devient très difficile.'

d. A middle-aged man was suffering from unspecific abdominal complaints, weight-loss and fatigue. The barium enema showed a colon carcinoma. This diagnosis was confirmed at operation, but the surgeon added carcinosis of the peritoneum. The pathologist, on the other hand, was of a totally different opinion; he reported tuberculosis of the peritoneum. Adequate therapy was given with good results.

THE SIGNIFICANCE OF A POLYP

In the context of this presentation we cannot do without mentioning the clinical significance of the polyp in rectum and colon. Every clinician, active in this field, is confronted with this phenomenon.

The concept that most carcinomas of the colon originate in adenomatous polyps was virtually unchallenged until just a few years ago. Prophylactic radical sleeve- or even bowel-resection, merely for atypical changes in a polypoid lesion, was a common procedure. Recurring polyps and polyps in clusters would seem to lend strength to the above-mentioned supposition. Along with the more recently expressed opinion that the potentiality of malignant change in adenomatous polyps is greatly exaggerated ... is it really? ... there has been a trend towards a much more conservative approach in the treatment of polypoid lesions in general.

Other speakers in this course will go into this subject more extensively; I am very anxious to hear their point of view.

SPECIAL MARKERS FOR COLON CARCINOMA

The clinical evaluation of the symptomatology is so complicated that the doctor must always be on his guard, in the interest of the patient. Furthermore, in the initial period of the disease, there is no simple diagnostic test which can help. Even now there is no specific marker available yet for colon cancer. From a diagnostic point of view, the CEA-test has some value, especially in the follow-up. It is not up to me to tell you about this technique and its value.

Recently it has been shown that cancers of the colon, the pancreas and the stomach have organ-type specific neo-antigens. These neo-antigens are able to stimulate tumor-specific immunity in the host which may be detected by 'tube leucocyte adherence inhibition assay'. These findings need to be confirmed. Unfortunately, at present we shall have to be satisfied with conventional methods such as radiological examinations and fiber-optical methods.

PARANEOPLASTIC SYNDROME

Paraneoplastic phenomena are non-metastatic peripheral manifestations of internal malignancy. Acanthosis nigricans, dermatomyositis, paraneoplastic hypertrophic osteoarthropathy are some of the syndromes described in patients suffering from colon carcinoma.

To conclude, it must be noted that we still have a long way to go – and we shall have many disappointments! We are penetrating into the fundamental principles of the cell. Let us not deviate from our goals. The war against cancer requires coordination, dedication, tenacity and phantasy with backcoupling to reality. This reminds me of a statement by Sir Winston Churchill: 'There is only one thing certain about war, that it is full of disappointments and also full of mistakes.' This famous sentence fits exactly to the crusade against colon cancer and in a broader perspective to clinical medicine in general.

REFERENCES

1. Miller LB: Unpublished observation. Cited in: *Gastrointestinal Disease* by Sleisinger H.H. and Fordtran JS, 2nd edition, p 1787 (Saunders).
2. Dieulafoy G: *Manuel de la pathologie interne*, 14th edition, 1904.

4. PROGNOSTIC FACTORS IN STAGING OF COLORECTAL CANCER

C.B. WOOD

INTRODUCTION

An accurate staging classification, which is essential for good management of any cancer, should highlight the major factors which influence survival. Cancer of the colon and rectum spreads in a predictable fashion through successive layers of the intestinal wall and spreads to lymph nodes or distant organs. In 1932 Dukes used this pattern in tumour spread as the basis for the staging classification of colorectal cancer, which bears his name. He reported the results of 215 patients with operable rectal cancer and staged them into 3 categories – A, B and C – according to the extent of bowel wall penetration by tumour and the presence or absence of lymph node metastases. A few years later Gabriel et al. (1) modified the classification by subdividing stage C (positive lymph nodes) into types 1 and 2 depending on the level of lymph node involvement. Although the Dukes' classification originally was applied to carcinoma of the rectum, it was implied what the staging could also be used for colonic tumours.

A major modification of the Dukes' classification was recommended in 1949 by Kirklin et al. (2). They subdivided category B into 2 types, B_1 in which tumour had spread into, but not through, the muscularis propria and B_2 in which tumour had penetrated through muscularis. In 1954 Astler and Coller (3) made additional alterations to the Kirklin modification of the Dukes' classification. They subdivided category C into C_1 to describe lymph node involvement but where tumour had not penetrated the muscularis propria, and C_2 in which tumour had both spread through the muscularis and to lymph nodes. This modification of the Dukes' classification gained wide acceptance, particularly in the United States of America. However, there has developed a dichotomy of opinion in the staging of colorectal cancer with British authors tending to use Dukes' original classification whilst in the American literature the Astler-Coller modification is usually preferred. Major differences exist between the two classifications in that the anatomical boundary for spread in the original Dukes' classification was the bowel wall, or for the colon, the serosa whilst in the Astler-Coller modification, the muscularis propria was the important boundary line, the transgression of which by tumour, produced a significant fall in prognosis. Furthermore, the subdivision of category C proposed by Gabriel et al. (1) defined the level of lymph node spread whereas Astler and Coller had related lymph node spread to the depth of bowel wall penetration. Despite these essential differences between the staging systems the eponym of Dukes' classification has often been maintained regardless of the actual classification used. This has led to increasing confusion regarding the use of Dukes' classification. Several authors (Goligher (4); Beart et al. (5)) have highlighted the difficulty in comparing one reported series with another because of the many classifications and modifications in current use.

The purpose of this paper is to describe some of the prognostic factors on which Dukes' classification, or its modifications, have been based and to discuss the relevance of other prognostic indices.

LOCAL TUMOUR INVASION

In addition to the problems of existing classifications outlined above, other more fundamental defects exist (5). Dukes' classification deals specifically with the spread of tumour across the bowel wall but does not make special allowance for tumours that are resectable but which have spread beyond the bowel wall into surrounding tissues or organs. It would be reasonable to expect poorer survival for patients with tumours invading beyond the bowel wall compared with those in which tumour was confined to the wall. Dukes and Bussey (6) found that extensive local invasion was indeed a critical factor in determining prognosis. When they categorised their patients into those with no extra rectal spread of tumour and those with varying degrees of extra rectal invasion, they found that the extent of local spread was as important as lymphatic metastases, histological grading, or vein invasion by tumour and was closely related to all these factors. Positive lymph nodes were present in only 14.2% of cases with no extra rectal spread but in 74.6% of patients with extensive extra rectal spread of tumour. It is somewhat surprising therefore that having shown the importance of local invasion, this was omitted from the staging classification.

A recent study (7a) has also highlighted the importance of local tumour invasion. A total of 404 patients with cancer of the colon and rectum were prospectively studied and the presence of local tumour invasion was assessed at laparotomy and the extent of invasion of surrounding structures, including fat, mesentery or adjacent organs was noted. Tumour invasion was confirmed histologically to distinguish patients with inflammatory adhesions rather than tumour spread. Of the patients with Dukes B tumours, in whom the primary tumour was resected, 19% had some degree of macroscopic local invasion. By comparison 36% of resected Dukes C_1 tumours showed invasion of adjacent structures or organs, a difference that was statistically significant ($P < 0.05$). By definition, Dukes A tumours did not show local tumour invasion and the number of patients in the Dukes C category was too small for meaningful analysis. All patients in this study were followed regularly after operation for a mean period of 42 months. Table 1 shows the crude 4-year survival rate for patients staged according to Dukes' classification and a significant difference exists between each tumour stage. In particular, a clear difference in survival is seen between Dukes B and C_1 categories. However, table 2 shows the crude survival rates for patients with Dukes B and C_1 tumours, subdivided according to the presence of absence of local tumour invasion. The presence of macroscopic extramural spread produced a significant fall in survival rate for both B and C_1 stages.

The effect of local tumour invasion was also shown by Gunderson and Sosin (7b) who reported on the areas of failure in 74 patients who underwent 'second look' laparotomy after apparently curative surgery for adenocarcinoma of the rectum. They modified the Astler-Coller staging system so that tumours were placed in either the B_2 or C_2 categories on the basis of microscopic examination or gross bowel wall penetration seen at laparotomy. Lesions which were adherent, or invading adjacent tissues or organs were categorized with the notation of B_3 and C_3. For C_3 tumours, the recurrence rate at re-operation was 100%. For C_2 tumours with gross extension of the primary tumour, the failure rate was 91.3%. By comparison, the tumour recurrence rate for C_2 tumours with only microscopic extension through the

Table 1. Crude % 4 year survival according to Dukes' classification.

Dukes' classification	Crude % 4 yr survival
A	100
B	76
C_1	50
C_2	18
D	5

Table 2. Crude % 4 year survival related to local tumour spread in Dukes B and C_1 categories.

	Dukes classification	4 yr survival
No local invasion	B	85%
	C_1	83%
Local invastion	B	42%
	C_1	20%

bowel wall was 75%. A similar pattern was seen for tumours in which lymphatic spread had not occurred. From these results, Gunderson and Sosin concluded that survival rates decreased and local regional failures increased when lesions extended completely through the bowel wall and the poorer prognosis was related, in part, to the degree of extra rectal involvement. Similar results were found by Moossa et al. (8) who studied the incidence of local recurrence after abdomino-perineal resection for rectal cancer. In their study, the recurrence rate was significantly higher in patients who had spread of tumour into perirectal fat. The Cancer Surveillance Epidemiology and End Results (SEER) reporting file at the National Cancer Institute (9) included 11,374 cases of colorectal cancer collected from over 100 centres in the United States. This study, which analysed a large number of variables found that the patients with 'limited extension' of tumour had almost a 50% improvement in 5 year survival compared to those with 'further' direct extension. The report concluded that the local extent of disease was the variable with the largest impact on survival.

Clearly, local tumour invasion is a major prognostic factor and should either be included in existing staging systems or form the basis of a new classification for colorectal cancer. A modified staging classification, based not on lymph node spread but on the extent of local tumour invasion was proposed by Wood and his colleagues (10):

Stage 1 – tumour confined to bowel wall;

Stage 2 – tumour penetrated bowel wall but no gross local invasion; irrespective of lymph node spread;

Stage 3 – macroscopic extramural tumour invasion, irrespective of lymph node status;

Stage 4 – distant mestastases. Inoperable primary tumour. Peritoneal seeding. Extensive lymph node metastases.

The crude survival curves for patients in each of these stages is shown in Figure 1 and illustrates the dramatic effect on survival caused by local tumour invasion.

LYMPHATIC METASTASES

There has never been any doubt that the presence of lymph node metastases is an important prognostic determinant. However, in discussing the relevance of lymph node spread, it should be noted that other factors have to be taken into consideration. Dukes and Bussey (6) found a close correlation between lymphatic spread and the extent of local tumour invasion, tumour histology and vein invasion. They warned that the Dukes' classification tended to exaggerate the prognostic significance of lymphatic spread and to disguise

New Classification

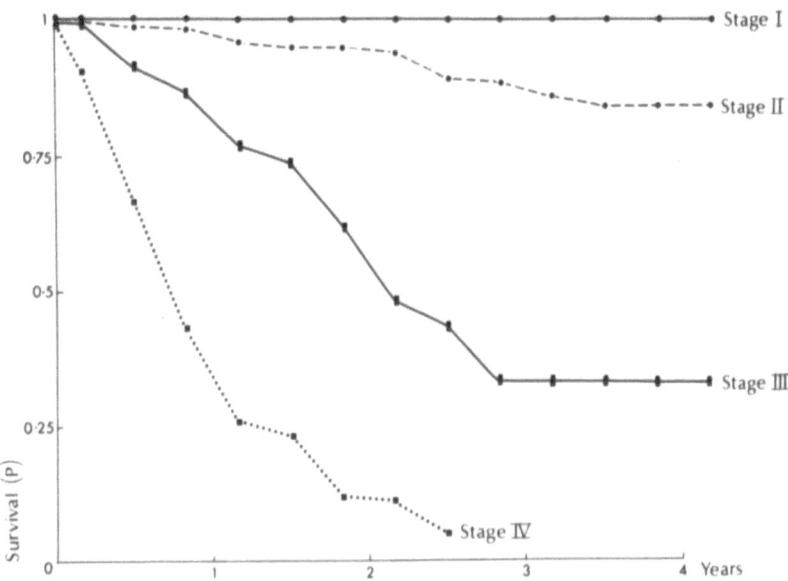

Fig. 1. Probability of survival for patients staged according to the proposed classification – see text.

the fact that if lymphatic invasion was still at an early stage, prognosis may be relatively good. Gunderson and Sosin (7) also found no difference in the tumour recurrence rate between patients with positive or negative lymph nodes. Instead, the recurrence rate in their study was more closely related to the degree of spread by the primary tumour beyond the bowel wall. Similar results were obtained in my study of 404 patients with colorectal cancer. Patients with Dukes C_1 tumours had a significantly poorer prognosis ($P < 0.05$) than patients with Dukes B cancers (table 1). However, when patients were subdivided according to the presence or absence of extramural tumour invasion of adjacent tissues or organs, the difference in survival between B and C_1 categories desappeared (table 2). The reason for the decreased survival for Dukes C_1 patients shown in table 1 may be the significantly higher proportion of locally invasive tumours in this group which would produce an unfavourable bias on the survival figures. Thus, there is evidence to suggest that local tumour invasion may be a more important prognostic factor than early lymphatic spread.

The number of involved nodes may be important since an increasing number of positive nodes is associated with a progressive decrease in survival. Dukes and Bussey (6) reported a correct 5-year survival rate of 53.6% when only 1 lymph node was involved, 36.5% when 2-5 lymph nodes were invaded and 21.9% when 6-10 nodes were involved. The survival rate fell to only 2.1% when more than 10 nodes were replaced by tumour. Spratt and Spjut (11) found that for patients with 1-5 nodes involved, the 5-year survival rate was 24% compared with 9% when 6-10 positive nodes were recovered. Several authors have found similar results in breast cancer. McLaughlin et al. (12) found that patients with breast cancer and less than 4 nodes involved had a long-term survival pattern almost identical to that of patients with negative nodes. Clearly, when there is an extensive lymph node spread, particulary if lymphatics are involved beyond the surgical resection line, then the prognosis must be adversely affected.

TUMOUR GRADING

There is a broad correlation between the histological characteristics of a tumour and its malignant potential. Many systems of histological tumour grading have been devised, the most well known being that of Broders (13) whose staging system was based on the proportion of undifferentiated cells and mitotic figures within a tumour. Many modifications to the Broders' classification have been proposed but there is general agreement amongst them all that patients with poorly differentiated carcinomas have a worse prognosis than those with well differentiated tumours (14, 15, 16, 17).

The major problem with all these classifications is the lack of specific reproducible criteria for classification. Histological grading is therefore dependent, at least in part, on the subjective impression of the Pathologist with the result that grading is often arbitrary and comparison of results from different sources is difficult (18). It has also been shown that varying histological grades can be found from different areas of the same tumour (19, 20).

Table 3 summarises the results of my own study of 222 patients who underwent resection of primary colorectal cancer. Patients with poorly differentiated tumours had a significantly poorer survival compared to those with well differentiated lesions. The proportion with distant metastases was the same in each group but there was a higher incidence of local invasion associated with poorly differentiated cancer (P <0.05). This would be enough

Table 3. Crude % 4 year survival related to tumour grading.

Tumour grading	Crude 4 yr survival
Well differentiated	68%
Moderately well differentiated	63%
Poorly differentiated	54%

to account for the difference in survival between patients with well or poorly differentiated tumours. Thus, tumour grading cannot be considered in isolation but must be taken in conjunction with other factors.

Distant metastases are found in 20% or more of patients with colorectal cancer at initial diagnosis (21). Since metastatic spread occurs mainly from tumour emboli carried in venous circulation from a tumour, the finding of venous invasion within a primary cancer is relevant. Indeed, several studies have shown that venous invasion is associated with a high incidence of distant metastases and a significant reduction in survival rate (15, 17, 22, 23). Venous invasion is found in between 17-28% of large bowel cancers (16, 24) although Brown and Warren (22) found microscopic evidence of vein invasion in 61% from an autopsy study of 165 patients.

Dionne (23) studied 1592 patients with rectal cancer and found that in patients with venous invasion, the incidence of metastases was 47% compared to only 27% of patients in whom the vein was free of tumour. Grinnell (25) found metastases in 27% of cases with venous invasion but only 7% of those without invasion.

Although the finding of venous invasion is important, it does not indicate distant metastases in all patients. In the study by Dionne (23) 53% of patients showing gross invasion did not have evidence of blood borne metastases. He found that other factors produced as high an incidence of visceral metastases as did vein invasion. For example, Dukes C tumours had a 44% incidence, poorly differentiated tumours 40%, extensive local spread 43% and stenosing tumours 45%. Dukes and Bussey (6) observed that invasion of veins was not present until the tumour had completely penetrated the bowel wall and rarely occurred in the absence of regional lymph node metastases.

The importance of the extent of venous invasion has recently been highlighted by unpublished work from St Mark's Hospital, London (26). A study of 703 patients with colorectal cancer was made, of which 108 had intramural venous spread and 248 extramural venous invasion. The corrected 5-year survival rates were 65.7% and 33% respectively. The survival rate for the 328 patients without evidence of venous spread was 73% (P <0.001). The incidence of distant metastases was 49.6% in patients with extramural venous invasion but only 21.9% in those without spread to veins. The presence of intramural spread did not significantly increase the incidence of distant metastases. The results of this study also showed that venous spread progressed in parallel with local invasion of tumour.

One factor which has not yet been fully established is whether or not the presence of venous invasion indicates patients at high risk of developing distant metastases after surgery, and who might benefit from adjuvant therapy.

LIVER METASTASES

The most common site for distant metastases from colorectal cancer is the liver. Of all the factors known to influence survival the presence of liver metastases has the most dramatic effect. The average survival rate is approximately 6 months after diagnosis and most patients with untreated liver metastases are dead within 2 years (28, 29).

Although the overall prognosis is very poor, the pattern of survival is related to the extent of secondary spread within the liver. In a study of patients with liver metastases from tumours of pancreas, biliary tract, stomach and large bowel, Jaffe et al. (30) found a median survival time of 136 days for patients with solitary liver metastases, 93 days for metastases localised to a single liver lobe, and 72 days for patients with widespread liver metastases. Nielsen (31) showed that patients with 'few' liver metastases had a mean survival rate of 18 months whereas patients with 'several' metastases had an average of 9 months and patients with multiple metastases survived on average for only 5 months. In a retrospective study of patients with liver metastases from colorectal cancer (29) the one year survival rate was 5.7% for those with widespread liver metastases, 27% for metastases localised to a segment or lobe of liver and 60% for patients with solitary metastases. In this study the mean survival was 25 months for patients in whom solitary liver metastases were the only evidence of metastatic spread.

In recent years there has been considerable interest in the treatment of liver metastases. Chemotherapeutic agents, whether administered systemically (32) via the hepatic artery (33) or by infusion into the portal vein (34) have been reported to produce objective tumour regression and improved survival rates. Other techniques, such as hepatic artery ligation, have also been advocated (35). When assessing the results of these various treatment modalities, it is important to take account of the degree of secondary spread within the liver since survival is closely related to this factor. Cady and Oberfield (36) studied 55 patients with liver metastases who had infusion with 5 fluoro-2-deoxyuridine (5-FUDR) via the hepatic artery. When less than 25% of the liver was involved with secondary tumour, the median survival time was 16 months. When 50% or more of the liver was involved with tumour, the median survival was only 8 months.

Patients with solitary liver metastases should be considered for hepatic resection. The results of surgical removal of secondary liver tumours are not conclusive but some encouraging reports have been published. Foster (37) in a collected review of the literature, found 83 patients who had undergone liver resection for metastatic spread. Of these, 47% survived 2 years and 21% were alive 5 years after resection. An excellent study was performed by Wilson and Adson (38) at the Mayo Clinic. They reported 60 patients who had resection of hepatic metastases from colorectal cancer; multiple lesions were removed from 20 patients and solitary lesions from the remaining 40 patients. The results of surgical resection of solitary metastases showed 5 and 10 year survival rates of 42% and 28% respectively. No patients survived 5 years after resection of multiple secondary deposits. Wanebo et al. (39) found that of 25 patients with resected solitary liver metastases, 9 (36%) survived 4 years after resection whereas only 3 (17%) of 18 patients with unresected solitary metastases survived the same length of time. Of the 149 patients with unresected multiple liver metastases in this study, only 2 (1%) survived 4 years.

Of the patients who present with liver metastases, only about 10% have solitary or localised lesions and could be considered for hepatic resectional surgery. Thus, it is very difficult for any one surgeon to acquire the necessary skill, both in operative technique and post-operative management. However, in centres with specialist experience in liver surgery, resection carries an acceptable operative mortality (40, 41) and long-term results can be most encouraging.

TUMOUR MARKERS – CARCINOEMBRYONIC ANTIGEN (CEA)

In addition to the many pathological factors which may influence prognosis, some of which have been described above, there have been, in recent years, a range of tumour marker substances described. For large bowel cancer, the most well known of these tumour markers is carcinoembryonic antigen (CEA). This was originally described by Gold and Freedman (42) and since that first report, this substance has been extensively investigated. At first it was thought to be specific for colonic tumours but it soon became apparent that elevated CEA levels could be found in the serum and tissue fluids of patients with a wide range of malignant tumours as well as benign and inflammatory disorders (43, 44). For this reason CEA could not be used as a screening test for gastrointestinal malignancy and several large studies have confirmed its lack of specificity (45, 46).

The most important role for CEA is in the postoperative follow-up of patients after surgery for colorectal cancer. After successful resection of the tumour, CEA levels usually return to normal levels. A number of studies (47, 48, 49) have shown that CEA levels will become elevated again in patients who develop recurrent tumour, often with considerable lead time over clinical evidence of recurrence (50, 51). To take full advantage of this lead time it has been proposed that further treatment should be started on the basis of rising CEA levels. Martin et al. (52) reported 22 patients who had resection of primary large bowel cancers and who were submitted to 'second-look' surgery when two consecutively elevated CEA levels were recorded in the post-operative period. Recurrent tumour was found in 19 of these patients, 6 had resectable tumour and the remaining patients had distant metastases. A later report from the same group (49) gave results on an additional 14 patients, 11 of whom had localised recurrent tumour. All gross tumour recurrence was removed surgically at the time of the second-look operation in these patients. The improvement in the results in the later series was explained by the fact that the time interval between the first CEA elevation and second look operation was reduced from 7 months in the earlier study to 1.4 months in the later series. By shortening the time delay, they were able to increase the proportion of patients with resectable carcinoma from 27% to 78%. Thus, the use of CEA in post-operative monitoring must be combined with rapid early investigation and treatment of patients with rising levels if improved prognosis is to be obtained.

Recent work on the pattern of CEA elevation in patients developing tumour recurrence (53, 54) have shown two distinct patterns of CEA elevation. Rapidly rising CEA levels were characteristic of distant metastatic spread whilst patients with slowly rising levels had mainly local recurrence (table 4). Thus, in our study (54) 64% of patients with local recurrence had slow rising CEA titres compared to 37% of patients with rapid elevation. Staab and his colleagues (53) have suggested that second-look operation may be indicated only in those patients with 'flat' or slowly rising CEA levels since the majority of their patients with rapidly rising levels had developed metastatic disease by the time of second-look surgery. This would explain why Wood et al. (54) found that patients with rapid CEA elevation had a much poorer prognosis than those with very slow pattern of rise.

Table 4. Recurrent tumour site related to pattern of CEA rise.

Site of recurrence	Total	Pattern of CEA rise	
		Fast	Slow
Local	17	8	9
Local + liver	2	2	0
Local + bone	2	2	0
Local + 2nd primary	1	1	0
Liver	8	6	2
Bone	5	2	3
Lung	2	2	0
TOTAL	37	23	14

This differential pattern of CEA elevation may provide a valuable guid to the site of recurrent tumour and direct the need for appropriate investigations. Several authors (55, 56) have criticised the CEA test because of its apparent inability to predict local recurrence. In this respect, the differential pattern may also be important and it should be remembered that locally recurrent tumours are more likely to exhibit a slow rise in CEA levels, perhaps only marginally above the upper limit of normal for a considerable period of time. Recent evidence has suggested that the pre-operative CEA level may give an index of patients at risk of developing tumour recurrence. Lo Gerfo et al. (57) studied 150 patients with colorectal cancer. In the post-operative period, of the patients who died or were alive with the recurrent disease, 57% had elevated CEA levels pre-operatively, compared to only 32% of those patients who remained alive and well. Similar results were recorded by Herrera et al. (58) and Wanebo et al. (59). However, our own results did not show such a relationship and indeed there was no significant difference between the pre-operative CEA positivity for those developing tumour recurrence and those who did not (table 5). At least, part of the reason for the lack of agreement on the value of the CEA test as an indicator of tumour recurrence may be difference in techniques for CEA assay. The studies in which CEA does indicate those patients with high risk of tumour recurrence have used a Perchloric acid extraction technique whereas the technique used in our study was a double antibody non-extraction technique (60). MacKay et al. (50) using the same non-extraction technique also failed to find the pre-operative CEA level of any value in predicting tumour recurrence.

Table 5. Value of preoperative CEA assay in predicting tumour recurrence.

Clinical status		No.	No. with Pre-op CEA elevated
No evidence of recurrence		111	50 (45%)
Proven tumour recurrence		23	11 (48%)
	TOTAL	134	61

SUMMARY

Many factors are known to influence survival for patients with colorectal cancer. This paper has discussed some of the prognostic factors which form the foundation of existing staging classification systems and to mention other important factors which in the light of recent studies may justifiably deserve a place in the staging of the disease. Clearly, it is important to get as accurate a staging classification as possible in order to understand the natural history of the disease and to allow careful assessment of treatment.

40

REFERENCES

1. Gabriel WB, Dukes CE and Bussey HJR: Lymphatic spread in cancer of the rectum. *Br J Surg* 23: 395-413, 1935.
2. Kirklin JW, Dockerty MB and Waugh JM: The role of the peritoneal reflection in the prognosis of carcinoma of the rectum and sigmoid colon. *Surg Gynecol Obstet* 88: 326-331, 1949.
3. Astler VB and Coller FA: The prognostic significance of direct extension of carcinoma of the colon and rectum. *Ann Surg* 139: 846-852, 1954.
4. Goligher JC: The Dukes A, B and C categorization of the extent of spread of carcinomas of the rectum. *Surg Gynecol Obstet* 143: 793-794, 1976.
5. Beart RW, van Heerden JA and Beahrs OH: Evolution in the pathologic staging of carcinoma of the colon. *Surg Gynecol Obstet* 146: 257-259, 1978.
6. Dukes CE and Bussey HJR: The spread of rectal cancer and its effect on prognosis. *Br J Cancer* 12: 309-320, 1958.
7b Gunderson LI and Sosin H: Areas of failure found at reoperation (second or symptomatic look) following 'curative surgery' for adenocarcinoma of the rectum. *Cancer* 34: 1278-1292, 1974.
7a Wood CB: Tumour Staging. Boerhaave International Course on colorectal cancer, University of Leiden. Conference proceedings p 11-16.
8. Moossa AR, Ree PC, Marks JE, Levin B, Platz CE and Skinner DB: Factors influencing local recurrence after abdomino-perineal section for cancer of the rectum and rectosigmoid. *Br J Surg* 62: 727-730, 1975.
9. Godwin JD and Brown CC: Some prognostic factors in survival of patients with cancer of the colon and rectum. *J Chronic Dis* 28: 441-454, 1975.
10. Wood CB, Gillis CR, Hole D and Blumgart LH: Prospective study of the natural history of patients with synchronous liver metastases from colorectal cancer, 1980 (in preparation).
11. Spratt JS, Jr and Spjut H: Prevalence and prognosis of individual clinical and pathological variables associated with colorectal carcinoma. *Cancer* 29: 1976-1985, 1967.
12. McLaughlin CW, Jr, Coe JD and Adwers JR: A thirty year study of breast cancer in a consecutive series of private patients. Is axillary nodal study a valuable index in prognosis. *Am J Surg* 136: 250-253, 1978.
13. Broders AC: Grading of carcinoma. *Minnesota Med* 8: 726-730, 1925.
14. Dukes CW: Cancer of rectum; an analysis of 1000 cases. *J Path Bacteriol* 50: 527-539, 1940.
15. Sunderland DA: The significance of vein invasion by cancer of the rectum and sigmoid; a microscopic study of 210 cases. *Cancer* 2: 429-437, 1949.
16. Dunning EJ, Jones TE and Hazard JB: Carcinoma of the rectum. A study of factors influencing survival following combined abdomino-perineal resection of the rectum. *Ann Surg* 133: 166-173, 1951.
17. Copeland EM, Miller LD and Jones RS: Prognostic factors in carcinoma of the colon and rectum. *Am J Surg* 116: 875 881, 1968.
18. Buckwalter JA, Jr and Kent TH: Prognosis and surgical pathology of carcinoma of the colon. *Surg Gynecol Obstet* 136: 465-472, 1973.
19. Grinnell RS: The grading and prognosis of carcinoma of the colon and rectum. *Ann Surg* 109: 500-533, 1939.
20. Qualheim RE and Gall EA: Is histologic grading of colon carcinoma a valid procedure? *Arch Pathol* 56: 466-472, 1953.
21. Bengmark S and Hafstrom L: The natural history of primary and secondary malignant tumours of the liver. *Cancer* 23: 198-202, 1969.
22. Brown CE and Warren S: Visceral metastasis from rectal carcinoma. *Surg Gynecol Obstet* 66: 611-621, 1938.
23. Dionne L: The pattern of blood-born metastasis from carcinoma of rectum. *Cancer* 18: 775-781, 1965.
24. Dukes CE: The surgical pathology of rectal cancer. *Proc Roy Soc Med* 37: 131-144, 1944.
25. Grinnell RS: The lymphatic and venous spread of carcinoma of the rectum. *Ann Surg* 11: 200-216, 1942.

26. Talbot IC, Ritchie S, Leighton M, Hughes AJ, Bussey HJR and Morson BC: The clinical significance of invasion of veins by rectal cancer. *Br J Surg*, 1980 (in press).
28. Oxley EM and Ellis H: Prognosis of carcinoma of the large bowel in the presence of liver metastases. *Br J Surg* 56: 149-152, 1969.
29. Wood CB, Gillis CR and Blumgart LH: A retrospective study of the natural history of patients with liver metastases from colorectal cancer. *Clin Oncol* 2: 285-288, 1976.
30. Jaffe BM, Donegan WL, Watson F and Spratt JS, Jr: Factors influencing survival in patients with untreated hepatic metastases. *Surg Gynecol Obstet* 127: 1-11, 1968.
31. Nielsen J, Balslev I and Jensen HE: Carcinoma of the colon with liver metastases. Operative indications and prognosis. *Acta Chirurgica Scand* 137: 463-465, 1971.
32. Ariel IM: Systemic 5-fluorouracil in hepatic metastases from primary colon or rectal cancer. *N Y State J Med* 72: 1041-1044, 1972.
33. Watkins E, Jr, Khazei AM and Nahra KS: Surgical basis for arterial infusion chemotherapy of disseminated carcinoma of the liver. *Surg Gynecol Obstet* 130: 581-605, 1970.
34. Taylor I: Cytotoxic perfusion for colorectal liver metastases. *Br J Surg* 65: 109-114, 1978.
35. Murray-Lyon IM, Parsons VA, Blendis LM, Dawson JL, Rake MO, Laws JW and Williams R: Treatment of secondary hepatic tumours by ligation of hepatic artery and infusion of cytotoxic drugs. *Lancet* ii: 172-175, 1970.
36. Cady B and Oberfield RA: Regional infusion chemotherapy of hepatic metastases from carcinoma of the colon. *Am J Surg* 127: 220-227, 1974.
37. Foster JH: Survival after liver resection for cancer. *Cancer* 26: 493-502, 1970.
38. Wilson SM and Adson MA: Surgical treatment of hepatic metastases from colorectal cancers. *Arch Surg* 111: 330-334, 1976.
39. Wanebo HJ, Semoglou C, Attiyeh F and Stearns MJ, Jr: Surgical management of patients with primary operable colorectal cancer and synchronous liver metastases. *Am J Surg* 135: 81-85, 1978a.
40. Adson MA and Sheedy PF: Resection of primary hepatic malignant lesions. *Arch Surg* 108: 599-603, 1974.
41. Blumgart LH, Drury JK and Wood CB: Hepatic resection for trauma, tumour and biliary obstruction. *Br J Surg* 66: 762-769, 1979.
42. Gold P and Freedman SO: Specific carcinoembryonic antigens of the human digestive system. *J Experim Med* 122: 467-481, 1965.
43. Reynoso G, Chu TM, Holyoke D, Cohen E, Nemoto T, Wang J-J, Chuang J, Guinan P and Murphy GP: Carcinoembryonic antigen in patients with different cancers. *JAMA* 220: 361-365, 1972.
44. Booth SN, King JPG, Leonard JC and Dykes PW: Serum carcinoembryonic antigen in clinical disorders. *Gut* 14: 794-799, 1973.
45. Costanza ME, Das S, Nathanson L, Rule A and Schwartz RS: Carcinoembryonic antigen. Report of a screening study. *Cancer* 33: 583-590, 1974.
46. Hansen HJ, Snyder JJ, Miller E, Vandevoorde JP, Miller ON, Hines LR and Burns JJ: Carcinoembryonic antigen (CEA) assay. A laboratory adjunct in the diagnosis and management of cancer. *Hum Pathol* 5: 139-147, 1974.
47. Dhar P, Moore T, Zamcheck N and Kupchick HA: Carcinoembryonic antigen (CEA) in colonic cancer. Use in preoperative and postoperative diagnosis and prognosis. *JAMA* 221: 31-35, 1972.
48. Zamcheck N: The present status of CEA in diagnosis, prognosis and evaluation of therapy. *Cancer* 36: 2460-2468, 1975.
49. Minton JP, James KK, Hurtubise PE, Rinker L, Joyce S and Martin EW, Jr: The use of serial carcinoembryonic antigen determinations to predict recurrence of carcinoma of the colon and the time for second-look operation. *Surg Gynecol Obstet* 147: 208-210, 1978.
50. Mackay AM, Patel S, Carter U, Laurence DJR, Cooper EH and Neville AM: Role of serial plasma CEA assays in detection of recurrent and metastatic colorectal carcinomas. *Br Med J* 4: 382-385, 1974.
51. Sorokin JJ, Sugarbaker PH, Zamcheck N, Pisick M, Kupchik HZ and Moore FD: Serial carcinoembryonic antigen assays. Use in detection of cancer recurrence. *JAMA* 228: 49-53, 1974.

52. Martin EW, James KK, Hurtubise PE, Catalano P and Minton JP: The use of CEA as an early indicator for gastrointestinal tumour recurrence and second-look procedures. *Cancer* 39: 440-446, 1977.
53. Staab HJ, Anderer FA, Stumpf E and Fischer R: Slope analysis of the postoperative CEA time course and its possible application as an aid in diagnosis of disease progression in gastrointestinal cancer. *Am J Surg* 136: 322-327, 1978.
54. Wood CB, Ratcliffe JG, Burt TW, Malcolm AJH and Blumgart LH: The clinical significance of the pattern of elevated serum carcinoembryonic antigen (CEA) levels in recurrent colorectal cancer. *Br J Surg* 67: 46-48, 1980.
55. Go, VLW: Carcinoembryonic antigen. Clinical application. *Cancer* 37: 562-566, 1976.
56. Moertell CG, Schutt AJ and Go VLW: Carcinoembryonic antigen test for recurrent colorectal carcinoma. Inadequacy for early detection. *JAMA* 239: 1065-1066, 1978.
57. Lo Gerfo P and Herter FP: Carcinoembryonic antigen and prognosis in patients with colon cancer. *Ann Surg* 181: 81-83, 1975.
58. Herrera MA, Chu TM and Holyoke D: Carcinoembryonic antigen (CEA) as a prognostic and monitoring test in clinically complete resection of colorectal carcinoma. *Ann Surg* 183: 5-9, 1976.
59. Wanebo HJ, Rao B, Pinsky CM, Hoffman RG, Stearns M, Schwarts MR and Oettgen HF: Preoperative carcinoembryonic antigen levels as a prognostic indicator in colorectal cancer. *New Engl J Med* 229: 448-451, 1978b.
60. Laurence DJR, Stevens U, Bettleheim R, Darcy D, Leese C, Tuberville C, Alexander P, Johns EW and Munro Neville A: Role of plasma carcinoembryonic antigen in diagnosis of gastrointestinal, mammary and bronchial carcinoma. *Br Med J* 3: 605-609, 1972.

5. CYTOLOGY OF COLORECTAL CARCINOMA

P. LOPES CARDOZO

INTRODUCTION

Colorectal cytology is a neglected field in clinical cytology. Yet it was already being advocated in the years 1949-1959 (1-12).

In those early days the material was generally obtained by colonic washings, performed after the same preparative procedures used in colonic roentgenology.

With careful examination about 90% of the cancers could be diagnosed cytologically by experienced cytologists. However the method was unduly time-consuming (13). A considerable simplification was proposed later (14). Apart from being laborious there must have been other reasons for the lack of popularity of colonic cytology. Certainly the fact that a suspected colorectal carcinoma usually was sent immediately to the surgeon and not to the gastroenterologist had considerable influence. Surgeons tend to perform a sigmoidoscopy, take some histological biopsies and order X-rays of the colon. Then they operate. Up to now most (but not all!) clinicians (apart from hematologists, gynecologists and pulmonologists) often looked upon cytology as some minor form of morphology, instead of the most refined range of methods available to detect malignancy. This therefore may have been a psychological reason why colonic cytology as a rule did not even get a chance to demonstrate its usefulness.

A second psychological factor is the well-known 'law of the daily rounds': 'so far we have not used cytology and we think we are doing reasonably well, why then should we make additional efforts?'. And perhaps one sometimes is not encouraged to do so, because the average cytological department is already overloaded with vaginal smears, sputa, etc. Most cytologists therefore have not been looking for extra work, which might in fact be cumbersome to organize, the more so as the diagnostic gain over the usual methods was only moderate.

Perhaps for these four reasons cytology of the colorectum never achieved the place it deserved. Indeed it was neglected so thoroughly that Raskin and Pleticka (11) spoke of '15 years of lost opportunity'. This is the more regrettable as colorectal carcinoma is the most frequent of all cancers of the gastroenterological tract (15).

K. Welvaart et al. (eds.), Colorectal Cancer, 43-52. All rights reserved.
Copyright © 1980 by Martinus Nijhoff Publishers, The Hague/Boston/London.

However things should change now, because at present several easy sampling techniques are available for colorectal carcinomas.

METHODS

1. The simpliest method is to scratch the bottom and wall of (an ulcerous) cancer rather vigorously with the gloved finger (fig. 1). One then gets some bloody mucus, which can be smeared on a slide and stained with the instant Giemsa stain or by means of the quick Papanicolaou (e.g. Szczepanik (16)) technique. The diagnosis can then be available at the same session, if necessary even often within 15 minutes. We usually did this as a routine office procedure during the patient's first visit and it never failed. But it must be said once again: the scratching must be done rather vigorously, so that it is abrasive and somewhat hemorrhagic.

2. The usual sampling techniques nowadays are twofold and they are often combined: one makes *imprint smears of all endoscopic biopsies* and also takes *aimed swabs and brushes* (it is usually advised that the latter be taken before the biopsies are obtained, because otherwise the material is bloody; but we get both). In contrast to the tiresome lavages (which are hardly ever used anymore) these direct procedures are quick and easy, both for the clinician and

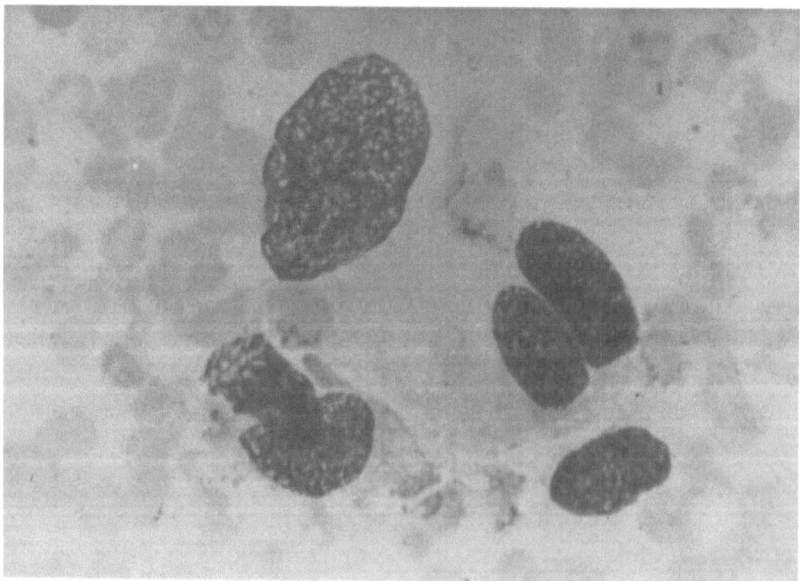

Fig. 1. Scraping tumor cells with a gloved hand. Tumor cells scratched off of an ulcerating rectal carcinoma. Note the hemorrhagic background, caused by the scraping.

the cytologist. The multiplicity of the specimens is useful since occasionally some materials are positive whereas others are not. It may also give some indication of the extent of the process.

Because these modern techniques provide material from the lesion, analysis is quick and the yield and reliability are very high, well over 95%. Generally the cytological findings match the correctly chosen histological biopsy, but sometimes cytology is positive when histology is not (rarely also the reverse may be true). There can be false-negative histological reports for various reasons. The process may also be a papilloma with malignant degeneration that has not yet reached the stage of infiltrative growth. In the latter case it is some form of incipient carcinoma. One might call it 'carcinoma-in-situ', but this concept is perhaps not yet as well-defined and well-known in proctology as it is in gynecology (cervix uteri).

In such noninfiltrative cases careful excision of the whole papilloma is adequate therapy. Probably however follow-up should be more intense as the patient's proclivity to colorectal carcinoma has been demonstrated by the cytologist. As a matter of fact we have had several such cases, that began with a degenerated noninfiltrating papilloma which was followed by a true colorectal carcinoma later.

3. Finally we must look into the possibility of a *needle aspiration biopsy* of colorectal carcinomas (figs. 2 and 3). Sometimes the carcinoma can be palpated from outside as a lump and therefore the needle can be inserted directly through the abdominal wall. Although this harmless intervention can be easily and quite rapidly performed it is usually not done when an endoscopic examination must still be carried out. Sometimes perhaps the transabdominal fine needle aspiration may save the patient this uncomfortable endoscopic examination, notably if the X-rays provide the surgeon with enough general information. If a lesion is situated far from the sphincter ani, the unequivocal proof provided by an experienced cytologist that the lesion actually is a carcinoma should be enough in many cases.

The second use for a fine needle aspiration biopsy is during the *laparotomy* itself (17). Although this is certainly possible, the aim of every surgeon should be to have the diagnosis of carcinoma before he embarks on an operation. So this type of cytology, which is sometimes useful, e.g. in carcinomas of the pancreas, should be restricted to special emergency cases in carcinoma of the colorectum.

The third indication for a fine needle aspiration biopsy is the various forms of f.n.a.b. cytology in *metastatic carcinoma* of the colon. This develops in a vast proportion of the colorectal cancers, and then the cytologist accompanies, as it were, both the clinician and the patient. It includes needle aspiration of *lymph glands anywhere*, even supraclavicular ones, and lymph node aspiration biopsies under fluoroscopic control after lymphadenogra-

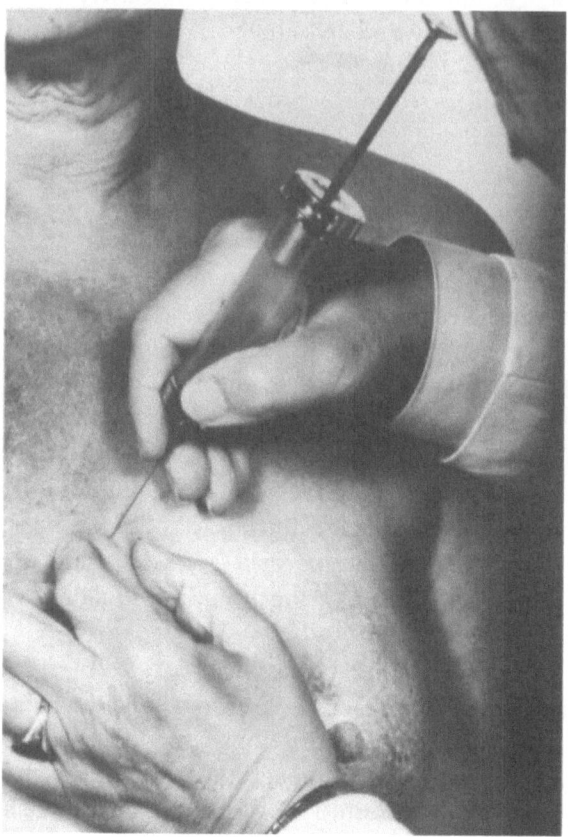

Fig. 2. The most refined needle aspiration technique is with a syringe which can be locked in the aspiration position. The needle (and syringe) are held like a pencil. The movements are as subtle and flexible as in handwriting. Also palpatory information about the aspirated lesion is recorded.

phy, ultrasound or sometimes C.T. It also includes f.n.a.b. of the *liver*, guided by palpation, ultrasound, scintigraphy or rarely C.T. (18). Of course examinations of *effusions*, generally *ascites* but sometimes *pleural fluid*, are regularly required. Also the metastatic tumor cells can be obtained by precision fine needle aspiration biopsies of *bone, lung tissue* or indeed any site.

Although not falling within the scope of this Boerhaave Course we wish to point out briefly the remarkable and considerable usefulness of cytology in *benign colonic diseases* (19). Many lesions other than carcinoma of the colon are readily recognized or at least hinted at with our Giemsa cytology. We regularly find benign papillomas, ulcerative colitis and colitis granulomatosa (Crohn's disease) – the latter even several times when the concomitant histology was negative and had to be repeated. Also cytology is a very refined tool for evaluating the results of therapy in such inflammatory diseases. Sometimes the cytologist can diagnose infectious diseases, such as amebiasis,

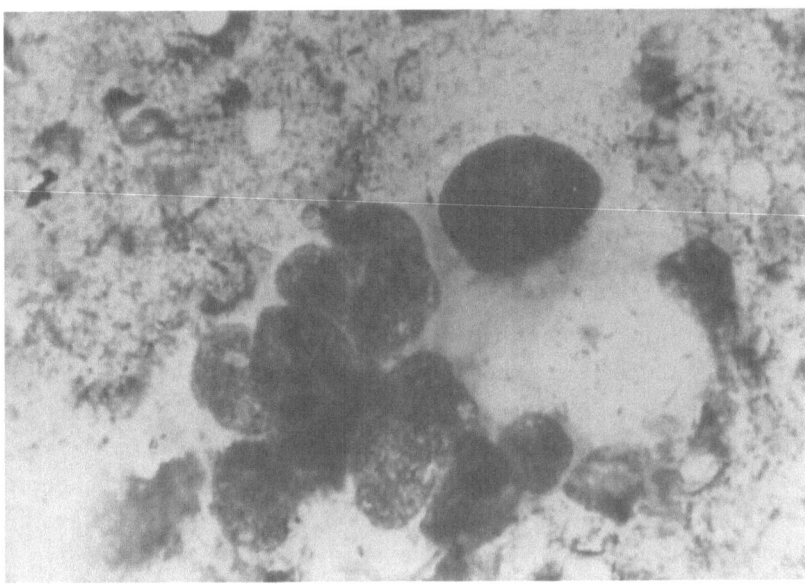

Fig. 3. Transabdominal fine needle aspiration biopsy. This is a harmless and quick procedure if the tumor is felt as a lump through the abdominal wall. Note the fecal flora in the background. Usually however material collected via the sigmoidoscope is preferred.

lambliasis or candidiasis. Also salmonellosis, shigellosis and cholera can be seen with the Giemsa technique (20). Amyloid is seen more easily in smears of the liver, bone marrow and other nonmucinous material stained with Giemsa (not with the Papanicolaou or Hematoxylin-Eosin staining methods). In exceptional cases we have encountered noncolonic tumors such as metastatic or infiltrative carcinoma of the uterus, ovary, bladder or prostate, some forms of malignant lymphoma, and even other sarcomatous diseases.

Good clinical information is often very helpful for the cytologist in these cases.

CYTOLOGICAL PATTERNS IN COLORECTAL CARCINOMA

In smears the benign villous papilloma is composed of small slim cylindrical cells, which are tightly grouped like palisades. The elongated and slim cytoplasm is diminished in size. The nuclei are also elongated and their chromatin pattern is granuloreticular, which is transparent due to the rather fine pattern of the meshes. There are two to four slightly irregular greyish-blue nucleoli. Mitotic figures are unusual. The papillomas can degenerate toward carcinoma. In such cases the cells demonstrate one or more features of dedifferentiation (figs. 4 and 5). The first characteristic suggesting colorectal carcinoma is the rounding and enlarging of the nuclei. The nuclei and the cells lose their slim shape, which is so obvious in benign papillomas. Anisokaryosis develops. The nucleoli too increase in size and may even become a prominent feature. The nuclear-cytoplasmic ratio may increase. Mitotic figures can appear. The palisade arrangement of the nuclei becomes less stringent and may even disappear in highly dedifferentiated cases. In the latter the intercellular cohesion may diminish to such an extent that many cells lie separately.

It is interesting to note that in breast cytology this extreme loss of the intercellular cohesion exhibited by nondegenerated highly viable cells (dissociated carcinoma type) has proven to be an ominous feature, indicating proclivity of the tumor to rapid metastatic spread (21).

In a minority of cases several giant cells may appear. My (vague) impression is that an average nuclear diameter of over 15 μ is also an unfavorable phenomenon. A very rare case is the 'nearly small cell anaplastic' type of rectocolonic carcinoma. Once I saw a filiform type of nuclei and cell bodies. It is a well-known fact that a medium-sized signet cell type of colonic carcinoma sometimes occurs. Squamous cell carcinomas can only arise in the perianal region.

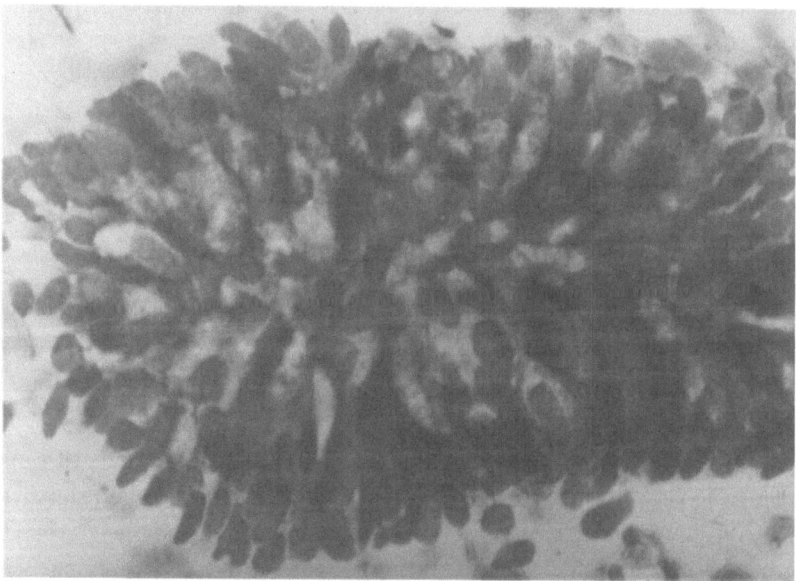

Fig. 4. Benign villous papilloma. Imprint smear of a biopsy taken endoscopically. Note the slim cylindrical cells arranged like palisades. The nuclei are slim and elongated, the nucleoli inconspicuous.

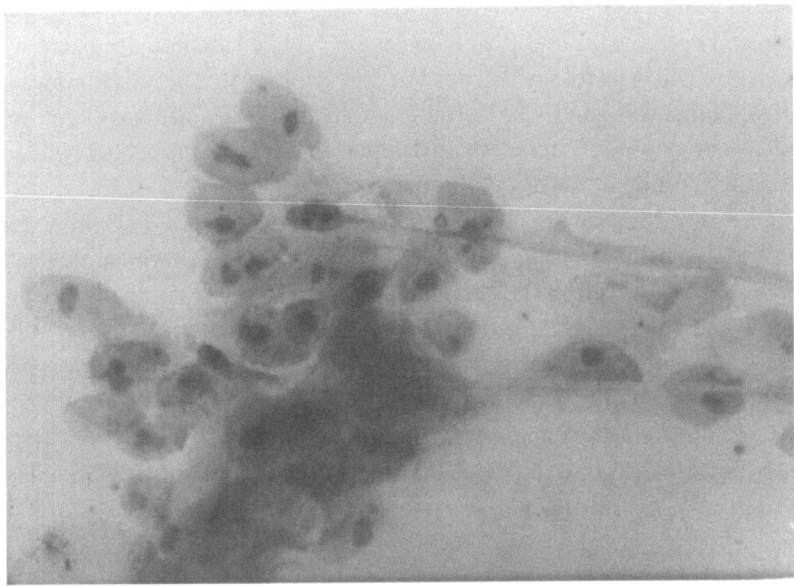

Fig. 5. Malignant villous papilloma. Imprint smear of a biopsy taken endoscopically. Aniso-cytosis, anisokaryosis, some pleomorphism, prominent irregular nucleoli.

RESULTS

We reviewed our cases of the last 7 years (5890 specimens in total). In the years 1972-1974 we obtained 2537 specimens:

596 were either benign papillomas or normal mucosa,

818 showed severe inflammatory processes,

985 had moderate or light inflammations (often clinical follow-up), and

57 were insufficient specimens.

The finding 'normal mucosa' was often clinically meaningful because it was either sent in to exclude organic disease, to check on therapy in inflammatory diseases or to follow a carcinoma after surgery.

A total of 19 patients (25 specimens) were suspect (class III). Histology was obtained in 18 of these cases and only 4 were reported suspect. The final diagnosis in 13 of the cytologically suspect cases however was carcinoma. This means that our material with a class III cytological staging but normal histological findings still had a 50% chance of being a colorectal carcinoma so that steps had to be taken, such as renewed examinations or even exploratory surgery (depending on the clinical case).

A total of 43 patients (56 specimens) were frankly positive for carcinoma; 23 of them proved to be noninfiltrative carcinoma.

In the years 1975-1978 we had another 3353 specimens; 110 of them were colorectal carcinomas and 2 were metastatic pelvic carcinomas. There was one case in which histology was positive and cytology was negative. However one papilloma was sent to the histologists and another – a benign polyp – was given to the cytologist, so the negative report in this case was probably due to the clinician and not to the cytologist.

There were 28 specimens (17 patients) which were suspect, 3 of which were also histologically 'atypical'. Of these 17 patients, 1 had, both cytologically and histologically, a class V carcinoma upon a second examination. Clinically, 2 had colitis, 6 were benign, 6 were malignant with infiltration and 3 were, in my opinion, incipient carcinomas. Again a suspect cytological report was an indication for further action.

The findings for the remaining 3200 benign cases, though often of clinical importance, are beyond the scope of this article and have already been dealt with in general terms.

DISCUSSION

In reviewing our cases, it appears that for colorectal carcinoma cytology was useful for many reasons, in both benign and malignant cases. As for malignancy it gave a quick answer, routinely within 24 hr but if necessary within one hour, which meant a substantial gain in time. Moreover cytology yielded several extra positives. Of considerable importance were the cytologically doubtful and histologically negative cases. They comprised about 35% of our cases in the first years (1972-1974); in 1975-1978 about 15%.

Our results were achieved with a simple Giemsa stain on air-dried smears, requiring no special immediate fixation and no additional May-Grünwald stain. Immediate fixation may be quite an inconvenience although a floating problem, such as seen in urine with Papanicolaou stain, has not been reported so far. However with air-dried smears the floating problem does not exist at all.

More alarming is the fact that the brushes used in patients with a malignancy and cleaned in alcoholic solutions can cause false-positive reports (22). It has at any rate been found that fixed tumor cells from previous examinations can get mixed together with fresh material from the next patient. We wash the brushes with tap water. This destroys all remaining cells owing to the extreme hypotonia. Subsequently an extra cleansing is performed by washing the brushes in water with an enzyme-containing detergent. On checking the smears made from brushes cleaned in this routine manner, we found that not a single cell was left.

We had no true false-positive reports, although we had one suspected class

IV sarcomatous extrarectal tumor. After removal this tumor proved to be a fatty necrosis. An exceptional case indeed!

According to Rachail et al. (23) completely false-negative examinations do not exceed ½-2%. In our experience with 174 cases in 7 years the false-negatives were probably about 5%. They were no surprise to the clinician as he generally knew beforehand that he had been unable to get near enough to the lesion. Clinicians still send this material in, because a class III cytological report in such cases is an important alarm signal. One might consider the use of aimed lavage in such cases, but so far this is not done.

Finally one should mention the use of cytology for screening for colorectal carcinoma. At the present time there seems to be only one indication worth considering, i.e. the high-risk groups such as patients who have undergone surgery for colorectal carcinoma or the excision of several polyps, or in the event of definite familial heredity. This again would have to be done using a colonic lavage technique, according to DeLuca et al. (14).

Although false-positive reports did not occur, there is a small grey zone of doubtful findings which our histologists, because of the absence of infiltrative growth, look upon as doubtful positives and we cytologists consider as clear-cut 'prehistologic stages' of malignancy or carcinoma-in-situ with obvious malignant cells. This touches on the problem that modern experienced cytologists always encounter a few cases in which they do not accept the histologist's verdict. For me (being simultaneously a hematologist) this is only logical because it is a known basic fact, both from daily practice as well as on historical grounds, in the diagnoses of leukemia, pernicious anemia and other diseases (well-known hematological diseases). I also met this in some of my over 500 patients with Hodgkin's disease. Fortunately the discrepancy can usually be resolved in time.

REFERENCES

1. Wisseman CL, Lemon HM and Lawrence KB: Cytologic diagnosis of cancer of the descending colon and rectum. *Surg Gynecol Obstet* 89: 24-30, 1949.
2. Loeb RA and Scapier J: Rectal washings, technique for cytologic study of rectosigmoid. *Am J Surg* 81: 298-302, 1951.
3. Bader GM and Papanicolaou GN: The application of cytology in the diagnosis of cancer of the rectum, sigmoid and descending colon. *Cancer* 5: 207-314, 1952.
4. Rubin CE, Massey BW, Kirsner JB, Palmer WL and Stonecypher DD: The clinical value of gastrointestinal cytologic diagnosis. *Gastroenterology* 25: 119-137, 1953.
5. Galambos JT and Klayman MI: The clinical value of colonic exfoliative cytology in the diagnosis of cancer beyond the reach of the proctoscope. *Surg Gynecol Obstet* 101: 673-679, 1955.
6. Henning N and Witte S: *Atlas der gastroenterologischen Zytodiagnostik.* Thieme Verlag, Stuttgart, 1957.
7. Ayre JE: Colon brush: A new diagnostic procedure for cancer of the lower bowel. *Am J Dig Dis* 2: 74-90, 1957.

52

8. Oakland DJ: Exfoliative cytology of the colon and rectum. *Br Med J* 1: 1391-1394, 1957.
9. Oakland DJ: The diagnosis of carcinoma of the large bowel by exfoliative cytology. *Br J Surg* 48: 353-355, 1961.
10. Raskin HF, Palmer WL and Kirsner JB: Exfoliative cytology in diagnosis of cancer of the colon. *Dis Col Rect* 2: 46-57, 1959.
11. Raskin HF and Pleticka S: Exfoliative cytology of the colon, fifteen years of lost opportunity. *Cancer* 28: 127-128, 1971.
12. van Esser JGM: Over de cytologische herkenning van het colon carcinoom. Thesis, Nijmegen, 1959.
13. Prolla JC and Kirsner JB: *Handbook and atlas of gastrointestinal exfoliative cytology.* The University of Chicago Press, Chicago, 1972.
14. DeLuca V, Eisenman L, Moritz M, Feldstein E, Bautista A, Macionus R, Carrillo H and Laborda O: A new technique for colonic cytology. *Acta Cytol* 18: 421-424, 1974.
15. Bemvenuti GA, Prolla JC, Kirsner JB and Reilly RW: Direct vision brushing cytology in the diagnosis of colo-rectal malignancy. *Acta Cytol* 18: 477-481, 1974.
16. Szczepanik E: Ergebnisse einer Schnellfärbung bei cytologischen Untersuchungen (1971-1976) in der Gynäkologie. *Frauenarzt* 6: 578-580, 1977.
17. Axelsson C Kirk and Francis D: peroperative fine-needle aspiration biopsy. *Dis Col Rect* 21: 319-321, 1978.
18. Lopes Cardozo P: The combined application of radiology, nuclear medicine and fine-needle aspiration biopsy cytology. *Proc. First EAR Internat. Symp. on Intervention Radiology, Algarve Portugal, 1979. Excerpta Medica, 1980.*
19. Miczbán I, Fehér M and Gallyas K: Klinisch cytologische Untersuchungen der Schleimhaut des Rektosigmoideums. *Tijdschr Gastroenterol* 18: 161-170, 1975.
20. Lopes Cardozo P: *Atlas of clinical cytology.* Leiden Univ. Press, Leiden, Heinemann, London, Lippincott, Philadelphia, Edition Medizin, Chemie Verlag, Weinheim, 1976.
21. Wallgren A and Zajicek J: Cytologic presentation of mammary carcinoma on aspiration biopsy smears. *Acta Cytol* 20: 469-478, 1976.
22. Keighley MRB, Makuria T, Moore J and Thompson H: Preventing malignant-cell transfer during endoscopic brush cytology. *Lancet* i: 298-299, 1979.
23. Rachail M, Bronde H and Rachail-Arnoux: L'apport de la cytologie rectale au diagnostic endoscopique des cancers rectosigmoidiens. *Sem Hop Paris* 49: 3061-3066, 1973.

6. PATHOLOGICAL ASPECTS OF COLORECTAL CARCINOMA

DIRK J. RUITER

INTRODUCTION

The annual incidence of malignant tumours of the digestive tract in The Netherlands is about 5400 for males and 4700 for females. In comparison, these figures are 5700 and 540 for the respiratory tract, and 4440 and 5525 for the urogenital tract, respectively. Further specification indicates that the Dutch incidence for colonic carcinoma is 1225 for males and 1560 for females, and for rectal carcinoma 1040 and 850 respectively. These figures are estimated from the number of cases of colorectal carcinoma admitted to 141 Dutch hospitals for the first time since 1975.

Expressed per 100.000 age-adjusted individuals of the average Dutch population the incidence becomes 17.9 males and 22.7 females for colonic carcinoma and 15.2 males and 12.4 females for rectal carcinoma. If one assumes a similar average population in the United States, the corresponding age-adjusted incidences of 32.9 males and 29.4 females for colonic carcinoma (2) and 17.5 males and 10.5 females for rectal carcinoma (2) are remarkably higher. Indeed there is a marked interpopulation variation in the age-adjusted incidence of colorectal carcinoma; Correa (3) reports high rates for Canada (Saskatchewan), the U.S.A. (Connecticut), New Zealand and Hawai (Japanese people), whereas low rates are found in Columbia (Cali), India (Bombay), Japan (Miyagi), Israel (Oriental Jews) and Puerto Rico.

The age-specific rate for colonic carcinoma rises much more rapidly for individuals over 55 years of age than that for rectal carcinoma, as indicated by Del Regato and Spjut (2).

LOCALIZATION

Because there is no exact demarcation between the colon and the rectum, the incidence rates for both may vary. According to most authors (2, 4, 5), half of the cases of colorectal carcinoma are found in the rectum and rectosigmoid, whereas about 25% are localized in the remaining sigmoid and 25% elsewhere in the colon, with a predilection for the cecum.

In 4 to 7% of the cases multiple (usually two) colorectal carcinomas are found simultaneously, whereas in 3.5% of the surgically treated patients another colorectal carcinoma is found in the residual colon/rectum after an average period of 6 yr (4). There is a much higher incidence of multiplicity in familial polyposis coli and ulcerative colitis ·(6). An epithelial polyp is associated with colorectal cancer in resected specimens, in 30% remote from and in 14% contiguous with the tumour (4, 6).

MACROSCOPICAL PATHOLOGY

The gross characteristics of colorectal carcinoma are (2, 4, 5) an exophytic, well delineated tumour with an ulcerated surface, eventually leading to a central necrotic crater with overhanging borders (fig. 1). The tumour usually shows partial circumferential growth and invades the bowel wall. On the cut surface, the tumour tissue is generally firm, solid and grey-white, but in 10 to 15% of the cases it appears colloid (4). The diffusely infiltrating scirrhous type of carcinoma is very rare (4).

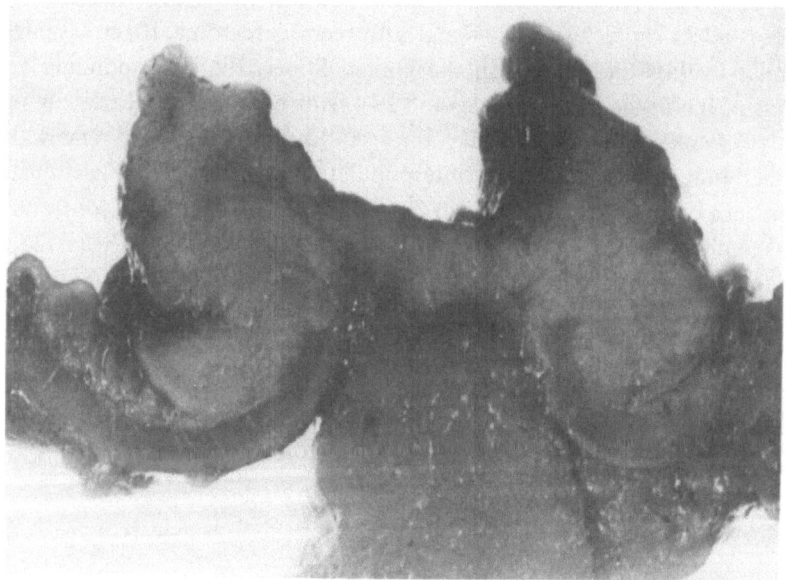

Fig. 1. Cut surface of ulcerating colonic carcinoma extending into the subserosal fat.

HISTOPATHOLOGICAL CLASSIFICATION

The WHO (1976) indicates the following classification (5):
– Adenocarcinoma,

- Mucinous adenocarcinoma,
- Signet-ring cell carcinoma,
- Squamous cell carcinoma,
- Adenocarcinoma with squamous differentiation,
- Undifferentiated carcinoma,
- Undetermined.

Adenocarcinoma of the tubular type (fig. 2) is seen in 85% of the cases (4). It shows a well-differentiated pattern in 20%, a moderate pattern in 60% and a poor one in 20% of the cases (4). Mucinous adenocarcinoma is found in 10 to 15% of the cases. Strictly speaking, there are two types of mucinous carcinoma: one with mainly extracellular mucin (lakes) and another with mainly intracellular mucin (signet-ring cell carcinoma). However, in the WHO classification signet-ring cell carcinoma is mentioned separately. It comprises about 2% of the cases (4). All the other types of carcinoma mentioned are very rare. Of these, only the undifferentiated carcinoma is noteworthy because of its relatively favourable prognosis (see the section on Prognostic Pathological Factors below).

Histologically, undifferentiated carcinoma shows a striking uniformity in cell appearance (4, 7). Its favorable prognosis and uniform histological pattern suggest an endocrine differentiation of the tumour, which is supported by positive argyrophilic staining in 6 out of 8 cases, as reported by Gibbs (7). However, occasional argyrophil and argentaffin cells may be found in a small proportion of all adenocarcinomas (7).

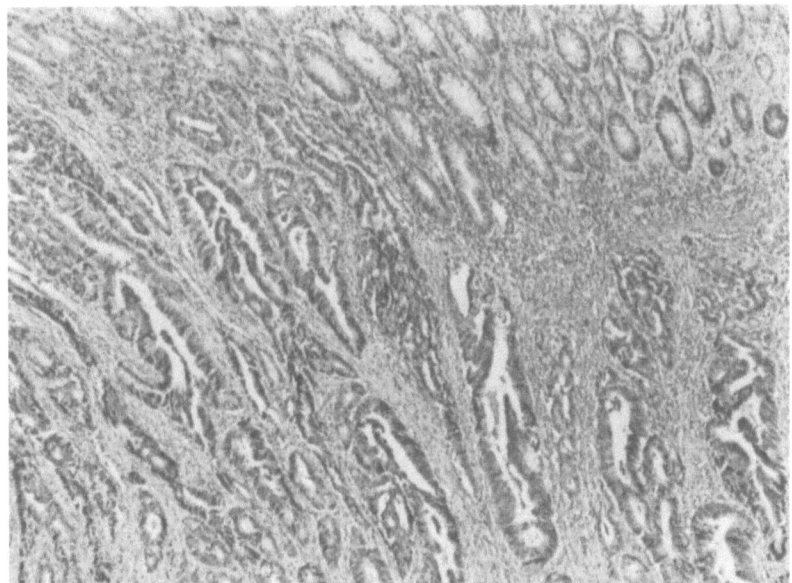

Fig. 2. Light microscopical aspect of a tubular adenocarcinoma in the mucosa and submucosa (Hand E, ×60).

EXTENTION OF THE CARCINOMA

Local spread and metastasis to regional lymph nodes are categorized according to the Dukes classification (8) and its variants (9, 10). Table 1 shows the original Dukes classification and the incidence for each category. Liver metastases are present at the time of diagnosis in approximately 20% of patients with colonic and 10% of those with rectal carcinoma. At autopsy, liver metastases are found in 76% and 62%, respectively (2).

Table 1. Extent of colorectal carcinoma in surgical specimens.

Dukes classification	Local extent of tumor	Regional lymph nodes	Incidence
A	not beyond muscularis propria	negative	15%
B	into pericolic or perirectal fat	negative	35%
C	as A or B, or further	positive	50%

(After Dukes (8), and Morson and Dawson (4)(.

PROGNOSTIC PATHOLOGICAL FACTORS

Different prognostic factors are known from the literature (see table 2). Most of the pathological factors are interrelated; they show a good correlation with the pre-operatively assessed level of carcino-embryonic antigen (11). Furthermore, a combination of the two sets of data gave a better prognostic index than either alone (11). Because mesocolic lymph node histology is not correlated with the Dukes classification, it gives additional prognostic information (12).

Dukes Classification

According to Morson and Dawson (4), cases classified as Dukes A have an excellent (i.e. 98% 5-year survival), Dukes B a reasonable (70%) and Dukes C a bad (33%) prognosis.

Number of Positive Lymph Nodes

The same authors (4) found that 80% of the cases survived 5 years if no positive lymph nodes could be found but that as the number of positive nodes increased, this percentage dropped to 60% (one positive node), 35% (two to six positive nodes) and 20% (six or more positive nodes). However, much lower figures were found by Falterman et al. (10) in a study of over 2000 cases,

Table 2. Prognostic pathological factors in colorectal carcinoma.

Prognostic pathological factors	References
Dukes classification	4, 8
Number of positive lymph nodes	4
Histological grade	4
Histological type	4, 7
Local cellular immune reaction	11
Vaso-infiltrative growth	4, 11
Mesocolic lymph node histology	12

i.e. only a 45% 5-year survival rate if no positive lymph nodes were found and only 13% if there were positive nodes (number not stated).

Histological Grade

By evaluating the degree of tubular differentiation, nuclear arrangement and nuclear atypia, colorectal carcinoma can be graded histologically as highly, moderately and poorly differentiated (4). According to Morson and Dawson (4), 80% of the first group survives 5 years, while 60% of the second and 25% of the third survive.

Histological Type

Patients with signet-ring cell carcinoma have a grave outlook, being unlikely to survive two years from the time of diagnosis (4). The presence of much mucin tends to worsen the prognosis slightly (4). As reported by Gibbs (7), 5 of his 8 patients with undifferentiated colonic carcinoma survived 6 years or longer.

Local Cellular Immune Reaction

Scoring the amount of lymphoplasmocellular infiltrate at the tumour periphery on the basis of three classes (nil, moderate, marked), Zamchek et al. (11) found in a small series of 55 patients that the percentage of patients developing metastases (alive or dead) was significantly lower for the groups with marked (0%) and moderate (31%) infiltration than for those with none (77%).

Vaso-Infiltrative Growth

In the same study mentioned above Zamcheck et al. (11) found that a low percentage of patients developed metastases (alive or dead) when there was no

58

lymphatic, vascular or perineural invasion (5%); for patients with some kind of invasion this percentage varied from 46 to 100.

Mesocolic Lymph Node Histology

Mesocolic lymph node histology is an important prognostic parameter, according to Patt et al. (12). They found that for a group of 19 patients with abundant paracortical immunoblasts the 5-year survival rate was 74% versus only 35% for a group of 17 patients with fewer immunoblasts. Furthermore, they showed a 77% 5-year survival for a group of 18 patients with sinus histiocytosis versus 50% for another group of 18 patients without sinus histiocytosis. Moreover, the presence of both of these findings had an extremely good prognostic implication, 83% of 13 patients were alive 5 years or longer after surgery.

REFERENCES

1. Centraal Bureau voor de Statistiek in samenwerking met Stichting Medische Registratie: *Kanker. Morbiditeit en Mortaliteit 1975/1976.* Staatsdrukkerij, The Hague, 1979.
2. Del Regato JA and Spjut HJ: *Ackerman and del Regato's Cancer. Diagnosis, Treatment and Prognosis.* St. Louis, Mosby. Cy (5th edition) 1977, p 510-547.
3. Correa P: Epidemiology of Polyps and Cancer. In: *The Pathogenesis of Colorectal Cancer* (Vol. 10 in the series Major Problems in Pathology), Morson BC (ed), Saunders, Philadelphia, 1978, p 126-152.
4. Morson BC and Dawson JMP: *Gastrointestinal Pathology,* Blackwell, Oxford, London, 1972, p 539-573.
5. Oehlert W: *Klinische Pathologie des Magen-Darm-Traktes. Histologische Diagnose und Differentialdiagnose am gastroenterologischen Biopsiematerial.* Schattauer Verlag, Stuttgart, 1978, p 452-457.
6. Morson BC: Polyps and Cancer of the Large Bowel. In: *The Gastrointestinal Tract* (International Academy of Pathology Monograph). Yardley JH, Morson BC and Abell MR (eds), The Williams & Wilkins Cy, Baltimore, 1977, p 101-108.
7. Gibbs NM: Undifferentiated carcinoma of the large intestine. *Histopathology* 1: 77-84, 1977.
8. Dukes CE: Pathology of Colorectal. Cancer. In: *Cancer of the rectum.* Smithers DW and Dukes CE (eds), Livingstone Ltd.. Edinburgh and London 1960, p 59-68.
9. Wood CB: Tumour staging. In: *Colorectal Cancer.* Welvaart K, Blumgart LH and Kreuning J (eds), Leiden University Press. The Hague, 1980, p 29-42.
10. Falterman KW, Hill CB, Markey JC, Fox JW and Cohn Jc J: Cancer of the colon rectum and anus: A review of 2313 cases. *Cancer* 34: 951-959, 1974.
11. Zamcheck N, Doos WG, Prudente R, Lurie BB and Gottlieb LS: Prognostic factors in colon carcinoma: Correlation of serum carcinoembryonic antigen level and tumor histopathology. *Hum Pathol* 6: 31-45, 1975.
12. Patt DJ, Brynes RK, Vardiman JW and Coppleson LW: Mesocolic lymph node histology is an important prognostic indicator for patients with carcinoma of the sigmoid colon: an immunomorphologic study. *Cancer* 35: 1388-1397, 1975.

PART II

DIAGNOSTIC PROCEDURES

7. SCREENING WITH OCCULT BLOOD TESTING

P. FRÜHMORGEN AND L. DEMLING

INTRODUCTION

While in 1953 16 of every 100,000 inhabitants of the Federal Republic of Germany died of a colorectal carcinoma, in 1975 this figure had risen to 36 per 100,000 inhabitants, that is, 22,302 people (fig. 1). With respect to mortality, carcinoma of the colon had become the most frequent malignancy in man. Moreover, as a result of improved roentgenological (double contrast technique) and endoscopic (colonoscopy) examination methods and the fact that the potential malignancy of adenomas (70% of all colonic polyps) has now been confirmed, colorectal carcinoma moved into the foreground of medical and socio-political interests. Only early diagnosis and timely therapy can, at the present time, effectively improve the poor prognosis of colorectal carcinoma.

The question which should be clarified in a prospective study is: is the search for occult blood in the stools within the framework of a screening examination (high degree of accuracy, great sensitivity, simply and rapidly performed) a suitable method for the selection of patients for subsequent X-ray and endoscopic examinations?

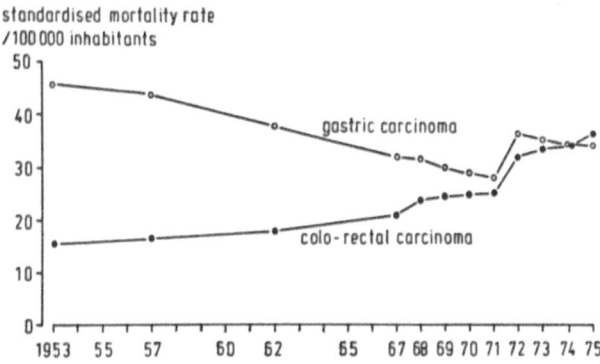

Fig. 1. Incidence of colorectal and gastric carcinoma in the Federal Republic of Germany.

METHOD

In a prospective field study, we investigated the efficacy of a modified guaiac test (Haemoccult, Röhm Pharma) in 6,007 subjects over forty years of age. The evaluation was carried out at room temperature, 30 s after the application of a few drops of the stabilized developer solution. Whenever occult bleeding was discovered, the person involved was subjected to a thorough diagnostic work-up on an in-patient basis (rectal digital palpation, recto-sigmoidoscopy, double contrast enema, colonoscopy, oesophago-gastroduo-denoscopy). Every participant in the study was given three 'test envelopes'. Dietary measures were limited to avoiding raw and half-cooked meat for the three days prior to the test as well as the three days of the test, when a small stool specimen was to be placed in one of the test envelopes.

RESULTS

Of the 6,007 participants, each of whom had been provided with three test envelopes, 5,016 (83.5%) returned test envelopes which could be evaluated so that a total of 15,048 envelopes were evaluated. For 136 (2.7%) of the subjects, one, two or three positive findings were established. Subsequently 117 individuals with demonstrated occult bleeding were hospitalized for further examination.

In 90% of these cases, a source of bleeding was found in the colon after an intensive search (table 1). The diagnostic yield was astonishingly high. In addition to other pathological findings, we were able to diagnose 13 carcinomas, 2 adenomas with severe cellular atypia (so-called focal carcinomas) and 83 polyps (49 adenomas) (table 2).

The probability of finding a carcinoma increased markedly with the number of positive test results (table 3). A comparison of the diagnostic methods has shown that none of the polyps and none of the carcinomas were detected by rectal digital palpation. The high degree of diagnostic reliability of colonoscopy is obvious (table 4).

Table 1. Detection of a source of bleeding in patients with occult peranal bleeding (117 patients).

Certain or probable source of bleeding	69×1
	29×2
	5×3
	2×4
Improbable sources of bleeding	9×1
No source of bleeding	3

Table 2. Pathological findings in patients with occult bleeding (117 patients).

Carcinomas		13
radical surgery	8	
palliative surgery	2	
inoperable	3	
Polyps		83
adenomas	49	
adenomas with severe atypia	2	
hyperplastic	25	
pseudopolyps	7	
Polyposis coli		3
Haemorrhoids (7/13 ca!)		83
Miscellaneous (colon)		69
(upper GI tract)		65

Table 3. Positive findings.

×	86 (63.9%)	3 carcinomas (1/29)
× ×	36 (26.5%)	6 carcinomas (1/6)
× × ×	14 (10.3%)	5 carcinomas (1/3)

Table 4. Comparison of diagnostic methods.

Method	Carcinomas (n=13)	Polyps (n=83)
Rectal digital	0	0
Rectosigmoidoscopy	8	21/83 (25%)
Double contrast enema	8 (+2)	42/83 (51%)
Colonoscopy	13	82/83 (99%)

DISCUSSION

Since, for the future, no marked improvement in the prognosis of colorectal carcinoma can be expected from surgical methods, an effective prophylaxis coupled with early detection, which requires more than the rectal digital palpation used in Germany, is of considerable importance. This applies all the more since surgical treatment of Dukes A colorectal carcinoma yields a five-year survival rate of more than 90%, and the rigourous excision of colonic polyps significantly reduces the incidence of carcinoma.

With endoscopic and roentgenological examination techniques, colonic carcinoma can be found at a curable stage in *every* case; this also applies for initially benign but later malignant polyps (adenomas). The latter can, moreover, be removed during the primary diagnostic endoscopic examination in one and the same session, thus avoiding conventional surgical intervention. Colonoscopic polypectomy represents not only the initial diagnostic method; it is also a means of true prophylaxis of carcinoma, i.e. preventive care, in the event of adenomas with severe cellular atypia (so-called focal carcinoma) or with invasive carcinoma showing Grade I or Grade II malignancy, provided the process can be removed together with surrounding healthy tissue. In these cases it is also an adequate therapeutic measure. The mortality rate for radical surgery exceeds the 3% risk of existing lymphogenic metastases in adenoma with invasive adenocarcinoma at the time of polypectomy. Due to expenses of staff and equipment, high colonoscopy and X-ray examination are, however, not suitable as screening methods. The only alternative is the selection of high-risk groups. Our study has shown that the demonstration of occult blood in the stools is a highly selective means of screening out those patients and apparently healthy individuals who must be subjected to the proper diagnostic methods (radiology, endoscopy).

The percentage of positive test results in our group (2.7%) has also been confirmed by approximation by others, although the sensitivity of the test envelopes is not uniform (2, 3, 4, 5, 6). A comparison of the costs of various preventive examinations shows that the outlay for a carcinoma diagnosed after the demonstration of occult blood is relatively low (table 5).

The limitations of this method for the demonstration of occult blood in the stools are given by the number of false-negative and false-positive results and the fact that accuracy is obtainable only in cases of bleeding from the large bowel. Our experience points to some 10% 'false-positives' and some 20 to 30% 'false-negatives' in the case of carcinoma; for polyps, the figures are about 30-50%, depending upon the size of the polyp. False-negative findings are also observed after the oral intake of ascorbic acid (7).

In addition, the time interval between the sampling of the stools and the evaluation of the test envelopes, in particular in the case of borderline concentrations of blood, is of great importance. Thus, 21 days after the preparation of the test envelopes, we obtained negative results for a number of stools containing unknown concentrations of blood. In quantitative examinations, we established negative results in all cases when the blood concentration was 0.1%, and in some cases when the blood concentration was 0.6%, as of the 3rd

Table 5. Mass-screening examinations (costs).

1 pos. gynaecological-cytological finding	DM 15,000-16,000
1 confirmed ca. of the neck of the uterus	DM 40,000-80,000
1 ca. confirmed at rectoscopy	DM 45,000-50,000
1 ca. detected with Hemoccult	DM 9,000-12,000
(Erlangen study)	

day after sampling. The results for blood concentrations of 1.0% were always positive up to and including the 21st day.

On the basis of these facts, we recommend that no ascorbic acid be ingested for 3 days prior to, as well as for the duration of, the test, and that the test envelopes be examined within 14 days.

False-positive findings simulated by foodstuffs containing hemoglobin or myoglobin were of only secondary importance, and thus so was the question of whether certain foods should be avoided before and during the test. Feifel (1) was able to show that in test subjects under the age of 45 years, no positive findings were seen with either a normal diet or a 'provocative diet' (salami, raw beef, peanuts).

The search for occult blood in the stools (provided the test instructions are complied with), colonoscopy routinely carried out in selected persons and endoscopic polypectomy will permit us to take a considerable step forward in our efforts to provide prophylactic measures and to establish an early diagnosis in colorectal carcinoma.

SUMMARY

Due to the considerable time and effort required for staff and equipment, as well as the costs involved, endoscopy and radiology are not suitable for use in screening examinations. Thus, the only effective alternative is the selection of high-risk groups in the population.

In a prospective study, the demonstration of occult blood in the stools has been shown to be an effective method for the selection of patients from among apparently healthy individuals who can then be subjected to the more complicated (expensive) diagnostic measures. This situation has been clarified in a screening examination within the framework of a prospective study involving 6,007 people. In 117 out of 136 persons with demonstrated occult bleeding, we found, among other things, 13 carcinomas, 2 adenomas with severe cellular atypia and 83 polyps.

REFERENCES

1. Feifel G, Männer C and Liebe S von: Der Haemoccult-Test ohne diätetische Einschränkung. In: *Kolorektale Krebsvorsorge*, Goerttler K (ed), Wachholz, Nürnberg, 1978.
2. Glober GA and Peskoe SM: Outpatient screening for gastrointestinal lesions using guaiac-impregnated slides. *Am J Dig Dis* 19: 399, 1974.
3. Gnauck R: Okkultes Blut im Stuhl als Suchtest nach kolorektalem Krebs und präkanzerösen Polypen. *Z Gastroent* 12: 239, 1974.
4. Gnauck R: Dickdarmkarzinom-Screening mit Haemoccult. *Leber-Magen-Darm* 7: 23, 1977.

5. Gregor DH: Occult blood testing for detection of asymptomatic colon cancer. *Cancer* 28: 131, 1971.
6. Hastings JB: Mass screening for colorectal cancer. *Am J Surg* 127: 228, 1974.
7. Jaffe RM, Kasten B, Young DS, Maclowry JD: False-negative stool occult blood tests caused by ingestion of ascorbic acid (vitamin C). *Ann Int Med* 83: 824, 1975.

8. MASS SCREENING

P. DE RUITER

Wilson and Jungner formulated several criteria for mass screening. The first is: the condition sought should be an important health problem. This is certainly true for the individual patient with a carcinoma of colon or rectum: undoubtedly he will die from his disease without adequate treatment.

Figure 1 shows the most important causes of death from malignancy in The Netherlands during the year 1976. Carcinoma of the colon is fourth with 2,400 cases and rectal cancer seventh with more than 1,000 cases. If carcinomas of the colon and the rectum are added together they take second place, causing 12% of the deaths due to cancer or 3% of the total death rate. It is interesting to see that cervical cancer takes the 11th place and breast cancer the 3rd. For both of these types of malignancy mass screening programs have been initiated in several places in our country.

Figure 2 demonstrates the significant rise in mortality for colonic cancer during the period 1960-1975. This applies for both males and females. After

	male	female	total
lung	6308	479	6787
stomach	1819	1130	2949
breast	23	2479	2502
colon	1109	1291	2400
prostate	1577	—	1577
pancreas	750	581	1331
rectum	603	458	1061
leukaemia	518	410	928
ovaries	—	859	859
bladder	627	229	856
cervix (uteri)	—	400	400
body of uterus	—	367	367

total death due to cancer in The Netherlands (1976)   28.478
colon + rectum = 3461 cases
              = 2nd place
              = 12% of total deaths due to cancer
              = 3% of total death

Figure 1.

K. Welvaart et al. (eds.), Colorectal Cancer, 67-76. All rights reserved.
Copyright © 1980 by Martinus Nijhoff Publishers, The Hague/Boston/London.

Mortality for colorectal cancer in The Netherlands (CBS)

	1960	1975	1976	1977
colon	1530	2415	2400	2433
rectum	870	1089	1061	1019

Figure 2.

1975 the mortality rate seems to have stabilised. The increase in mortality for rectal cancer between 1960 and 1975 is not significant and is correlated with the rising average age. The mortality for rectal cancer seems to decrease after 1975.

Incidence rates are only known for some parts of our country. They show a tendency to increase for colonic cancer but not for rectal cancer. The same trend is seen in the United States, the United Kingdom and other countries in Western Europe. The number of new cases seen annually in The Netherlands can be derived from the known mortality figures and the overall 5-year survival rate which is about 40%. A rather rough calculation indicates that about 4,000 patients should present themselves each year with colonic cancer and about 1,800 patients with rectal cancer (fig. 3). Holland has about 600 practising general surgeons. They each see about 6 or 7 patients a year with colonic cancer and about 3 with rectal cancer. A general practitioner is confronted with one new patient with colonic cancer a year and one patient with rectal cancer every 3 years. 36% of our total population of about 14,000,000 people is older than 40 years of age. This means 1 to 2 new cases of colonic and rectal cancer per 1,000 persons older than 40 years of age annually. This number corresponds rather accurately with the findings of mass screening.

Estimated number of new cases seen annually in The Netherlands

	colon	rectum	total
mortality (1976)	2400	1061	3461
overall 5-year survival	± 40%	± 40%	± 40%
yearly number of new cases	4000	1800	5800
per surgeon	6-7	3	10
per general practioner	1	1/3	1-2
per 1000 persons ⩾ 40 years			1-2

Figure 3.

WHAT ARE THE RESULTS OF MODERN TREATMENT?

In about 10-20% of the cases excision of the tumour is not possible owing to invasion of non-resectable organs or to a poor general condition (fig. 4). About half of the resected tumours are still local upon surgery. We can offer these patients a good prognosis of a 70-90% 5- year survival rate. The chances for the other half are noticably worse because of nonresectable distant metastases or local recurrence.

	N	5-year survival
excision of tumor not possible	20	< 1%
excision possible:		
Dukes A + B	40	70-90%
Dukes C + D	40	20%
overall 5-year survival	100	40%

Figure 4.

Looking back over the last decades to what we have achieved, there are positive and negative points.

Positive:
– Compared with the past elective colorectal surgery may be considered fairly safe now.
– We have learned to prevent certain forms of iatrogenic recurrence.
– Small tumours can be treated locally by means of several techniques.
– Stapling devices can be a great help in performing a very low and safe anastomosis.
– We have learned that whenever possible an anterior resection must be performed instead of an abdominoperineal resection.
– Many problems with colostomies can be prevented.
– Chemotherapy, radiation, electrofulguration, etc. are good modalities for palliation.

Negative:
– The rising incidence of cancer of the colon is evident.
– Both the patients and the doctors delay too long.
– On studying literature no spectacular increase in the 5-year survival is noted. Most authors think there is no rise at all.

WHAT TO DO?

There are several theoretical possibilities for improving the prognosis: public education, proper training of our students and the organization Boerhaave Courses, such as like this one, are of unquestionable value. I do not think that alternative forms of surgical technique can bring about a significant improvement. Radiation, chemotherapy and immunotherapy are not expected to cure the patients. Curative endorectal radiation is a difficult technique, only suitable for selected small rectal cancers. It is possible that primary prevention must be sought in our food habits. Regular control of high-risk patients is important, but the great majority of the high-risk patients is formed by polyp carriers. And the question arises of how to detect these polyp carriers, because most of them are completely asymptomatic. In my personal opinion a real improvement in prognosis may only be expected with earlier diagnosis and treatment, preferably in an asymptomatic stage of the tumour.

IS EARLIER DIAGNOSIS POSSIBLE?

A lucky feature of carcinoma of the colon and rectum is that, normally, the tumour grows rather slowly with an estimated doubling time of 600 days. There are several studies available indicating that proctosigmoidoscopic examination of asymptomatic persons over 40 years of age will yield 1-4 patients with a carcinoma and 10% with other relevant pathology per 1,000 persons examined.

Most of these cancers are asymptomatic; about 80% are still local upon surgery and the 5-year survival is said to be 65-90%. When the neoplastic polyps seen in these patients are removed, the development of cancer in the follow-up period is much lower than expected. This indicates that not only the detection and treatment of evident carcinoma is important but also the removal of adenomas is of great prophylactic value! So, endoscopy can be a great help.

Proctosigmoidoscopic examination of 'asymptomatic' persons older than 40 years of age.

— *per 1000 persons: 1-4 carcinomas*
  mostly asymptomatic
  Dukes A−B: ±80%
  5-year survival: 65-90%!!
— *many adenomas found → treatment → fewer ca. developed than expected.*

Figure 5.

WHAT TYPES OF PERANAL ENDOSCOPY ARE AVAILABLE?

Rigid proctoscopy can be performed by a general practitioner. It is a quick and cheap method, but has the same disadvantages as a rectal examination: the working length is only 10 cm. and only 30% of all colorectal cancers can be seen at best (fig. 6).

A 25-cm rigid proctosigmoidoscope is rarely used by general practitioners. It is of much greater value when the entire length is inserted, but in practice the average length obtained is $\pm$ 18 cm; thus the total score of 60% that could be reached in theory is in reality much lower. An experienced flexible colonoscopist is able to inspect the entire left hemicolon in 90% of the cases and will detect 70% of all colorectal cancers and many, many adenomas.

Still better of course is a total colonoscopy and it is obvious that in theory the best method of detecting colorectal cancer would be a periodic total colonoscopy for the entire population starting at the age of 40 year. But I am afraid this is a little unrealistic.

In conclusion as far as endoscopy and mass screening are concerned, I would say that the cheap method is not effective and the most effective method is too expensive. Both rigid and flexible endoscopy have the great disadvantage of being disliked by patients and doctors alike. In theory all methods of endoscopy could be performed by specially trained paramedics. This could decrease the cost a little.

Endoscopy

method	working length	time	maximal score
rigid proctoscopy	10 cm	2 min	30%
proctosigmoidoscopy	25 cm	2- 5 min	60%??
flexible sigmoidoscopy	60 cm	5-30 min	70%
flexible coloscopy	150 cm	30-60 min	90%

Figure 6.

OTHER POSSIBILITIES OF EARLY DIAGNOSIS

Are there other possibilities of early diagnosis, preferably when the tumour is still asymptomatic?

We have already discussed endoscopy and rectal examination. A barium enema is an important diagnostic method in the investigation of symptomatic patients but most of the adenomas and 40% of the small cancers are missed by the radiologist. Acceptance by patient and doctor is rather poor, the method is labourious and expensive and has the disadvantage of repeated exposure to radiation. Cytological examination of the colonic washings is not suitable for mass screening. Tumour-associated antigens, such as CEA, are not helpful in detecting early colorectal cancer at the moment.

It has been known for many years that any ulcerating lesion in the gastrointestinal tract will increase the basal loss of blood in the faeces. Gregor from the U.S.A. was the first to use a commercially available test in clinical practice and he stated that an adenocarcinoma of the colon or rectum will bleed in more than 80% of the cases, even when the lesion is very small.

It is necessary to irritate the lesion by using a high-bulk diet and to avoid a false-positive reaction: red meat is forbidden during the test period. In the beginning 3 slides per person were used, nowadays with Haemoccult the use of 6 slides is advised.

In the U.S.A. and West Germany, countries with a high incidence of colorectal cancer, several mass screening programs with Haemoccult have been undertaken.

The average results are summarized in fig. 7. Something less than 3% of the persons on a high-bulk red meat-free diet showed one or more positive slides. These individuals were subjected to proctosigmoidoscopy and a barium enema. This means that out of 1,000 persons tested only 30 were subjected to specialistic diagnostic procedures. Of these 30, on the average, there were slightly less than 2 patients with a carcinoma, 6 with adenomas and 9 with other pathology such as piles, diverticulosis, colitis, ulcer, etc.

In about 7 patients no bleeding source was found, depending on the quality of the examination and fantasy of the examiner. In 6 cases no further examination could be performed.

The Haemoccult test did not indicate every carcinoma. There is a rate of

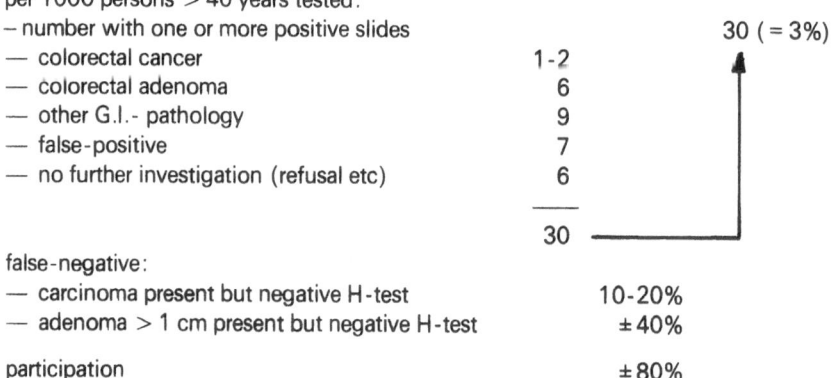

Average results of first mass-screening with Haemoccult

per 1000 persons > 40 years tested:
– number with one or more positive slides   30 (= 3%)
— colorectal cancer   1-2
— colorectal adenoma   6
— other G.I.- pathology   9
— false-positive   7
— no further investigation (refusal etc)   6
                                                                    ———
                                                                    30

false-negative:
— carcinoma present but negative H-test   10-20%
— adenoma > 1 cm present but negative H-test   ±40%

participation   ±80%

Figure 7.

false-negative reactions of about 10 to 20% for carcinoma and about 40% for adenomas larger than 1 cm. If the proper information is given to the public the level of participation is surprisingly high, about 80% for the first round.

Some characteristics of the detected neoplastic lesions (fig. 8)

The distribution over the colon and rectum is comparable to that seen normally, thus a predilection for the rectum, sigmoid and right colon. Normally about 5% of the patients with colorectal cancer are asymptomatic, their lesion being found by coincidence. In the case of mass screening about 30% of the patients with carcinoma and considerably more of the patients with adenomas are completely asymptomatic, the occult faecal bleeding being the only clue to their serious pathology. About 70% of the traced carcinomas are still local, whereas with current methods only 45% of the tumours are diagnosed early. 5-year survival rates are not known at the moment.

Some characteristics of the neoplastic lesions found:

— distribution of carcinomas and adenomas as expected
— ± 30% of the patients with proven carcinoma are completely asymptomatic
— ± 70% Dukes A or B

Figure 8.

Something about the costs involved (fig. 9)

One Haemoccult set costs about Dfl. 3.—; most of the work can be done by a secretary. Other costs include adressing Dfl. 1,000.—, stamps Dfl. 1,450.— and miscellaneous about Dfl. 150.—. Suppose 3% of the persons tested has one or more positive slides and is sent to a surgeon or a physician. On an outpatient basis a complete investigation of a patient with a positive slide will cost about Dfl. 400.—, which makes a total of about Dfl. 12,000.—.

In an area with a high incidence of colorectal cancer about one or two carcinomas and 6 adenomas can be expected. This means about Dfl. 9,000.— for every traced carcinoma and the prevention of another after removal of all important adenomas. Part of this amount, or possibly more, will be needed later anyway when the patient develops complaints. It has been calculated that the tracing of one cervical cancer costs about Dfl. 5,000.—.

On the basis of the Haemoccult studies done so far, there are positive and negative points. It makes it possible to identify those persons in the population in whom more agressive and expensive diagnostic procedures will give a high percentage of positive findings. About 30% of the patients with one or more positive slides harbour neoplastic lesions and about 40% relevant be-

First screening 1000 persons with Haemoccult

– H-test	Dfl. 3,000.—
— 2-weeks salary secretary	Dfl. 900.—
— addressing	Dfl. 1,000.—
— stamps	Dfl. 1,450.—
— miscellaneous	Dfl. 150.—

Dfl. 6,500.—

suppose: 30 persons ❽ slides ➞ surgeon.

— authorization – card	Dfl.	35.—
— laboratory (BSE, HB, SeFe)	Dfl.	30.—
— barium enema	Dfl.	80.—
— flexible proctosigmoidoscopy	Dfl.	240.—
— miscellaneous	Dfl.	15.—

Dfl. 400.— × 30   Dfl. 12,000.—

cost of detection 1-2 carcinomas and 6 adenomas	Dfl. 18,500.—
cost per person tested	Dfl. 18.50

Figure 9.

nign pathology of the digestive tract. The older the population is, the higher the predictive value of a positive Haemoccult test.

About one-third of the carcinomas detected is completely asymptomatic and at surgery the tumour is usually in an early stage. That is why it is not unrealistic to expect a better overall survival for these cases, but it is not certain that the overall prognosis for the whole population will improve by mass screening. It could be that screening selectively identifies those persons with localised disease. There are negative points too: 10-20% of the colorectal cancers are Haemoccultnegative and 40% of the adenomas larger than 1 cm. The test is not reliable for the higher gastro-intestinal tract. Several months after obtaining 3 negative Haemoccult slides we found large ulcerating adenocarcinomas of the stomach in two patients.

It is clear that a negative test for occult blood in the faeces does not exclude a serious disease of the digestive tract, so it is not a substitute for proper investigation of symptomatic patients.

Although the Haemoccult test itself is rather cheap, screening the whole population of The Netherlands for occult faecal bleeding is expensive.

Figure 10 shows a very rough calculation. We have five million inhabitants older than 40 years of age. With a presumed response rate of about 80% this means a cost of Dfl. 74,000,000.—.

Suppose one carcinoma is found per 1,000 persons tested, thus a total of 4,000 detected cancers of the rectum and colon. The overall 5-year survival at

First screening of the population of the Netherlands with H-test

±5,000,000 inhabitants > 40 years.
suppose: response 80% → 4,000,000 × Dfl. 18.50 = Dfl. 74,000,000.—
       1 carcinoma per 1000 persons → 4000 ca. detected
normal overall 5-year survival 14%   1600 patients
suppose: 70% early stages → overall
       5 year survival *could* increase to 60%   2400 patients
                                                  ————————
       more 5-year survivors   800 patients
Cost of one 5-year survival and prevention of several ca.
Dfl. 74,000,000 : 800 = Dfl. ±100,000.—

Figure 10.

the moment is about 40% or 1,600 patients. Suppose that about 70% of the carcinomas detected by screening is still local. This *could* mean that the overall 5-year survival will increase to 60% or 2,400 patients or 800 more 5-year survivors.

The cost of one 5-year survival and the prevention of one or several other colorectal cancers is therefore about Dfl. 100,000.—. I want to emphasize that these figures are speculative.

It is obvious that we need more data from controlled trials about the gain in survival rate and the economic feasibility because before offering screening to an asymptomatic population we must be certain that a definite improvement in overall prognosis is guaranteed at a reasonable price.

Other points to be considered are the expected drop in response rate in the following rounds and a reduction in the number of neoplastic lesions detected.

CONCLUSIONS

At the moment there is no place for a nation-wide screening program for colorectal cancer, although there may be one in the near future. Screening an entire population at regular intervals will require a tremendous and expensive organisation, for instance in the form of establishing screening centres where several important diseases can be traced. Furthermore it must be a proven fact that early diagnosis and treatment are possible and will improve survival or the quality of life significantly. The most elegant method would be to give the general practitioner the tools he needs for more preventive work and early diagnosis within the population he knows as nobody else does. In the meantime he can start by making occult faecal bleeding tests part of every periodic medical examination of patients older than 40 years of age. Surgeons and physicians should be obliged to control their high-risk patients carefully, preferable by means of periodic colonoscopy.

At present we are spending much energy and money on patients who come for curative treatment too late. It could be that a reorientation in medical thinking to a more preventive approach will be less expensive and more successful in the long run.

REFERENCES

1. Gilbertsen, V.A. and Nelms, J.M. The prevention of invasive cancer of the rectum. *Cancer* 41, 1137-1139 (1978).
2. Goertler, K. *Kolorektale Krebsvorsorge.* Wachholz, Nürnberg 1978.
3. Hertz, R.E., Deddish, M.R., Day E. Value of period examination in detective cancer of the rectum and colon. *Postgrad. Med* 27, 290-294 (1960).
4. Ruiter, P. de. Occult bloedverlies en vroege diagnostiek van colon- en rectumcarcinoom. *Ned. T. Geneesk.* 122, 365-369 (1978).
5. Wilson, J.M.G. and Jungner, G. Principles and practice of screening for disease. Public Health Papers Nr. 34, WHO, Genève, 1968.

9. COLONOSCOPY AS A SCREENING PROCEDURE?

CHRISTOPHER B. WILLIAMS

Had the invention of fibreoptic viewing bundles and the development of fibre-endoscopes come at the beginning of this century, when radiology was in its infancy, it is not difficult to imagine that present arrangements for screening or investigation of patients for gastrointestinal cancer might be very different. The organisation and the budgets of established X-ray departments cannot be equalled by the gastrointestinal endoscopy units in most centres, and there are insufficient medical staff to perform multiple screening endoscopies.

SCREENING BY ENDOSCOPY

The essential of any screening programme is to combine patient acceptability, cheapness, a worthwhile pick-up and low false-positive and negative score.

In the upper gastrointestinal tract, where the use of small diameter 'paediatric' gastroscopes has made it possible to perform rapid examinations without sedation of the patient, a few centres are starting to undertake gastroscopy as the initial investigation, largely owing to the relative inaccuracy of most European barium radiology. In comparison mass-screening programmes for stomach cancer in Japan are based on mobile high-quality barium X-ray units because even the relatively cheap 'gastro-camera' examination is felt to be unacceptable and more expensive. Fibre-endoscopy of any kind also has the great disadvantage of not providing any permanent overall record of the examination, except for the written opinion of the endoscopist and a few selected views or biopsies. This means that the validity of the examination depends on the manual dexterity and visual skills of the endoscopist and that, unlike X-ray, there is no way of looking back to check on the accuracy of the opinion given.

Presumably, with technical developments and the advent of competitive marketing between endoscope companies, the costs of instrumentation will fall, with relatively cheaper and certainly less fragile endoscopes. Endoscopy will always remain an assault on the person, and it is difficult to imagine that individuals will ever welcome the passage of a tube, however skilled and enthusiastic its passer.

K. Welvaart et al. (eds.), Colorectal Cancer, 77-82. All rights reserved.
Copyright © 1980 by Martinus Nijhoff Publishers, The Hague/Boston/London.

SCREENING COLONOSCOPIES?

Colonoscopy has, in addition to the other difficulties of fibre-endoscopy the added disadvantage that the colon is technically difficult to intubate. Compared with the constant anatomy and fixed attachments of the oesophagus and stomach, the loops and bends of the colon present a considerable mechanical problem (1). In the 'normal' colon, unattached by adhesions from previous surgery or diverticulitis, a screening examination in skilled hands will take only 15-20 min, which is comparable to the time for an air-contrast barium enema. The textbook idea of a 'normal' colon, attached in its pelvic, descending and ascending portions, and mobile only in the sigmoid and transverse colon, is not infrequently varied by the lack of conventional retroperitoneal attachments so that the colonoscope will force the bowel into unpredictable loops which make the examination difficult and painful. This difficulty cannot be anticipated before starting the procedure, so in starting a colonoscopy the endoscopist must always be prepared either to abandon the examination or to use sedation and/or fluoroscopy if he is to examine the whole colon without hurting the patient. A patient who has once proved difficult to examine is unlikely to be much easier on another occasion and it is useful to mark his records to that effect.

COMPROMISES – 'FIBRE-SIGMOIDOSCOPY', LIMITED COLONOSCOPY AND COMBINED ENDOSCOPY-ENEMA

All evidence, including the distribution of polyps removed at colonoscopy, shows that the majority of colonic pathology occurs distally, the incidence rising steadily towards the rectum. The sigmoid colon is also the area least well seen by the radiologist, mainly because of its tortuosity, but also because of the frequent occurrence of deforming diverticular disease and the technical difficulties of barium enema, as when the terminal ileum is overfilled with barium and obscures the view of the sigmoid.

Rigid procto-sigmoidoscopy, especially if the clinician attempts to examine more than the rectum, can be an excruciating experience and is frequently the most resented part of a 'colonic work-up'. By contrast fibreoptic sigmoidoscopy is normally quite painless to the proximal sigmoid colon and there is often little trouble in reaching around the sigmoid-descending junction to the splenic flexure. To achieve this a disposable phosphate enema is administered 20-30 min before the examination.

Limited examination can be equally well achieved with a conventional long colonoscope and this raises the interesting possibility of following endoscopy, if it proves difficult, with radiology. After normal colonoscopic air insufflation the colon remains considerably distended, often a source of discomfort and inconvenience to the patient, and a technical hazard for the radiologist, who has difficulty in getting the bowel wall adequately coated with barium. If the endoscopist uses carbon-dioxide for insufflation all the gas is normally re-absorbed within 30-40 min since CO_2 has 30 times the permeability of air. No air must be used at any stage of the examination and to be sure of this the air-pump is switched off and any water-cleansing of the lens performed manually by syringe. The endoscopist then has the option of doing as extensive a colonoscopy as is technically and humanely possible (perhaps without seda-tion) and if he cannot reach the caecum the patient is sent shortly after for X-ray. In particularly high risk patients or those with strictures or malignant lesions needing very precise demonstration it may even be desirable to com-bine total colonoscopy with immediate barium enema as a planned proce-dure.

'HIGH-RISK PATIENTS' REQUIRING COLONOSCOPY

Although an air contrast barium enema is for many clinical situations a perfectly acceptable screening procedure there are others where for various technical reasons the chance of radiological error is unacceptably high and the clinical risk is also relatively great – the two factors together providing a prime indication for colonoscopy. Patients with abdominal pain provide a good contrast in this respect from those with rectal bleeding: if the pain is colonic in origin it must derive either from a major lesion causing obstruction or from deep ulceration, either of which show up radiologically. In contra-distinction, it is accepted on the basis of a number of endoscopic series (2) that in at least 40% of patients referred for colonoscopy because of *persistent rectal bleeding* pathology is found in spite of a normal barium enema. This radio-logical failure is often due to errors of technique or interpretation, but some-times due to radiologically undemonstratable lesions such as flat telangi-ectases or radiation colitis or to situations such as diverticular disease in which the configuration of the colon makes X-ray interpretation largely a matter of guesswork. Patients with persistent, dark or 'mixed-in' bleeding are therefore excellent candidates for 'screening' colonoscopy on the grounds that if X-ray is negative, something may have been missed and if X-ray is positive colonoscopy will normally be indicated to provide biopsy proof or to attempt polypectomy. A patient with pain and known diverticular disease exemplifies the position: if there is no bleeding, barium enema is safer and will establish whether there is co-existent obstruction; if there is bleeding as well as pain a barium enema is a waste of time and the technical difficulty of colono-scopy entirely justified.

In the *operated patient* there are a number of situations where colonoscopy might come first. In the immediate post-operative phase if the anastomosis is to be checked to exclude a 'leak', barium contrast films give a much better chance of making a full functional assessment than endoscopy. Subsequently, however, for examination of the *anastomosis* to exclude the presence of recurrence it is illogical to use X-ray; endoscopy gives a more accurate colour view with the ability to take cytology brushings or biopsies of any suspicious area, whereas the radiological view cannot discriminate between surgical deformity, granulation tissue masses and actual tumour.

Any patient with a tumour is at high risk for development or recurrent missed synchronous or metachronous lesions and merits careful post-operative review and follow-up. After sigmoid resection the shortened and straightened colon should be extremely easy to examine endoscopically, probably without any sedation; if this proves to be the case, the extra accuracy of colonoscopy suggests its use rather than X-ray.

Colostomy patients can be very difficult to prepare and X-ray satisfactorily because of mechanical difficulties in avoiding leak-back at the stoma combined with the presence of faecal residue. Colonoscopically, such patients are usually rather easy to examine, the obstacle of the sigmoid colon having been removed, and visual discrimination between faecal masses and other lesions not presenting the same difficulty to the endoscopist in colour as it does to the radiologist in black and white.

The group with the highest potential cancer risk are the members of a *polyposis coli* family. Not surprisingly such patients have a keen interest in accurate diagnosis and it is desirable to give a definite 'yes' or 'no' diagnosis with a view to prophylactic resection in late adolescence. If a positive diagnosis and histological proof can be made on proctosigmoidoscopy and rectal biopsy, a screening barium enema may be sufficient to demonstrate the state of the rest of the colon whilst planning surgery. When few polyps or no polyps at all are present in the rectum however, limited colonoscopy or fibre-sigmoidoscopy will give a larger sampling area and a close-up mucosal view. The wide-angle objective lens and high resolution of modern fibre-optic instruments will demonstrate 1-2 mm lesions with the same accuracy as a hand-lens. Such tiny mucosal lesions are however, transparent and the endoscopist must expect to look carefully, particularly concentrating on reflections or 'highlights' on the mucosal surface thrown up by the illuminating bundles of the endoscope. A better method is the 'dye-spraying' technique in which a catheter is used to spread a thin film of dilute blue dye over the mucosal surface, through which any minute excrescences will project as white islands which can be biopsied. Indigo-carmine 0.2% in water is suitable but fountain pen ink is more easily available. Other patients such as those with a strong *family history of colon cancer* or having 6-8 larger polyps may be better

assessed with dye-spray in order to exclude the presence of tiny lesions, por-
tents of trouble in the future.

The other large group of patients requiring anti-cancer screening in the
colon is those with an over 10-year history of *extensive ulcerative colitis*
(3). Because colon cancer in colitis patients is not infrequently *sub*mucosal
there seems little point in relying on X-ray for screening purposes, whereas
Morson's demonstration of a pre-cancerous phase in the mucosa gives every
reason to take routine rectal biopsies (4). Our colonoscopic experience to date
has been that at least 90% of patients show no evidence of such dysplastic
change, and that 90% of those that do will also have similar abnormality in the
rectal biopsy, so colonoscopy is a mainly negative exercise in reassurance. It
would be very desirable to be able to select the most likely areas for biopsy,
and since severe pre-cancer often shows an irregular villous surface, the dye-
spray technique seemed worthy of trial. Unfortunately, the mucosal surface
in such patients is often highly irregular without pre-cancer, so there seems no
alternative to the taking of 10 or more biopsies in each patient. Fortunately,
insertion of the colonoscope is usually easy in chronic colitis patients because
of the shortening effect of the disease process on the colonic musculature.

COLONOSCOPY AS A SECOND-LINE PROCEDURE AFTER BARIUM ENEMA

Total colonoscopy is a sufficiently unpredicatable art that, for the foreseeable
future and with the above exceptions, that it seems likely to be used mainly
where X-ray has demonstrated probable abnormality requiring more precise
diagnosis. Where such abnormality is a polyp, colonoscopy is *always* indicated because of the high probability that the lesion will be adenomatous; 5%
of adenomas will consist wholly or partly of carcinoma (5). Colonoscopy will
frequently reveal other polyps and, even if these are only 6 mm or less in
diameter, 70% in our series are proven on biopsy to be adenomas and are
therefore simultaneously destroyed using the 'hot-biopsy' forceps (6). Only in
a patient of 80 or more years and in poor health is there no need for colonoscopy if X-ray shows a small colonic polyp; in younger patients the alternative
of repeated barium enemas seems worse than a single colonoscopy. If 3 or
more polyps are found in the left colon it is desirable to do a total colonoscopy, whereas if only one is present in the left colon it is most unusual to find
any pathology in the right colon, and limited colonoscopy may be sufficient.

CONCLUSION

As more physicians and surgeons are trained to use fibre-endoscopes colonoscopy will be increasingly often used, especially for limited colonoscopy,
covering a 'high-risk area' of the colon with ease in most patients. Liaison
with radiology departments, and technical tricks such as the use of CO_2 for
colonoscopic insufflation will make a combined endoscopy-enema assess-
men practical if endoscopy proves impossible or the patients merits very
careful study. Any patient may be difficult or impossible to examine technically, so that in any individual it is valuable to record whether colonoscopy is
easy or not – it may be more realistic in the technically difficult patients to
settle for X-ray follow-up, with endoscopy in reserve. Particularly high-risk
patients meriting initial colonoscopy include those with dark or persistent
rectal bleeding, members of polyposis coli or colon cancer families and those
with chronic extensive ulcerative colitis or previous surgery for cancer, all of
whom may justify initial screening colonoscopy.

REFERENCES

1. Cotton PB and Williams CB: *Practical gastrointestinal endoscopy*, Blackwells Scientific
   Publications, Oxford, 1980.
2. Hunt RH: Colonoscopy in unexplained rectal bleeding. *Clin Gastroent* 7: 719, 1978.
3. Williams CB and Waye JD: Colonoscopy in Inflammatory Bowel Disease, *Clin Gastroent* 7:
   701-717, 1978.
4. Lennard-Jones JE, Morson BC, Ritchie JK, Shove DC and Williams CB: Cancer in Colities:
   assessment of the individual risk by clinical and histological criteria. *Gastroent* 73: 1280, 1977.
5. Gillespie PE, Chambers TJ, Chan KW, Doronzo F, Morson BC and Williams CB: Colonic
   adenomas – a colonoscope survey, *Gut* 20: 240-245, 1979.
6. Williams CB and Riddell RH: Chapter: Colonoscopic polypectomy. In: *Topics in gastrointestinal endoscopy*, Salmon PR and Schiller KFR (ed), Heinemann Medical, London, 1976.

PART III

INDIVIDUALS AT RISK

10. DIETARY, ENVIRONMENTAL, AND HEREDITARY FACTORS IN THE DEVELOPMENT OF COLORECTAL CANCER*

MARTIN LIPKIN

Recent studies have attempted to identify factors that are associated with the development of colorectal cancer both in population groups with genetic predisposition to neoplasia and in individuals in the general population who are at high risk. Environmental and dietary elements suspected of inducing or promoting colon carcinogenesis and abnormalities observed in colonic cell development are under investigation. Colorectal cancer poses a major health problem in the United States and many other countries, and is currently responsible for a high proportion of the malignant neoplasms found in the United States. Recent figures have indicated over 80,000 new cases annually in the United States and high mortality (1). The proportion of individuals who survive the disease varies with the stage at which it is detected, success being higher with earlier detection (2).

ENVIRONMENTAL AND DIETARY FACTORS

There is reasonably strong evidence to indicate that environment has a role in the development of colorectal cancer; however, the most important elements involved are not clear because of conflicting findings. Numerous studies have shown a correlation between colon cancer, economic status, and geographic and dietary exposure. In industrialized countries, including those of north-west Europe and North America, a great deal of animal fat, protein, and refined carbohydrate is consumed; in these geographic regions, the incidence of colon cancer is much higher than in the developing countries of Africa, South America (except Argentina and Uruguay, whose populations are meat-eaters), rural India, and Japan, where much less meat is consumed and the diet is higher in vegetable fiber (3-7). These variations in incidence are not believed to be related to genetic differences because certain migrant groups tend to assume the colon cancer incidence rates of their adopted countries (6). For example, in studies of Japanese Issei (first generation) and Nisei (subsequent generation) migrants to Hawaii, a higher incidence of large bowel cancer was observed in individuals who no longer continued the practice of eating at least

* Reprinted with permission from *The Cancer Bulletin*, volume 30, number 6, pp 196-201, 1978.

one Japanese-style meal daily (3). A rise in the consumption of meat was the major difference in diet between residents of Japan and Hawaii, and the increase in beef consumption paralleled the higher risk of bowel cancer among Japanese migrants. A correlation between the daily consumption of meat and the incidence of colon cancer also has been noted in individuals from many countries, suggesting an etiological role (7, 8).

Observations of this type have led investigators to postulate that diets high in animal protein and fat, characteristic of high-risk populations, are responsible for colon cancer. In one study of 28 countries, positive correlations were found between the incidence of colon cancer and the amount of meat the various populations consumed (9). On the basis of epidemiologic findings of this type it has been postulated that colon cancer is associated with intestinal flora, which might possibly synthesize carcinogenic or promotor elements from both food and secretions in the intestine, such as bile acids. Diet might be expected to influence not only the composition of the intestinal flora but also the quantity of substrates available for the production of carcinogens. Further studies have led to the concept that low fiber content of the diet also may be associated with the development of colon cancer (10). Of recent interest are studies that have correlated the content of trace metals in the soil with the incidence of colon cancer; here, selenium has been emphasized (11-15).

A problem with epidemiologic data is that other factors in the environment could contribute significantly to the incidence of colon cancer. For example, the prevalence of infectious diseases and other chronic illnesses varies greatly among these populations who are at high and low risk, and these variations can also be correlated with the incidence of colon cancer. Other factors not related to food also change simultaneously with dietary habits, as populations undergo industrial and economic development. Even in dietary habits do discrepancies exist; for example, in certain countries, and in the Mormon population of Utah, high meat and beef intake are associated with relatively lower risk of colon cancer than among other groups (16). The epidemiological evidence available on the role of diet has therefore suggested that further studies be carried out; however, it has not supplied definite proof that any given dietary factors are causally related to variations in the incidence of colon cancer.

In attempting to explore the leads noted above, studies have been carried out to examine the fecal flora and related metabolic constituents obtained from individuals in different parts of the world. In an early analysis, fecal samples were obtained from individuals residing in England, Scotland, and the United States, regions having high incidence of colorectal cancer, and from Uganda, India, and Japan, where low incidences of colorectal cancer occur. Some differences in relative numbers of several bacterial groups were

observed. The British and American subjects had more gram-negative anaerobes than did the Ugandans, Indians, and Japanese, while the latter
groups had larger amounts of aerobic bacteria. As a result, the ratio of
anaerobes to aerobes was higher in individuals consuming a Western-style
diet than in those consuming largely vegetarian diets (17).

Concentrations of acid and neutral steroids in the feces also differed when
individuals on high and low meat diets were compared. Fecal specimens from
British and Americans on high meat diets contained higher amounts of
steroids than feces of Ugandans, Indians, and Japanese, whose diets contained little or no animal fat and protein. The amounts of neutral steroids
were low in the feces of Ugandans and Indians, intermediate in the feces of
Japanese, and high in the feces of British and Americans. Microbial conversion products of cholesterol, coprostanol, and coprostanone also contributed
a smaller amount to the total neutral steroid content of the feces of the
Ugandans, Indians, and Japanese than to the feces of the Western group.
Acid steroid concentrations were greater in the feces of British and Americans
than in the Ugandans, Indians, and Japanese, and the extent of conversion of
acid steroids also appeared to be higher in the British and Americans than in
other groups. The daily fecal excretion of cholesterol metabolites also was
believed to be greater in Americans who consume a diet containing meat than
in Americans on a meatless diet (17, 18).

In further attempts to elucidate mechanisms of colon carcinogenesis, other studies have suggested no significant differences in bacterial counts or
species isolated from the feces of volunteers on high meat or meatless diets.
Although minor quantitative variations were present, unique organisms in
high- or low-risk groups were not observed; organisms present in individuals
on high-risk diets were also found in individuals on low-risk diets. It was thus
suggested that taxonomic grouping of bacteria is not important in analyzing
the effects of diet on intestinal flora; rather, the effect of altered diet on
bacterial metabolic activity might be of greater interest, and in fact more
useful, in trying to understand the real factors contributing to colon cancer
development (19, 20). It was also of interest that alterations in flora were
believed to be affected by situations producing anger or stress in the host.
Some individuals in the general population, and also those with the high-risk
disease familial polyposis, excreted significantly higher amounts of cholesterol than the others (21-23).

In related studies, secondary bile acids in the feces were found to be higher
during fatty meat ingestion when concentrations of total bile acids were high,
leading to the concept that secondary bile acids are products of the de-
hydroxylation of primary fecal bile acids by intestinal bacteria (18, 24). In
further support of the above, high-fat, high-meat mixed Western diet and
non-meat diet, for which protein contents were similar, were compared in

human volunteers for steroid content of feces (25). The findings indicated that total anaerobic microflora count and fecal excretion of secondary bile acids and cholesterol metabolites were greater during consumption of the mixed Western diet than of the non-meat diet, supporting a role of dietary fat in the composition of intestinal flora and level of steroid conversion products in feces.

Individuals with colon cancer thus have been reported to have higher amounts of steroids and steroid conversion products such as deoxycholic acids, lithocholic acid, and cholesterol metabolites in their feces than controls without cancer. It has also been reported that the activity of fecal 7 α-dehydroxylase is higher in patients with colon cancer compared to controls, in association with the conversion of cholic and chenodeoxycholic acids to deoxycholic and lithocholic acids. A high frequency of individuals with cancer of the large bowel were reported to have greater concentrations of bile acids in their feces than did patients with other diseases (25, 26); the colon cancer patients also had greater amounts of acid steroids in the form of secondary bile acids than did the other patients.

These findings continue to support the view that there may be an association between fecal steroids and the production of cancer. However, since normal North Americans appear to show two patterns of neutral sterol conversion as measured by fecal analysis (22), important genetic factors may be operative in this area: 'high converters' have a stable pattern of extensive conversion of cholesterol, sitosterol, and campesterol by the intestinal flora to degradation products, while 'low converters' produce little or no such conversion.

Animal studies have been quite useful in attempting to elucidate the role of genetic, dietary, and environmental elements in the etiology of colon cancer. For example, an experiment has indicated a greater susceptibility to colon tumor induction by 1,2-dimethylhydrazine in rats fed high-fat diets, compared to animals fed a diet containing a normal amount of fat (27). Fecal excretion of acid and neutral steroids was also greater in animals fed high-fat diets than in animals on low-fat diets.

Among concepts believed to be relevant to cancer development, the multi-stage evolution of neoplasms and the presence of 'promoting' agents in addition to direct or indirect acting carinogens have been important. In the experimental work just cited, bile acids appear to have a potentiating effect in inducing colon carcinoma in laboratory animals and are believed to be promoting agents. The development of colonic tumors in rats exposed to the carcinogen N-methyl-N'-nitro-N-nitrosoguanidine was increased by instilling lithocholic or taurodeoxycholic acids intrarectally (28); the carcinogenic effect of azoxymethane in rats was increased by increasing the concentration of bile reaching the colon, by feeding cholestyramine, and by diverting the bile flow to the lower section of the small intestine (29, 30). Cholestyramine has been reported to increase the frequency of intestinal neoplasms induced by 1,2-dimethylhydrazine in germ-free rats (31). Of interest is the report that vitamin A-deficient rats had increased susceptibility to dimethylhydrazine-induced colon cancer (32, 33).

In a further attempt to understand the possible role of biliary metabolites in the development of colon cancer, the question of significant conversion of bile acids and cholesterol by bacteria is being assessed. In one area of investigation, fecal bacterial containing the enzymes 7-hydroxycholanoyl dehydroxylase and 3-oxocholanoyl Δ 4 dehydrogenase are being studied. These enzymes can convert primary bile acids to secondary ones and produce double bond formation on the bile acid nucleus. Thus, the possibility has been considered that both unsaturated and saturated bile acids contribute to the etiology of colon cancer, fulfilling roles of co-carcinogen and carcinogen (34).

In a further area of investigation, it has been postulated that cholesterol metabolites may be the important compounds in the pathogenesis of colon cancer, since fecal microbial 7-hydroxy-cholanoyl dehydroxylase and cholesterol dehydrogenase activities were noted to be higher in cancer patients compared to controls. Anaerobic intestinal bacteria contain enzymes that might induce the production of secondary bile acids and cholesterol metabolites.

Thus, it is believed by some investigators that metabolic products of biliary metabolism, low dietary fiber content, and bacterial and intestinal cellular enzymes are key factors increasing colon cancer risk. However, lack of a clear understanding of environmental relationships to colon cancer, highlighted by discrepancies in current data, remains. For example, Mormon and Seventh-Day Adventist populations have similar colorectal cancer standardized mortality rates despite greatly different rates of consumption of meat and beef. In Finland, the correlations also are poor. In animal and human studies, no specific bowel carcinogens have so far been detected. Work on additional factors that may be operative but have not been studied is needed.

Here, genotypic variability among individuals and population groups may be important, with the possibility that these may be greater than heretofore suspected; variability also may occur in the interaction of dietary elements with cells having different genotypic predispositions to neoplasia.

INCREASED SUSCEPTIBILITY WITH GENETIC PREDISPOSITION

The development of colorectal cancer has been shown to be influenced by genotypic predisposition. This is known to occur in a small percentage of total cases; it also has been postulated that genotypic predisposition may be responsible for a larger fraction of total colon cancer incidence than previously shown. The degree to which interactions among dietary elements and colonic cells may be enhanced by genotypic factors is unknown. Recent findings have indicated that familial associations in colon cancer in the general population are higher than in control groups, suggesting that inherited factors may well have a greater role in the genesis of colorectal cancer than has been generally believed. In addition to earlier ones, recent studies have shown a significant increase in the number of deaths due to colorectal cancer among first-degree relatives of index cases compared with the expected incidence. Factors associated with the increased risk were early age of onset, the presence of adenomas or other carcinomas in the operative specimen, and a history of previous carcinoma (35).

The genetic origin of several varieties of precancerous colorectal disease involving polyp formation has been well described. Inherited adenomatosis of the colon and rectum (familial polyposis, ACR) is associated with innumerable colonic adenomas. For this disease, it has been possible to estimate population frequency, relative fitness, and mutation rate. In inherited adenomatosis, carcinomas and the largest adenomas most often occur in the distal colon; this is similar to the occurrence of adenomas and carcinomas in the general population. Recent studies have shown that early abnormalities can be detected in colonic cells (36, 37), in cutaneous cells (38), and in stool contents (21, 22, 39, 40) of affected individuals and of some of their asymptomatic progeny.

Gardner's syndrome has been identified as a variant of familial polyposis, an autosomal dominant disorder showing a high degree of penetrance (42). Adenomatous polyps of the colon, and occasionally of the small intestine, are formed, and there is a propensity for adenocarcinomas to develop within the polyps. Other characteristic features include sebaceous cysts, desmoid tumors, fibromas, facial bone osteomas, and abnormal dentition. These conditions may appear singly or in combination. An increased susceptibility to other carcinomas, including lesions of the thyroid, ampulla of Vater, duodenum, and adrenal gland, has been reported to be associated with Gardner's syndrome and with familial polyposis. It has been estimated that one in seven cases of inherited familial polyposis is identifiable as Gardner's syndrome. Frequency in the population is estimated as approximately one in 8,000 for familial polyposis and one in 14,000 for Gardner's syndrome.

Variants of familial polyposis and Gardner's syndrome include Turcot syndrome (43), i.e., polyposis coli associated with tumors of the central nervous system. In addition, the Oldfield syndrome has been described, with extensive familial sebaceous cysts, polyposis coli, and adenocarcinoma. An additional autosomal dominant inherited disease with variable expression is the Peutz-Jeghers syndrome (44, 45), characterized by melanin pigmentation of the buccal mucosa, lips, face, fingers, toes, vagina, and anus. Polyps of the gastrointestinal tract, specifically in the small intestine, are found, with additional polyps appearing in the colon and rectum. However, these polyps are usually hamartomas rather than adenomas (46). The disorder appears to have very little malignant potential compared to familial polyposis or Gardner's syndrome, but some associated stomach and duodenal carcinomas have been reported.

One or more adenomas occur in 5% to 10% of the general population; these, too, can be associated with the development of adenocarcinoma, particularly when villous structures develop. Kindreds have also been reported to show an association of single and multiple adenomas with adenocarcinomas, a link that appears to be genetically influenced. Studies by Woolf et al. showed that 45% of the adult members of one generation had solitary adenomas and demonstrated the occurrence of adenomas in multiple generations (47). That family also had a high incidence of colon carcinoma, and the disease appeared to have an autosomal dominant mode of inheritance. Another inherited disorder is juvenile polyposis of the colon, in which the polyps are hamartomas and are not viewed as potentially malignant. Relatives of these juveniles do, however, express an above-normal rate of adenomas and colorectal adenocarcinomas.

The disease hereditary adenocarcinomatosis also has been observed in familial aggregates. The disease is inherited as an autosomal dominant with 90% penetrance (48), with a striking incidence of primary malignancies at multiple anatomic sites including the colon and an early age of onset in families highly predisposed to cancer (49). The general concept of 'cancer families' has now been broadened to include neoplasms of different types, in addition to those affecting a single organ such as the colon. The neoplasms in those families appear to be influenced by genetic predisposition and affect diverse organs, especially the colon and endometrium. They tend to develop earlier in life than usual and may occur separately or as multiple cancers in family members. Since adenocarcinomas of the colon and reproductive sites are known to coexist excessively in studies of multiple primary cancers, the familial syndrom may represent a scattering over the family tree of tumors that share etiologic influences (50).

PHENOTYPIC EXPRESSIONS OF INHERITED DISEASE

Specific abnormalities have been observed in the cells and in the intestinal contents of individuals with hereditary predisposition to colorectal cancer that are now serving as indices for experimental studies in two areas relevant to phenotypic expression of inherited disease. One is in the identification and

Table 1. Phenotypic characteristics recently reported in population groups with increased susceptibility to colon cancer.

Characteristics	Reference
Adenomatous morphology leading to adenoma-cancer sequence	52, 53
Abnormal proliferation of colonic epithelial cells in high frequency in colonic biopsies from individuals with familial polyposis and Gardner's syndrome	36, 37, 51
Immunologic response with inappropriate suppression of normal lymphocyte response to allogeneic stimulus in nonpolyposis familial aggregates	56
Heteroploidy of cutaneous epithelial cells in individuals with Gardner's syndrome	54
Growth modifications of cutaneous fibroblasts in familial polyposis and Gardner's syndrome	55
Decreased fecal degradation of cholesterol in familial polyposis and in some individuals in the general population	21, 39, 40
Mutagen activity in feces of human subjects in the general population	57

Adapted from Chait and Lipkin (41).

definition of population groups at high risk for colorectal cancer; another is in studies attempting to define interactions that may occur between cells genotypically predisposed to neoplasia and carcinogenic or promotor elements. These abnormalities are enumerated in table 1. In individuals with familial polyposis and Gardner's syndrome, proliferative abnormalities in colonic epithelial cells have aided identification of early disease and affected individuals. Proliferating colonic epithelial cells that have inherited the germinal mutation fail to repress DNA synthesis, and they undergo abnormal maturation as they migrate through the colonic crypts. Morphologically identifiable adenomatous cells that fail to repress proliferative activity develop and accumulate in the mucosa, and malignant cells evolve as these accumulations of adenomatous cells enlarge (36, 37, 51) (fig. 1). The development of villous components in the polypoid lesions is associated with the development of malignancy (52, 53).

Recent studies also have indicated that abnormal phenotypic expressions of inherited familial polyposis extend to cutaneous cells. A recent study reported increased heteroploidy in cutaneous epidermal cells derived from individuals with Garner's syndrome (54). In cutaneous fibroblasts, various abnormalities, including overgrowth and cytoskeletal structure defects have been detected (55). Abnormal ploidy in cells of polyps also has been observed.

An immunological abnormality associated with increased susceptibility to colon cancer in asymptomatic progeny of non-polyposis familial aggregates has recently been observed. It manifested itself as an inappropriate suppres-

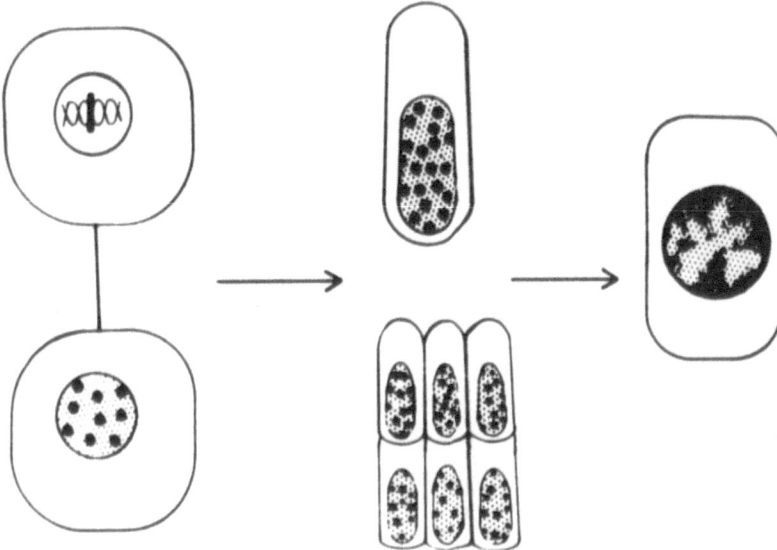

Fig. 1. Sequence of events believed to lead to malignancy in inherited adenomatosis of the colon and rectum (familial polyposis). Proliferating colonic epithelial cells that have inherited the germinal mutation fail to repress DNA synthesis (left side of diagram). Additional events are then believed to occur, giving rise to new abnormal clones from original cell population. These accumulate as adenomas (center of diagram), from which malignant cells then arise (right side).

sion of a potentially normal lymphocyte ability to respond to an allogenic stimulus. This defect in recognitive immunity appeared to be the same defect that was demonstrated in individuals with established malignancies (56). Studies to extend these various findings to additional familial aggregates and to related disorders leading to colon cancer are now under way and offer the possibility of new means for the early detection of susceptible population groups.

Related studies also are in progress to identify abnormal constituents of feces and to examine their potential carcinogenic activity in colon cells. Specifically, in the high-risk group with familial polyposis, several recent reports compared fecal neutral steroids and bile acids in patients with familial polyposis with those in controls (21, 39, 40). Individuals with familial polyposis excreted higher amounts of undegraded cholesterol than controls. Non-degraded cholesterol was also found in a small fraction of individuals in the general population (22). Further studies are in progress to assess the utility of these variations in cholesterol and its metabolites in screening high-risk population groups for disease, and to determine their possible role in the development of colon cancer. Similarly, a wide variety of analyses (including neutral sterols and bile acids, metabolic activity of fecal microflora, mutagens in feces, and nitroso-group exchange reactions in fecal bacteria) are presently under way to evaluate the fecal contents of high-risk groups and to attempt to determine significant parameters in these populations. The application of findings of this type to colon cancer prevention awaits more definite data on the effect of dietary and other modes of intervention on both fecal chemistry parameters and the neoplastic transformation of colonic cells.

REFERENCES

1. Silverberg E and Holleb A: Major trends in cancer: 25 years survey. *Ca – A Cancer Journal for Clinicians* 25: 8-22, 1975.
2. Gilbertsen V: Proctosigmoidoscopy and polypectomy in reducing the incidence of rectal cancer. *Cancer* 34: 936-939, 1974.
3. Doll R: The geographical distribution of cancer. *Br J Cancer* 23: 1-8, 1969.
4. Berg JS: Proceedings of the Second National Conference on Cancer of the Colon and Rectum. American Cancer Socity, Bar harbor, Fla, Sept 26-29, 1973.
5. Haenzel W, Berg J, and Sezi M et al.: Large bowel cancer in Hawaiian Japanese. *J Natl Cancer Inst* 51: 1765-1779, 1973.
6. Haenzel W and Kurihara M: Studies of Japanese migrants: I. Mortality from cancer and other diseases among Japanese in the United States. *J Natl Cancer Inst* 40: 43-68, 1968.
7. Wynder EL and Shigematsu T: Environmental factors of cancer of colon and rectum. *Cancer* 20: 1520, 1967.
8. Armstrong B and Doll R: Environmental factors and cancer incidence and mortality in different countries with special reference to dietary practices. *Int J Cancer* 15: 617-631, 1975.
9. Gregor O, Tomon R and Provosa F: Geographical distribution of stomach cancer in Czechoslovakia. *Gut* 10: 1031-1034, 1969.
10. Burkitt DP: Large bowel cancer: An epidemiologic jigsaw puzzle. *J Natl Cancer Inst* 54: 3-6, 1975.
11. Andrews ED, Hartley WJ and Grant AB: Selenium – responsive disease of animals in New Zealand. *New Zealand Vet J* 16: 3-10, 1968.
12. Harr JR, Exon JH and Weswig PH et al.: Effect of dietary selenium on N-fluorenyl-acetamide (fAA)-induced cancer on vitamin E supplemented rats. *Clin Toxicol* 6: 287-293, 1976.
13. Jacobs MM, Jansson B and Griffin AC: Personal communication.
14. Jansson B, Malahy MA and Seiburg GB: *Prevention and detection of cancer.* New York, Marcel Dekker, 1976.
15. Schrauzer GB and Ishmael D: Effects of selenium and of arsenic on the genesis of spontaneous mammary tumors of inbred C3 mice. *Ann Clin Lab Sci* 2: 441-447, 1974.
16. Enstrom JE: Cancer mortality among Mormons. *Cancer* 36: 825, 1975 (See also Lyon et al.: *Cancer* 39: 2608, 1977.)
17. Hill M, Drasar B and Aries V et al.: Bacteria and aetiology of cancer of large bowel. *Lancet* i: 95-100, 1971.
18. Reddy B and Wynder E: Large bowel carcinogenesis: Fecal constituents of populations with diverse incidence rates of colon cancer. *J Natl Cancer Inst* 50: 1437-1442, 1973.
19. Feingold S. Atteberg H and Sutter V: Effect of diet on human fecal flora: Comparison of Japanese and American diets. *Am J Clin Nutr* 27: 1456-1469, 1974.
20. Moore W and Holdeman L: Discussion of current bacteriological investigations of the relationships between intestinal flora, diet, and colon cancer. *Cancer Res* 35: 3418-3420, 1975.
21. Reddy BS, Mastromarino A and Gustafson C et al.: Fecal bile acids and Neutral sterols in patients with familial polyposis. *Cancer* 38: 1694-1698, 1976.
22. Wilkins T and Hackman A: Two patterns of neutral steroid conversion in the feces of normal North Americans. *Cancer Res* 34: 2250-2254, 1974.

23. Watne AL and Core S: Fecal steroids in polyposis coli and ileorectostomy patients. *J Surg Res* 19: 157-161, 1975.
24. Hill M: The effect of some factors on the faecal concentration of acid steroids, neutral steroids, and urobilins. *J Pathol* 104: 239-245, 1971.
25. Reddy B, Weisberger J and Wynder E: Effects of high risk and low risk diets for colon carcinogenesis on fecal microflora and steroids in man. *J Nutr* 105: 878-884, 1975.
26. Hill M, Drasar B and Williams R: Fecal bile acids and clostridia in patients with cancer of the large bowel. *Lancet* i: 535-538, 1975.
27. Reddy B, Narisawa T and Maronpot R et al.: Animal models for the study of dietary factors and cancer of the large bowel. *Cancer Res.*35: 3421-3426, 1975.
28. Narisawa T, Magadia N and Weisburger J et al.: Promoting effect of bile acids on colon carcinogenesis after intrarectal instillation of N-methyl-N'-nitro-N-nitrosoguanidine in rats. *J Natl Cancer Inst* 55: 1093-1097, 1974.
29. Chomchai C, Bhadrachari H and Nigro H: The effect of bile on the induction of intestinal tumors in rats. *Dis Colon Rectum* 17: 310-312, 1974.
30. Nigro N, Bhadrachari N and Chomchai C: A rat model for studying colonic cancer: Effect of cholestyramine on induced tumors. *Dis Colon Rectum* 16: 438- 443, 1973.
31. Asano T, Pollard M and Madsen Dij Effects of cholestyramine on 1,2-dimethylhydrazine-induced enteric carcinoma in germ-free rats. *Proc Soc Exp Biol Med* 150: 780-785, 1975.
32. Rodgers A, Herndon B and Newberne P: Induction by dimethylhydrazine of intestinal carcinoma in normal rats and rats fed high or low levels of vitamin A. *Cancer Res* 33: 1003-1009, 1973.
33. Rodgers A and Newberne P: Dietary enhancement of intestinal carcinogenesis by dimethylhydrazine in rats. *Nature* 246: 491-492, 1973.
34. Hill M: The role of colon anaerobics in the metabolism of bile acids and steroids and its relation to colon cancer. *Cancer* 36: 2387-2400, 1975.
35. Lovett E: Familial factors in the etiology of carcinoma of the large bowel. *Proc R Soc Med* 67: 751-752, 1974.
36. Deschner EE, Lewis CM and Lipkin M: In vitro study of human rectal endothelial cells: I. Atypical zone of H3 thymidine incorporation in mucosa of multiple polyposis. *J Clin Invest* 42: 1922-1928, 1963.
37. Deschner E and Lipkin M: Study of human rectal epithelial cells in vitro: III. RNA, protein and DNA synthesis in polyps and adjacent mucosa. *J Natl Cancer Inst* 44: 175-185, 1970.
38. Pfeffer LM and Kopelovich L: Differential genetic susceptibility of cultured human skin fibroblasts to transformation by KiMSV. *Cell* 10: 313-320, 1977.
39. Drasar BS, Bone ES and Hill MJ et al.: Colon cancer and bacterial metabolism in familial polyposis. *Gut* 16: 824-825, 1975.
40. Watne AL, Lai HL and Mance T et al.: Fecal steroids and fecal flora in polyposis coli patients. Proceedings of the Society for Surgery of the Alimentary Tract. San Antonio, Texas, May 1975.
41. Chait M and Lipkin M: Predisposition to large bowel neoplasia. In: *Carcinoma of the Colon and Rectum*. Chicago, Year Book Medical Publishers, Inc, 1978.
42. Gardner EJ: Follow-up study of a family group exhibiting dominant inheritance for intestinal polyps, osteomas, fibromas, and epidermal cysts. *Am J Human Genet* 14: 376-390, 1962.
43. Turcot J, Despres JP and St Pierre F: Malignant tumors of the central nervous system associated with familial polyposis of the colon: Report of two cases. *Dis Colon Rectum* 2: 265-268, 1959.
44. Jeghers H, McKusick VA and Katz KH: Generalized intestinal polyposis and melanin spots of the oral mucosa, lips, and digits. *N Engl J Med* 241: 993-1005, 1031-1036, 1949.
45. Peutz JLA: Over een zeer merkwaardige, gecombineerde familiaire polyposis van de slijmvliezen van den tractus intestinalis met die van de neuskeelholte en gepaard met eigenaardige pigmentatie van de huis en slijmvliezen. *Ned Maandschr Geneesk* 10: 134-146, 1921.
46. McKusick VA: Genetic factors in intestinal polyposis. *JAMA* 182: 271-277, 1962.
47. Woolf CM, Richards RC and Gardner EJ: Occasional discrete polyps of colon and rectum showing inherited tendency in kindred. *Cancer* 8: 403-408, 1955.

96

48. Anderson DE: Genetic varieties of neoplasia. In: *Genetic Concepts and Neoplasia.* A collection of papers presented at the 23rd Annual Symposium on Fundamental Cancer Research, 1969. Williams and Wilkins Co, Baltimore, 1970, pp 85-109.

49. Lynch HT: Hereditary factors in carcinoma. In: *Recent results in cancer research.* Springer-Verlag, New York, 1967, vol 12, pp 67-85.

50. Fraumeni JF Jr: Genetic factors. In: *Cancer medicine,* Holland JF and Frei E (eds). Lea and Febiger, Philadelphia, 1973, pp 7-13.

51. Lipkin M: Growth kinetics of normal and premalignant gastrointestinal epithelium. In: *Growth kinetics and biochemical regulation of normal and malignant cells.* A collection of papers presented at the 29th Annual Symposium on Fundamental Cancer Research, 1976. Williams and Wilkins, Baltimore, 1977, pp 569-589.

52. Morson BC and Bussey H Jr: Predisposing causes of intestinal cancer. In: *Current problems in surgery.* Ravitch M (ed). Year Book Medical Publishers Inc. Chicago, 1970, pp 1-50.

53. Spjut H: Malignant potential of large bowel polyps (adenomatous and villous). In: Program and Abstracts of Papers of the 1977 Workshop on Large Bowel Cancer, Modern Methods of Biomedical and Clinical Research Toward Control and Cure of Large Bowel Cancer. Houston, Jan 21-23, 1977, p 61.

54. Danes BS: The Gardner syndrome: A family study in cell culture. *J Natl Cancer Inst* 1977.

55. Kopelovich L, Colon S and Pollack R: Defective organization of actin in cultured skin fibroblasts from patients with inherited adenocarcinoma. *Proc Natl Acad Sci USA* 74: 3019, 1977.

56. Berlinger NT, Lopez C and Vogen J et al.: Defective recognitive immunity in family aggregates of colon carcinoma. *J Clin Invest* 59: 761-769, 1977.

57. Varghese AJ, Land P and Furrer R et al.: Evidence for the formation of mutagenic N-nitroso compounds in the human body. *Proc AACR* 18: 317, 1977.

11. THE PATHOLOGY OF POLYPS OF THE LARGE BOWEL

DAVID W. DAY

The word polyp is used clinically to describe any circumscribed lesion that projects above the surface of surrounding mucosa and used alone conveys nothing about the nature of such a lesion. Polyps vary in their shape, size and surface and may or may not have a stalk, that is they may be pedunculated or sessile. Although the naked eye appearances of some polypoid lesions are reasonably characteristic, it is only by microscopic examination that their true nature is determined. The several histological types of polyps differ in their clinical significance and particularly in their malignant potential. Thus the management of the individual patient with a polyp depends on accurate histological diagnosis. In practice it is of great help to the pathologist if the polyp is removed complete, if the stalk of any pedunculated lesion has been identified by a thread and if larger sessile polyps are pinned out on a flat piece of cork board. In this way the polyp can be correctly orientated and sections cut in the right plane. This can be of crucial importance not only in diagnosis of the type of polyp but in the case of neoplastic polyps in the interpretation of whether or not malignant change is present.

Polyps of the large bowel can be broadly divided into *non-epithelial* and *epithelial*. The *non-epithelial* polyps include those derived from lymphoid tissue, smooth muscle, fat and nervous tissue. The only one I wish to mention in any detail is the benign lymphoid polyp. This occurs as a usually solitary, sub-mucous, sessile polyp anything from a few millimetres to a few centimetres in size in the lower third of the rectum mostly in people in the third and fourth decades of life. It is commonly symptomless and usually an incidental finding. Histologically it consists of normal lymphoid tissue, usually with prominent follicular differentiation, which lies mainly in the submucosa and is covered by attenuated mucous membrane. Benign lymphoid polyps are harmless lesions, unrelated to malignant lymphomas, and probably a result of local inflammation.

Epithelial polyps, which are those most commonly seen in clinical practice, can be classified into four groups (see fig. 1).

The most important because they have the potential to become malignant tumours are the neoplastic group of polyps or adenomas. The other classes of polyp, the hamartomatous, inflammatory and hyperplastic have no malignant potential.

K. Welvaart et al. (eds.), Colorectal Cancer, 97-101. All rights reserved.
Copyright © 1980 by Martinus Nijhoff Publishers, The Hague/Boston/London.

Histological Classification of Epithelial Polyps of the Large Bowel

---

| (i) | Neoplastic | – | adenomas ($\pm$ invasive carcinoma) polypoid carcinomas |

(ii)	Hamartomatous	–	juvenile polyps Peutz-Jeghers polyps
(iii)	Inflammatory	–	polyps in idiopathic IBD polyps in infective colitis
(iv)	Unclassified	–	metaplastic (hyperplastic) polyps

Figure 1.

Hamartomas are malformations composed of a haphazard mixture of tissues normally found in the affected part of the body and often with an excess of one particular tissue type. In the large bowel two types of hamartomatous polyp occur, the juvenile and the Peutz-Jeghers, and both are uncommon.

The juvenile polyp, as its name suggests, is usually, although not exclusively, found in children and the majority occur in the rectum within 5 cm of the anus. They are usually single or few in number but a juvenile polyposis syndrome occurs rarely in which numerous polyps are present in the stomach and small and large bowel. Macroscopically they are round lesions up to 2 cm in diameter with a smooth, bright red surface beneath which are white patches which represent mucin-filled cysts. Microscopically they consist of epithelial tubules, many of which are dilated and cystic but lined by normal mucosal cells, separated by a large amount of lamina propria in which there is a characteristic absence of elements of the muscularis mucosae. Many juvenile polyps are probably symptomless, symptoms being related to the tendency of the polyp to undergo inflammation, ulceration, torsion and auto-amputation.

The polyps in Peutz-Jeghers syndrome occur mostly in the small intestine but the colon is involved in about 15% of cases. However, isolated polyps of the Peutz-Jeghers type are found in individuals who show none of the stigmata of the fully developed syndrome. This type of polyp is pedunculated or sessile with a coarsely lobulated surface and may be several centimetres in diameter. The characteristic features seen histologically are of branching bands of smooth muscle derived from the muscularis mucosae covered by mucus-secreting crypts which are crowded together, elongated and not infrequently convoluted. The risk of malignant change developing in Peutz-Jeghers polyps is widely held to be negligible, although an association with tumours of the upper gastro-intestinal tract, ovary and other diverse multiple neoplasms has recently been recognised.

Inflammatory polyps are frequently seen in European and American clinical practice where they occur in idiopathic inflammatory bowel disease (IBD), that is in Crohn's disease and more particularly in ulcerative colitis. In both conditions they are more prominent in the colon than the rectum. They may be single or numerous, segmental or diffuse. Their occurrence is related to at least one previous severe attack of colitis, in particular a total colitis, and a positive association with toxic dilatation has been noted. It is thought that during a severe episode of colitis there is extensive full thickness mucosal ulceration with undermining of the surviving epithelium, and re-epithelialisation occurs beneath these lengths of stripped up mucosa, leaving mucosal tags projecting into the lumen. They can have bizarre shapes and may stick to one another to form mucosal bridges across the lumen of the bowel. Grossly they project from the mucosa as finger-like outgrowths with little distinction between stalk and head. Histologically most consist of variably inflamed mucosa which may contain dilated glands, along with muscularis mucosae and submucosa, although some are composed of granulation tissue with little or no glandular component. They remain even when the inflammatory bowel disease has resolved. Inflammatory polyps may also occur in ischaemic bowel disease, in bacillary dysentery, and in such parasitic infestations as amoebiasis and schistosomiasis, when the responsible organism can be identified.

Hyperplastic or *metaplastic* polyps occur as multiple sessile lesions in about 75% of adults over the age of 40. They are most common in the rectum but can occur in all parts of the colon and occasionally in the appendix. They are usually below 0.5 cm in diameter and are the same colour or paler than surrounding normal mucosa with a flat or convex surface and tending to lie on the crest of mucosal folds. Histologically the crypts are elongated and dilated, with reduced numbers of normal goblet cells and a serrated appearance to the epithelium due to patchy flattening of cells. These polyps are symptomless and harmless and their only importance is that they can be mis-diagnosed as adenomas. Their pathogenesis is not known although kinetic studies have shown that the epithelial cells of the hyperplastic polyp grow more slowly and live longer than normal mucosal cells (1).

The remaining group of benign polyps and the most important because of their relationship to colo-rectal carcinoma are the *adenomas*. These vary considerably in macroscopic and microscopic appearance but they all have a common cytology which is the main reason for regarding them only as different growth patterns of the one disease. On the basis of their structure they may be split into three groups (2), the tubular adenoma at one end of the spectrum, the villous adenoma at the other and the tubulo-villous adenoma which, as the name suggests, has a structure intermediate between the other two. In a series from St. Mark's Hospital, approximately 75% were tubular adenomas, 15% tubulo-villous adenomas and 10% villous adenomas (3).

The typical tubular adenoma is small, spherical and pedunculated with a smooth surface broken into lobules by intercommunicating clefts. Microscopically it consists of closely packed epithelial tubules which grow and branch horizontally to the muscularis mucosae and which are separated by normal lamina propria. On the other hand the villous adenoma is usually large and sessile with a shaggy surface and histologically consists of finger-like processes each made up of a core of lamina propria covered by epithelial cells growing vertically towards the bowel lumen, the epithelium dipping down between the processes to rest on the muscularis mucosae. The tubulo-villous adenoma may consist of either a mixture of these two growth patterns or have an intermediate uniform pattern with broad and stunted villi below which are epithelial tubules similar to those in a tubular adenoma. However, adenomas with a tubular structure histologically may be large and sessile, and a small pedunculated lesion can have a typical villous configuration. Common to all adenomas are hyperchromatic nuclei and increased numbers of mitoses and on the basis of nuclear changes such as enlargement, pleomorphism, loss of polarity and stratification a subjective grading into mild, moderate and severe epithelial atypia or dysplasia may be made. Differences in degree of atypia are seen not only between individual adenomas but also within the same tumour. The terms carcinoma in-situ and focal carcinoma are used by some pathologists to describe the appearances in an adenoma in which there is respectively total or partial severe dysplasia. However, they are liable to misinterpretation and can lead to unnecessarily radical surgery. When a tumour is entirely superficial to the muscularis mucosae even though the tissue changes satisfy the cytological criteria for malignancy there is no potential for metastasis. This is because in the large bowel, lymphatics are not present in the colonic mucosa (4).

Apart from carcinoma arising in long-standing extensive ulcerative colitis, it appears that all or the vast majority of carcinomas of the large bowel arise from a pre-existing adenomas, a process referred to as the adenoma-carcinoma sequence. Thus when a series of adenomas is examined a proportion will show focal areas of invasive tumour, that is neoplastic cells deep to the muscularis mucosae. Alternatively if surgically resected large bowel carcinomas are studied carefully, residual adenomatous tissue may be identified at the margins of the tumour. The proportion increases the more limited the spread of the carcinoma through the bowel wall, implying that as a carcinoma grows, residual adenoma is encroached on and destroyed. Some polypoid lesions removed endoscopically consist entirely of carcinomatous tissue, so called polypoid carcinomas, and this presumably has been the sequence of events in these cases.

Autopsy studies on the prevalence of adenomas in areas where the incidence of large bowel carcinoma is high have shown that upwards of 50% of the population over the age of 50 can have these tumours. It is obvious therefore that the vast majority of adenomas behave in a benign fashion and do not progress into malignant tumours.

From studies of large series of adenomas the likelihood of malignant change has been found to be associated with increasing size, a villous growth pattern and severity of epithelial dysplasia (5).

REFERENCES

1. Hayashi T, Yatani R, Apostol J and Stemmermann GN: Pathogenesis of hyperplastic polyps of the colon: a hypothesis based on ultrastructure and in-vitro kinetics. *Gastroent* 66: 347-356, 1974.
2. Morson BC (ed): Histological typing of intestinal tumours, No. 15 in International histological classification of tumours, World Health Organisation, Geneva, 1976.
3. Muto T, Bussey HJR and Morson BC: The evolution of cancer of the colon and rectum. *Cancer* 36: 2251-2270, 1975.
4. Fenoglio CM, Kaye GI and Lane N: Distribution of human colonic lymphatics in normal, hyperplastic, and adenomatous tissue. *Gastroent* 64: 51-66, 1973.
5. Morson BC, Bussey HJR and Samoorian S: Policy of local excision for early cancer of the colorectum. *Gut* 18: 1045-1050, 1977.

12. POLYPOSIS COLI

E.A. VAN SLOOTEN

The factors of polyposis coli which have aroused so much interest are two-fold: its genetic characteristics and its biological behaviour.

GENETIC ASPECTS

Polyposis is one of the very rare neoplastic diseases with a dominant Mendelian genetic pattern. When one parent has polyposis, an average of 50% of the offspring may be expected to develop this disease. Applying the laws of chance to this pattern, there may be families with 5 children who are all free of disease or who are all affected. With a 1 in 32 probability for either of these possibilities, the law of chance must be considered the main reason why the disease disappears in some families.

The other factors leading to the disappearance of strong genetic traits, such as deformities resulting in social isolation of an affected individual or disorders that often cause death or invalidism before the reproductive age, do not apply to polyposis. Severe symptoms and death from cancer of the colon rarely occur before the age of 30 years and the patients have a completely normal outward appearance. The genetic trait is very strong. Instead of becoming less pronounced in successive generations it is more usual for symptoms to appear at an earlier age and for cancer to develop in younger individuals. Sometimes the disease seems to skip a generation. Very probably the penetrance of the genetic disturbance was less pronounced in the asymptomatic member, with late development of polyps and death from a cause other than cancer of the colon at a relatively young age. Every now and then an individual case is encountered whereby none of the patient's forbears has died of bowel cancer and even a very thorough search does not produce a family member with bowel disease. In such a case a new mutation must have occurred. As the disease is known to be hereditary, the mutation can only have occurred at a very early stage of development in order to have affected the entire colon, sometimes the gastric mucosa and the fore-runners of the germ cells in the reproductive system. In rare instances the polyposis is associated with proliferative mesodermal changes, cutaneous fibromas and osteomas (Gardner's syndrome) but usually only the colon and rectum are

104

affected. The changes have no predilection for a certain part of the large bowel, so that rectoscopy will as a rule suffice to detect the disease. There may, however, be cases in which the disease is more prominent in the proximal part of the colon.

BIOLOGICAL DEVELOPMENT

Before polyps become visible small areas of atypical proliferation can already be found in random biopsies of rectal mucosa (fig. 1). These develop into adenomatous polyps, usually during childhood (fig. 2). It is rare for an individual affected by polyposis not to have apparent polyps at the age of 15 years. They commonly remain completely asymptomatic for several years. Bleeding, the production of abundant mucus and tenesmus often herald the malignant transformation. As a rule thousands of polyps will form covering the entire surface of the mucosa, but sometimes they are found to be less numerous with apparently normal mucosa in between. Even then there will be at least one hundred polyps (fig. 3).

Although in some rare instances multiple polyps, e.g. more than 5, are found in people who do not belong to a polyposis family, they should not be regarded as spontaneous mutants with all the resulting consequences. There is a wide numerical gap between 'multiple' polyps and polyposis. Histological examination as a rule reveals the coexistence of nonprotuberant areas of

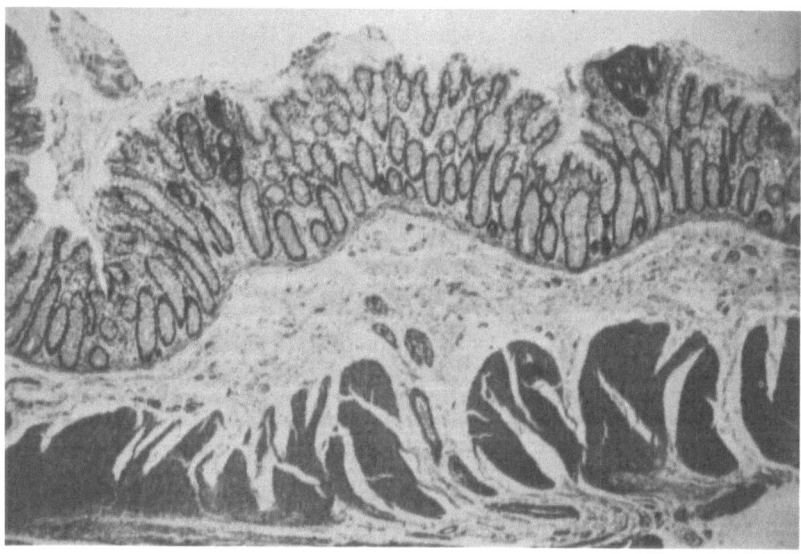

Figure 1.

atypical proliferation, polyps of all sizes with a relatively regular adeno-matous epithelium and polyps with highly atypical areas, suggesting carci-noma in situ. A thorough search will often show small spots of incipient infiltrating growth in a larger polyp. These spots and also evident malignant transformation are found more frequently with increasing age. The entire

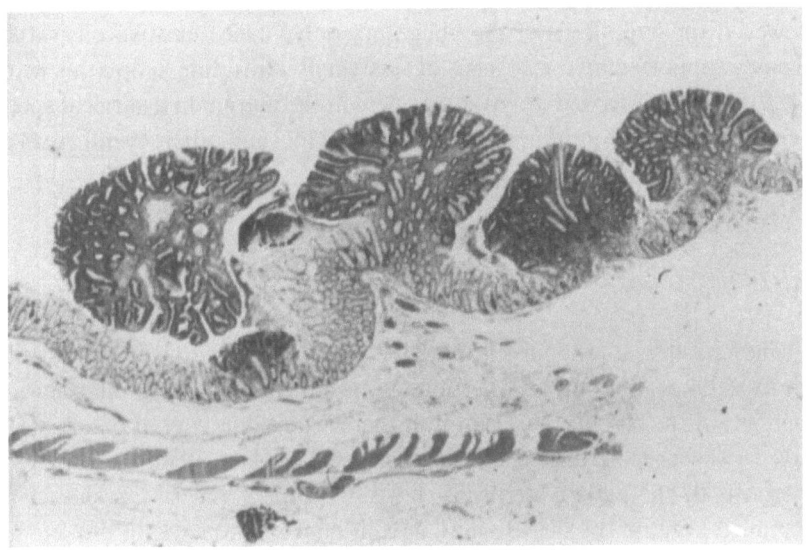

Figure 2.

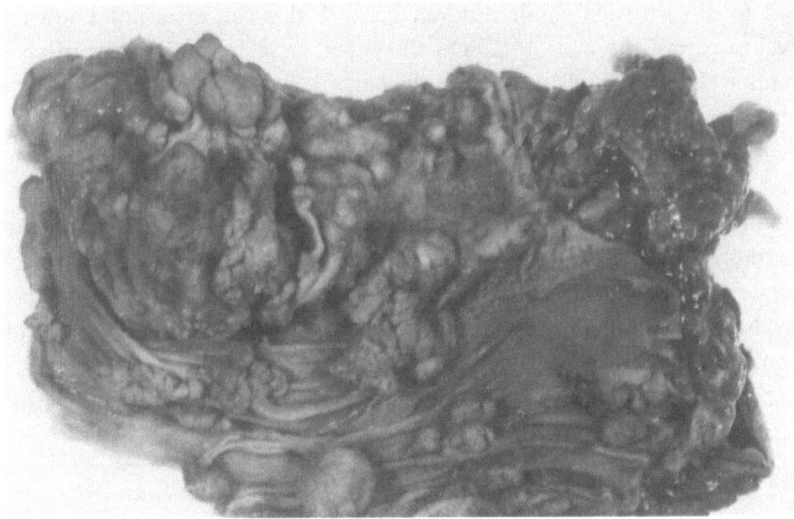

Figure 3.

picture of the polyp-cancer sequence can be found within a small area of mucosa in the polyposis patient, forming as it were a condensation of what happens in the general population – where at least a few thousand people would be needed to produce that seen in this one individual.

The question of whether cancer in the colon always develops in an area with usually polypoid adenomatous proliferation or also arises de novo in the mucosa with infiltrating growth right from the start has not yet been solved. However, the hypothesis of the obligatory polyp-cancer sequence is rather strongly supported by the absence of very small infiltrating neoplasms without a partially distroyed polyp somewhere in the margin in a surgical specimen which contains innumerable proliferative foci and often several areas of invasive growth in the larger polyps.

FAMILY SCREENING

Whenever a case of polyposis is detected, a very conscientious family history has to be taken, not only by questioning the patient but also by interviewing members of the parents' generation. If there is no single case of polyposis or large bowel cancer in this generation there is no need to extend the search for polyposis to the patient's cousins, but his brothers and sisters should be examined because the disease may have been asymptomatic in one of this parents. As a matter of course the patient's offspring must be examined. Whenever the family history is suggestive of polyposis, the implications are self-evident.

Although polyps may already be apparent in a child 4 years old, there is no need to disturb such small children because this cancer is not known to develop before the age of 12. On the other hand it is very rewarding to examine children at risk as soon as they are likely to be cooperative because the earlier adequate treatment is carried out, the better the adaptation to the new situation will be in later life.

No case has as yet been reported in which polyposis became apparent in a person over 35 years of age who had been followed up for several years. Therefore there is no indication for further examination if no signs of the disease are found in a person from a polyposis family who is over 35 years of age. From the foregoing it should be evident that the examination is not complete unless several (10 or more) random biopsies from different sites in the rectum and rectosigmoid have been examined, even when the mucosa is apparently normal.

TREATMENT AND FOLLOW-UP

There are two ways in which polyposis may be treated once the principle that no polyp should be allowed to progress to cancer has been clearly understood. As there are no other ways to inhibit growths or progression of innumerable polyps in the colon, surgical treatment is the only choice, either a total proctocolectomy or a colectomy with an ileorectal anastomosis at a distance of $\pm$ 15 cm from the anal verge preceded and/or followed by fulguration of the polyps in the remaining part of the rectum (fig. 4).

Since all the stages of development of polyps can be seen side by side, patient and doctor must be prepared to face a life-long follow-up with a visit at least every 6 months involving rectoscopy each time with fulguration of the polyps that have appeared during the interval.

Although recent surgical improvements and better stomal care and appliances have reduced the inconveniences of an ileostoma, it is still an object of concern and constant care for the patient and is often a social handicap. On the other hand total proctocolectomy relieves the patient of the fear that cancer may develop in the remaining part of the large bowel. The choice of the optimum treatment remains a very personal decision.

The experience of most physicans who have treated and followed patients who have undergone colectomy with ileorectostomy is by no means unfavourable on the condition that the operation has been carried out correctly.
– Nearly every patient is ready to keep the follow-up appointments regularly.
– Careful, selective and well-staged fulguration of polyps does not lead to fibrosis of the rectum or to strictures.
– As a rule the number of new polyps gradually decreases as follow-up proceeds.

Polyposis coli

Treatment

A. Total procto-colectomy,
        permanent ileostomy.
    Safe but very inconvenient.

B. Colectomy with ileorectostomy,
        satisfactory normal continence.
    Lifelong follow-up examination every
    6 months with fulguration of apparent
    polyps.
    Small chance of development of cancer.

Figure 4.

108

– If cancer develops, it is still very small and responds to local treatment.
– After an adaptation period of 6-12 months, normal or semi-normal stools are formed and defaecation takes place one to three times a day. There is no need for a special diet and occasional diarrhoea can easily be controlled by imodium, etc.

Total proctocolectomy is only strictly indicated when cancer has already developed at a site where abdomino-perineal excision would have been unavoidable anyway. Another indication is an unwillingness or inability of the patient to return regularly for follow-up examination.

In view of the possibility that polyps may also exist in the stomach, it is advisable to perform a gastroscopy and an X-ray examination. The procedure should be repeated every 2 to 3 years. When polyps are found they are usually few in number and can be removed endoscopically. Quite rarely polyps are also formed in the ileum. It is still not known whether they have the same tendency toward malignant change as the colonic polyps. It should be clear that the care for the individual polyposis patient, and for families afflicted by the disease, can only be carried out in an institution that has a watertight follow-up system and by specialists with a great interest in this rare condition.

Some figures may illustrate the importance of family screening: the average age of patients in whom polyposis was found after they visited their doctor because of symptoms often caused by malignant change is 35 years. The average age of members of polyposis families in whom the disease is detected by organized screening is 25 years. Malignancy is very rarely found in this group of people without or with only very slight symptoms (fig. 5).

Polyposis coli

35 yrs   Average age at which progressive complaints lead to diagnosis.

25 yrs   Average age at which disease is detected by screening relatives of polyposis patients.

Assumed average length of time needed for the polyp ⟶ cancer sequence   10 yrs.

Figure 5.

ACKNOWLEDGMENT

Figures 1-3 have been reproduced by kind permission of Afd. fotografie, Antoni van Leeuwenhoekhuis, Het Nederlands Kankerinstituut.

REFERENCES

1. Bussey JHR: *Familial polyposis coli.* 1978 John Hopkins Univ, Press Baltimore.
2. BusseyLorson BC: *Gastrointestinal tract cancer* 1978, p 275 Pleum Book Co. New York and London.
3. Schaupp WC and Volpe PA: Management of diffuse colonic polyposis. *Am J Surg* 124, 218, 1972.
4. Yonemoto RH, Slayback JB and Byron RJ Jr: Familial polyposis of the entire gastrointestinal tract. *Arch Surg* 99, 427, 1969.

PART IV

ADENOMAS OF THE COLON

13. CLINICAL SIGNIFICANCE OF A POLYP

J. KREUNING

When a clinician uses the term polyp, a broad range of histopathologic entities is included. Some are clearly benign and others are neoplastic with varying degrees of malignant potential. The word 'polyp' is purely a descriptive one, meaning a lesion which projects from a mucosal surface into the bowel lumen. To the surgeon and endoscopist, the shape and size of polyps are important, but the characterization of the histological features have greater importance. The clinical significance of a polyp and the management of the patient are directly related to the histologic type of the polyp. For this reason it is essential that all removed polyps should be given to the pathologist for microscopic examination.

Morson (1) has made a histologic classification of polyps in the large bowel. The different types of polyps fall into four main groups:
1. Hamartomas
   a. Juvenile polyp
   b. Peutz-Jeghers polyp
2. Inflammatory polyp
   a. Benign lymphoid polyp
   b. Inflammatory polyposis
3. Unclassified polyp
   Metaplastic or hyperplastic polyp
4. Neoplastic polyp
   a. Tubular adenoma
   b. Tubulo-villous adenoma
   c. Villous adenoma
The neoplastic polyp is the only type which has malignant potential.

The juvenile polyp occurs chiefly in childhood and approximately 72% of these polyps are situated in the rectum. Rectal bleeding immediately after defecation is the most common symptom. Furthermore they can present with abdominal pain and sometimes may prolapse out of the rectum. Most often these polyps will infarct through torsion of the pedicle and pass spontaneously. When there is continued rectal blood loss polypectomy can be done.

The Peutz-Jeghers polyp may occur as one or more polyps in the colon, but it is a part of a gastrointestinal polyposis in combination with mucocutaneous pigmentation and is known as the Peutz-Jeghers syndrome. The cutaneous

K. Welvaart et al. (eds.), Colorectal Cancer, 113-116. All rights reserved.
Copyright © 1980 by Martinus Nijhoff Publishers, The Hague/Boston/London.

pigmentation is usually located around the mouth, nostrils, palms, fingers, dorsum of the hands and soles of the feet. The mucosal pigmentation is found on the lips and on the buccal, nasal, rectal or anal mucosa. Severe recurrent colicky abdominal pain usually due to intussusception of the small intestine is the most common symptom. Furthermore rectal bleeding is common and hematemesis can occur with gastric or duodenal polyps. Although these polyps are benign and are not thought to undergo malignant transformation, adenocarcinoma of the gastrointestinal tract has been reported. Most of these are malignancies of the stomach, duodenum and proximal small intestine. Although colonic cancer in Peutz-Jeghers patients has also been reported, there is not sufficient evidence to regard it as a precancerous condition of the colon.

Benign lymphoid polyp is very rare, usually solitary and is mostly situated low down in the rectum. Differentiation from a malignant lymphoma is important.

Hyperplastic polyps are very common and very rarely larger than 0.5 cm. These are most common in the rectum and are nearly always multiple. These polyps are not neoplastic and are seen as incidental findings. In general these polyps give no clinical symptoms. On a macroscopic level, they have the same color as the surrounding mucosa and could be distinguished from adenomas. However, in practice this sometimes seems to be difficult and therefore they should be removed when encountered in order to distinguish them histologically from adenomas.

None of the polyps described above has malignant potential and for this reason regular follow-up examinations are not necessary.

Adenomas are localized neoplastic tumours of colonic epithelium and may undergo malignant transformation. I will restrict myself to the tubular adenoma, because the villous adenoma will be presented elsewhere. In the majority of instances patients with tubular adenoma are asymptomatic. Rectal bleeding, vague abdominal discomfort, flatulence or changes in the nature of bowel habits often lead to a diagnosis of tubular adenoma. Rectal bleeding is the most common presentation that can be attributed to tubular adenomas and may occur in 40 to 50% of the patients. The appearance of gross blood in the stool depends on the rate of bleeding and a distal location of the polyp. When noticed, the bleeding typically is fresh, intermittent and scanty. When there is occult blood loss, the patient can have an iron-deficiency anaemia. Melaena can rarely, if ever, be attributed to a tubular adenoma. Constipation may occur with large polyps in the distal colon which rarely give diarrhea. The colon is not so susceptible as the small intestine to intussusception by a pedunculated polyp because it is for the most part firmly fixed and has a wide lumen. Rarely a patient may call attention to a adenoma presenting at the anus and examination will disclose the prolaps of a polyp with a large stalk. However these symptoms should not be attributed to the polyp unless they disappear with polypectomy.

The detection of common polyps of the colon depends principally on certain special examinations, because polyps are seldom apparent on physical examination. Even rectal polyps can escape detection by the palpating finger because they are small, pliable and often movable. Feces in the rectum may obscure even larger polyps. Some polyps which bleed intermittently may be detected by repeated testing of stools for occult blood. The most important examinations are however proctosigmoidoscopy, barium-enema radiography and colonoscopy.

In different autopsy studies it was found that the likelihood of the presence of an adenoma rose with increasing age, and that in about half of these cases, they were multiple. Ekelund and Lindström (2) did a histopathological analysis of benign polyps in patients with carcinoma of the colon. They found polyps in 22% of the patients with a carcinoma and in 49% there were two or more polyps. 81% of these polyps were adenomas and three quarters of these were tubular adenomas. Due to the high incidence of multiple adenomas and adenomas with carcinomas, it is important that when a single adenoma has been discovered in a patient, the entire colon must be investigated.

The technologic advances in the area of colonoscopy has simplified the clinical approach to colonic polyps. In previous decades the decision to remove a polyp beyond the reach of a sigmoidoscope meant a major abdominal operation and in older patients it was not always without complications. It is generally recommended now that all polyps be removed by endoscopic polypectomy and given to the pathologist for microscopic examination. If there is a malignant change and after this has crossed the muscularis mucosae into the stalk, segmental colonic resection is recommended. Occasionally, even in expert hands the colonoscope cannot be advanced into the whole colon and lesions in the cecum or ascending colon cannot be reached even with repeated attempts. Furthermore there are instances in which the polyp can be reached, but where it is impossible to snare the polyp. In these cases the management of polyps poses a problem, especially when they are not larger than 1 cm. The chance of a carcinoma in polyps under 1 cm is low, namely 1% (1). Patients who have had one or more neoplastic polyps are more likely to develop further adenomas. Therefore a policy of regular follow-up examinations is recommended. When the whole colon is carefully examined and no additional polyps are detected, re-examination every two to three years is probably sufficient. Individuals in the high risk group, with multiple polyps or polyps with carcinoma, should have yearly examinations.

REFERENCES

1. Morson Basil C (ed): *The pathogenesis of colorectal cancer*, vol. 10 in the Series Major problems in pathology, W.B. Saunders Company, Philadelphia, London, Toronto, 1978.
2. Ekelund G and Lindström C: Histopathological analysis of benign polyps in patients with carcinoma of the colon and rectum. *Gut* 15: 654-663, 1974.

14. THE CLINICAL SIGNIFICANCE OF A VILLOUS ADENOMA

A. YORK MASON

NOMENCLATURE

It is important to define and to understand the meaning of the many and sometimes confusing names applied to benign epithelial neoplasms of the colon and rectum. 'Adenoma' is strictly a histopathological diagnosis, and, two distinctive growth patterns, tubular and villous, or an admixture of these two, are now internationally accepted by histopathologists. 'Villous' is a descriptive term used both by pathologists and by clinicians. 'Villous tumours', about which I propose to speak, do seem to constitute a recognisable clinical entity. An alternative nomenclature is villous papilloma. To the touch (and fortunately the majority are sited in the rectum within reach of the index finger) they feel soft and velvety; by endoscopy the slender branching villi can be seen, often floating in clear mucus, and this is a characteristic appearance, as illustrated in fig. 1.

CLINICAL PRESENTATION

Clinical details of the first patient with a large benign villous tumour of the rectum, treated successfully by surgical resection, were published by Quain (1) in 1855. Four years later, in 1859, he published a monograph (2) adding more facts about his first patient and including details of a second patient presenting with an almost identical growth and treated by him in similar manner.

I would like to base my talk on this original contribution by Quain because, although over the course of the next hundred years much was written about similar tumours, these publications have added little to our understanding of the nature of these growths, and in many instances have served only to obscure the very clear picture presented by Quain.

But first, a little about the man and his credentials: Richard Quain was Professor of Clinical Surgery, University College Hospital, London, and a president of the Royal College of Surgeons of England. In the tradition of Dr. Boerhaave, Professor of Medicine at Leyden University, 1714 to 1738, Quain was essentially a bed-side teacher. As a clinician he was meticulous in

K. Welvaart et al. (eds.), Colorectal Cancer, 117-130. All rights reserved.
Copyright © 1980 by Martinus Nijhoff Publishers, The Hague/Boston/London.

118

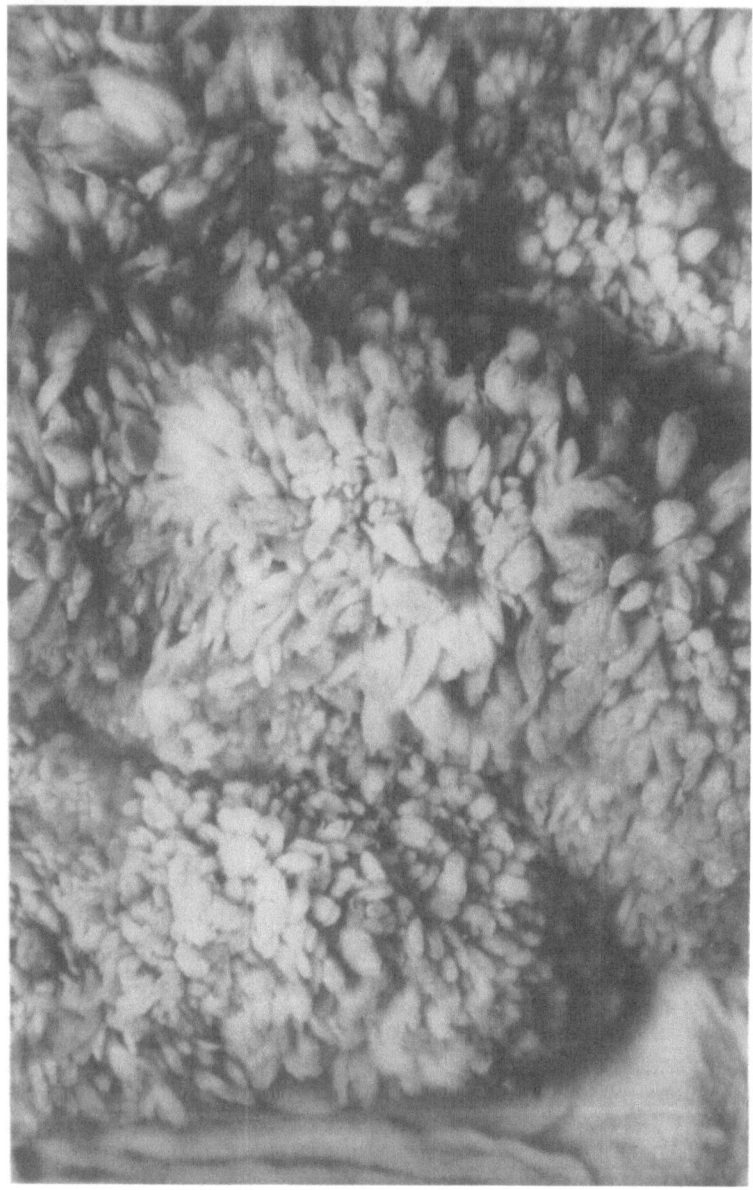

Fig. 1. The characteristic surface appearance of a villous tumour of the rectum.

his attention to detail, and he possessed, to a remarkable degree, the ability to observe and to record his observations with perfection (correct use and writing of the English language was a life-long hobby).

All these attributes are exemplified by his published case reports, parts of which I would like to quote.

His first patient 'a lady then aged 68 years ... had been suffering inconvenience in the bowel for seven years; and during two of those years she was in almost continual distress occasioned by the presence of a large mass and its protusion each time she had an evacuation, and even with the escape of flatus. It was replaced by a servant after each descent; in fact, a servant was kept exclusively to attend on this lady. There was much loss of blood. ... the patient had become much enfeebled ...'. His second patient presented with a ten year history of bowel trouble. 'She had frequent calls to evacuate their contents – as often as ten or twelve in a day, passing mostly nothing but mucus... This lady has been told from time to time, during several years, that she suffered from piles. From the various methods of treatment that had been resorted to for her relief, she derived no advantage'.

Quain thus recorded consisely in these two brief case reports the clinical presentation, since confirmed by learned theses based on the study of larger series, namely rectal bleeding, diarrhoea, painful defaecation, mucous discharge, prolapse and impairment of general health.

MORPHOLOGY AND PHYSICAL SIGNS

I come now to his description of the growths. Both tumours were within easy reach of the index finger. About the first he wrote: 'When partially prolapsed, was found to be a large, pulpy mass separable into several loosely connected lobes, consisting of pencil-like processes, the whole surface being covered over with blood and mucus... The pedicle was about 2 inches broad'; and about the second he recorded 'The tumour in the second case was in great measure similar', but he noted that it was sessile, growing from the mucous membrane but 'there was no connection with the muscular coat of the gut'. It felt soft throughout, and 'the bowel around the diseased out-growth was ... free from hardness ...'.

From his careful clinical assessment Quain concluded that both these large growths, one with a broad base and the other sessile, were benign neoplasms. 'The best evidence that upon which the surgeon can rely with most confidence as to the cancerous nature of a disease, is here wanting ...', and Quain was right; it is possible for an experienced clinician to decide, before treatment, that a particular growth is benign. Unfortunately, he became emotionally involved in an argument with Rokitansky. Quain concluded that all villous tumours of the rectum constituted a benign entity; Rokitansky took the opposite view, that they were all cancers. As a result of this argument, Quain changed his nomenclature and entitled his monograph *Illustrations of a peculiar Bleeding Tumour of the Rectum*. Fig. 2 is a reproduction of the single plate used by Quain to illustrate his monograph. Because of its unusual title this remarkable monograph is seldom, if ever, to be found in the very long list of references. Both had right on their side but both were wrong to generalise. We now know that villous tumours are all members of the adenoma family, and as such do have malignant potential. It is generally accepted that those adenomas with a villous growth pattern have a higher malignant potential, and also it is generally accepted that there is a relationship between size of adenoma and the chance of malignant change; also that there is a time relationship. Paradoxically, however, some very large villous carpets, known to have been in existence for more than ten years, and carpeting the entire rectum, are found still to be benign. Conversely, some small lesions, discovered perhaps because of a single rectal bleed, are deeply invasive cancers. It is interesting to speculate that these extensive villous carpets represent a wide 'field change', that their size and age should be measured by the depth of the pile of the carpet rather than by its surface area. However, we still do not know whether Quain's tumour constitutes a 'peculiar' clinical entity or whether it is an extreme variant.

PRE-TREATMENT CLINICAL ASSESSMENT

Returning to reality, it is the responsibility of the clinician to decide, before embarking on any form of treatment, whether invasive change has taken place. Surface biopsies, even multiple ones, are seldom of value, and may as illustrated by fig. 3, be misleading. Careful palpation, feeling for areas of hardness which characterise early invasive change, feeling and looking for an ulcer crater which is often conclusive evidence of carcinoma, are necessary. Ulceration may be preceded by baldness due to loss of villi. The real difficulties occur when the lesion has been damaged by deep biopsy or by previous attempts at unsuccessful piecemeal removal, especially by diathermy.

INCIDENCE OF INVASIVE CHANGE

The true incidence of invasive change is difficult to interpret from published series because there are so many variables, and because so much depends upon the thoroughness of examination of the resected specimen. In my personal series of 58 patients referred as having benign villous tumours 40 were assessed as benign, 6 as doubtful and 12 as definitely malignant. Peroperatively, one 'benign' tumour was thought to be doubtful, and histopathological examination of the resected specimen confirmed microscopic invasion in this patient and in four others of this benign group. 35 of the 40 benign group were thus correctly assessed with an accuracy rate of well over

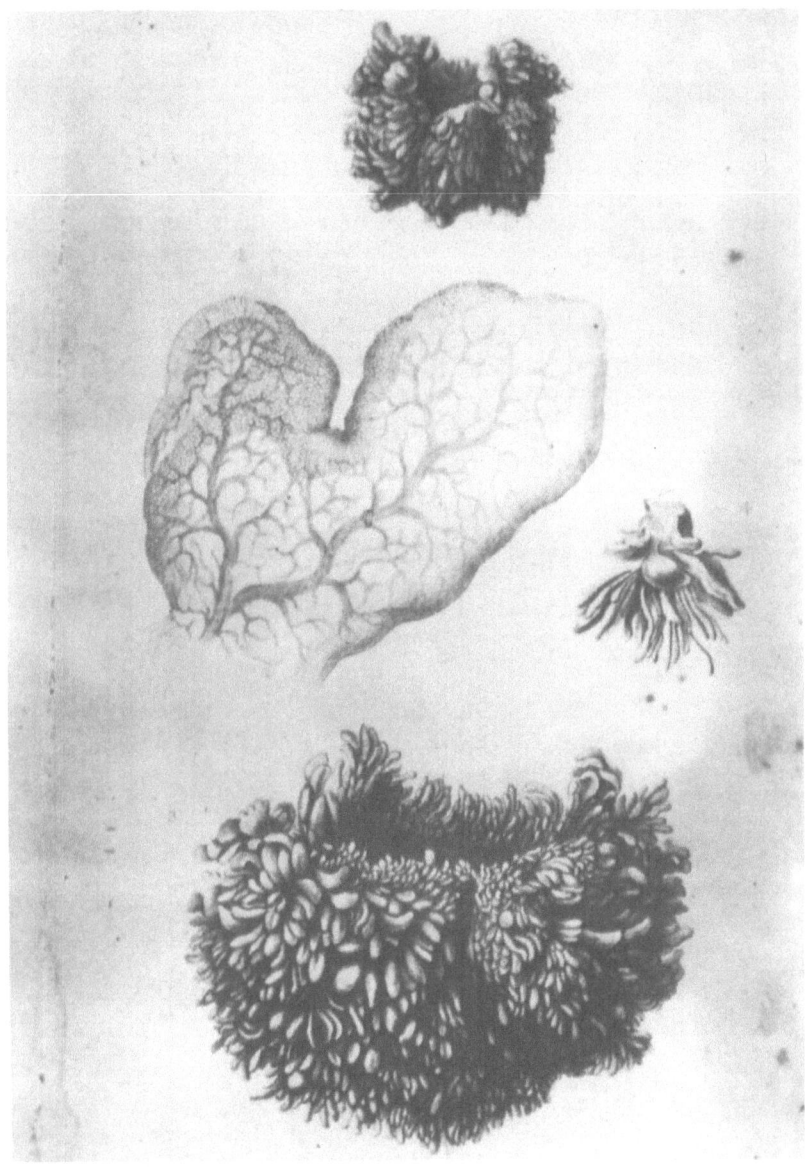

Fig. 2. This is the plate which Quain used to illustrate his monograph. Although somewhat discoloured around the edges by age, it still portrays the essential features of a villous growth with remarkable accuracy.

80%. Of the 12 patients in the cancer group, two were eventually classified as benign, an accuracy rate again of over 80%. In the 6 'doubtful' patients, invasive cancer was found during operation in 3, the growth was considered still to be confined to the mucosa in 2 patients, but there was still some doubt

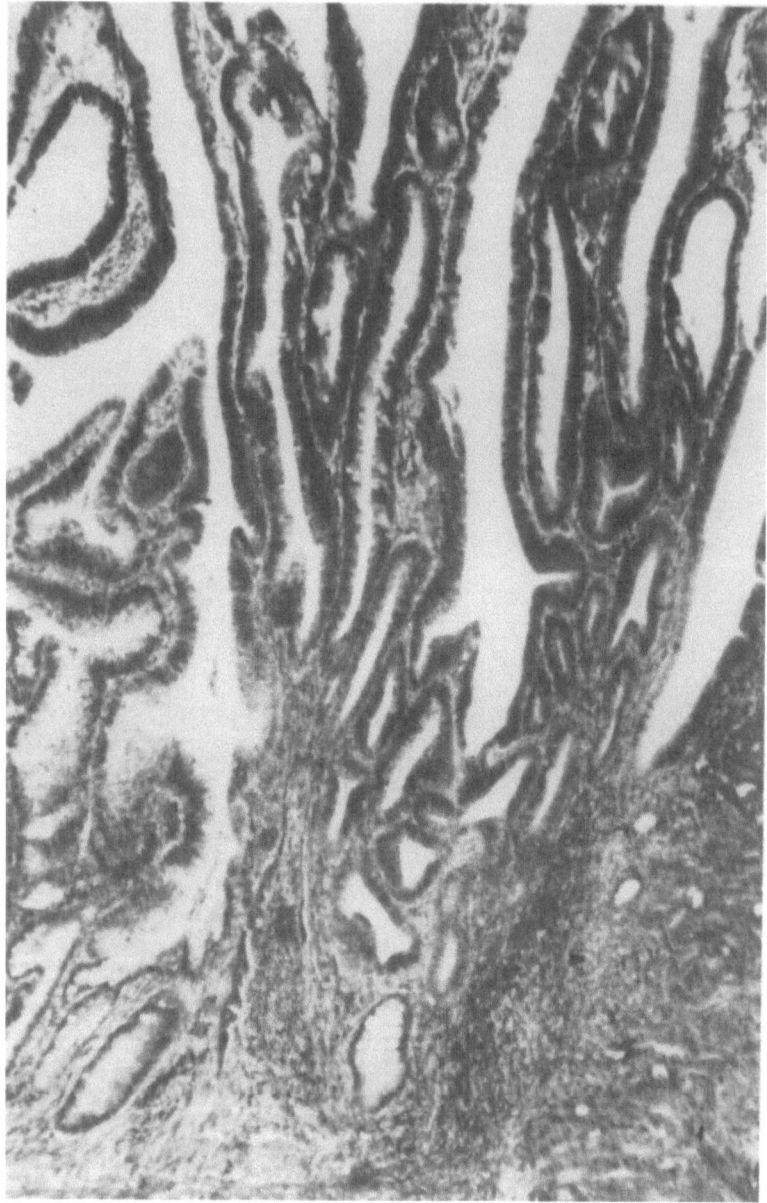

Fig. 3. Multiple surface biopsies showed benign adenoma: the index finger recognised the presence of this deeply invasive cancer.

about the last. However, microscopic invasion was found in this remaining doubtful case.

It is interesting that the final assessment of the overall incidence of invasive change, approximately 30%, corresponded closely with the overall pre-operative assessment, but only because of a cancelling out of over-assessment by under-assessment during or after operation.

Pre-treatment clinical assessment is, of course, not complete until the entire large bowel has been examined, because there is a significant incidence of synchronous epithelial neoplasms, benign or malignant. Good quality barium enema studies are essential, and, if there is still any doubt, then colonoscopy is necessary. In my personal series one patient had had partial colonic resection for an antecedent cancer; synchronous cancer was found in three patients and during the course of follow-up 'metachronous' cancers were found in three.

CONSTITUTIONAL EFFECTS

Following Quain's original contribution, nearly a century elapsed before we came to appreciate the significance of associated constitutional symptoms. These may be rather vague complaints of progressive muscle weakness, tiredness, weight loss and odd mental symptoms. Recognition of the true underlying cause may be very long delayed and patients wrongly diagnosed as suffering from a surprisingly wide variety of diseases. However, these symptoms are alleviated by correction of the associated hypokalaemia and cured by removal of the villous adenoma. Presentation may be more dramatic, emergency admission of the patient in a state of coma. Several papers were published about 100 years after Quain's first case report. In 1955 Fitzgerald (3) recorded extreme fluid and electrolyte loss in a patient admitted as 'diabetic coma', resuscitated with some difficulty. Some time elapsed before her large villous adenoma of the upper rectum was found and she was cured when her growth was eventually resected by Professor Bryan Brooke. Cooling and Marrack in 1957 (4), Roy and Ellis in 1959 (5), reported the measured excessive loss of potassium from their patients and so called their lesions 'potassium secreting tumours'. Lee and Keown (6) in 1970, however, considered that in their two cases, the primary fault was loss of sodium. The significance of an earlier report by Garis (7) was probably not appreciated, and there had been occasional earlier references to some odd features, and I have not referred to all the published reports.

The true incidence of what is now commonly referred to as the McKittrick. Wheelock syndrome (8) is difficult to assess. It is low in published series from specialist centres because the majority are admitted as emergencies to the nearest district hospital. The dehydration, hyponatraemia, hypokalaemia and pre-renal uraemia culminating in circulatory collapse will probably be recognised and most patients will respond well to large quantities of intravenous saline with added potassium. However, diagnosis of the underlying cause may again be long delayed and some patients may have died in coma.

In my personal series of 58, there are 6 patients who were originally admitted to another hospital with severe dehydration and electrolyte disturbance. The simple explanation should be that those patients with large villous growths present a very large surface area of villi lined with tall columnar mucus-filled cells. Although there does seem to be some correlation between size of tumour and electrolyte disturbance, this cannot be the simple answer: some patients known to have had very large villous growths with a copious loss of mucus over many years remain in fluid and electrolyte balance; conversely some comparatively small growths have caused severe disturbance. Various studies, notably that of Duthie and Atwell (9), have highlighted the role of colonic mucosa in the maintenance of fluid, potassium and sodium balance. We know something about its response to hormones and that there are complicated feed-back mechanisms. It is interesting to speculate that some of these tumours are hormone producers; possibly Quain was right when he renamed them 'Peculiar Tumours'.

TREATMENT

Clearly there can be no single best treatment for all patients found to have a villous tumour of the rectum. It is necessary to separate benign from malignant, and the choice of treatment will also be dictated by morphology, site and size of tumour. There are general factors such as age and general condition of the patient which need to be taken into consideration.

There has been a revival of interest in Quain's method for those growths which can be prolapsed through the anal canal and simply cut away. It is possible to excise smaller lesions through the dilated anus, and this can be extended to include larger carpets growths, by submucosal dissection after infiltration with a dilute adrenalin solution to expand this plane and to reduce bleeding (10). Faced with the problem of a very large villous growth, involving the entire rectum, many surgeons would reason, and perhaps rightly so, that the best solution is abdomino-perineal resection. Fig. 4 is an example of such a growth treated in this manner. (There were other reasons for this choice of treatment in this particular patient; after many years of diarrhoea, profuse mucus discharge and intermittent prolapse, she presented with acute large bowel obstruction due to a carcinoma of the sigmoid. She was old and her sphincter atonic.) However, as can be seen in fig. 5 it proved to be benign. Fig. 6 is of an almost identical growth treated by transsphincteric exposure and submucosal resection of a complete tube of growth. This has been opened up in the midline posteriorly and spread out and correctly orientated. 27 separate blocks of tissue were examined before the

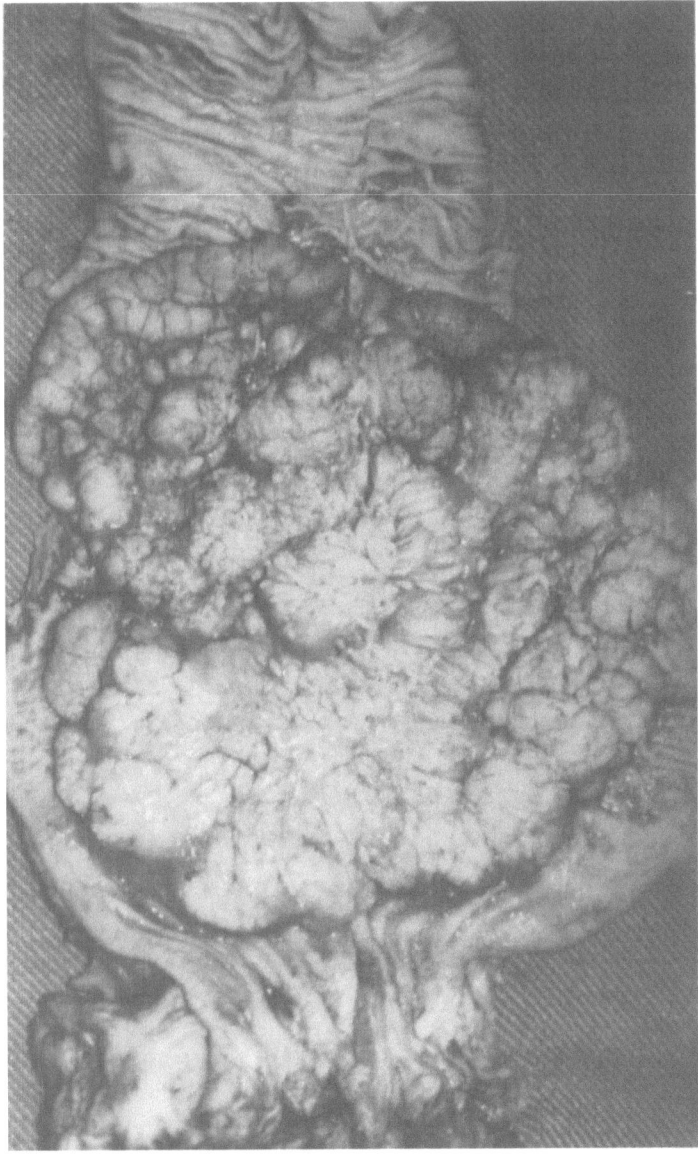

Fig. 4. A villous growth which had replaced all normal rectal mucosa; treated by abdomino-perineal resection.

pathologist was entirely satisfied that there was no suspicion of microscopic invasion. Normal defaecation was preserved in her case.

There are alternative combined techniques, particularly applicable if there is doubt about malignant change and fig. 7 shows a tumour treated by a combined trans-abdominal and trans-sphincteric procedure, with submucosal dissection of the lowest 3 cm. In fact this turned out to be a benign growth

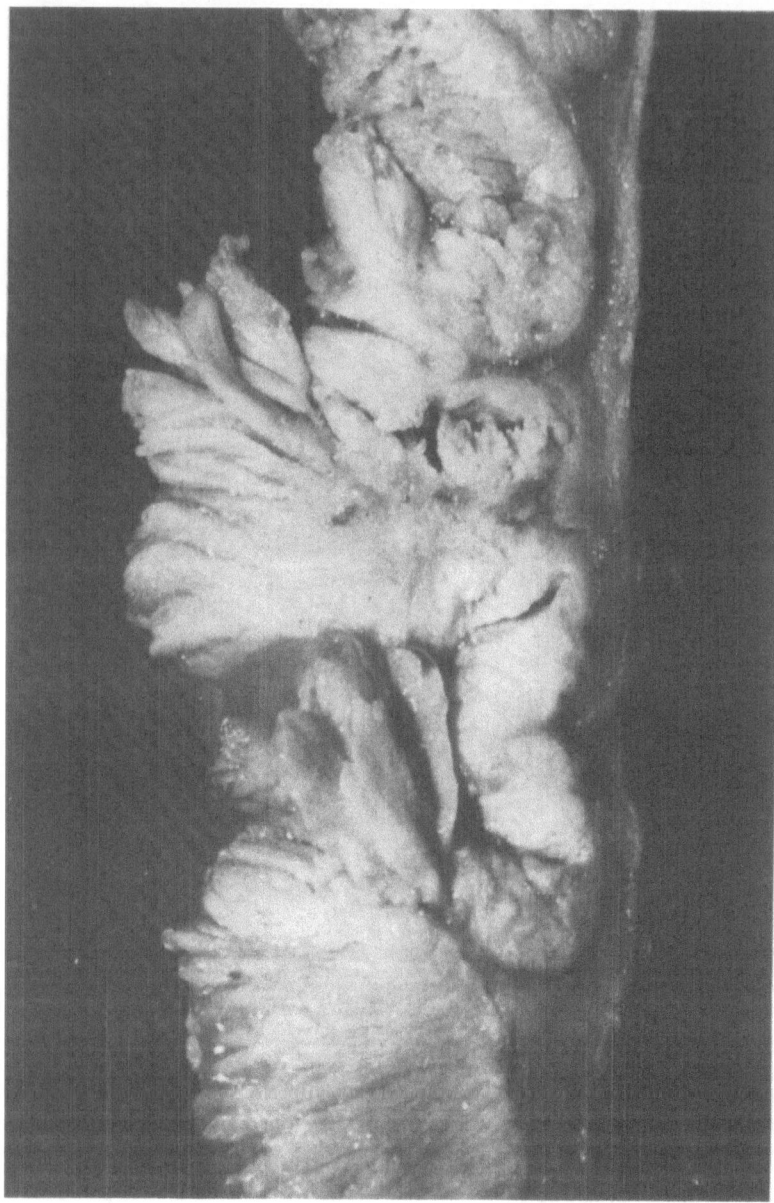

Fig. 5. A photograph of a longitudinal slice through the specimen (illustrated in fig. 4) showing that the villous growth is still confined to mucosa. Multiple sections confirmed that the muscularis mucosae was intact throughout.

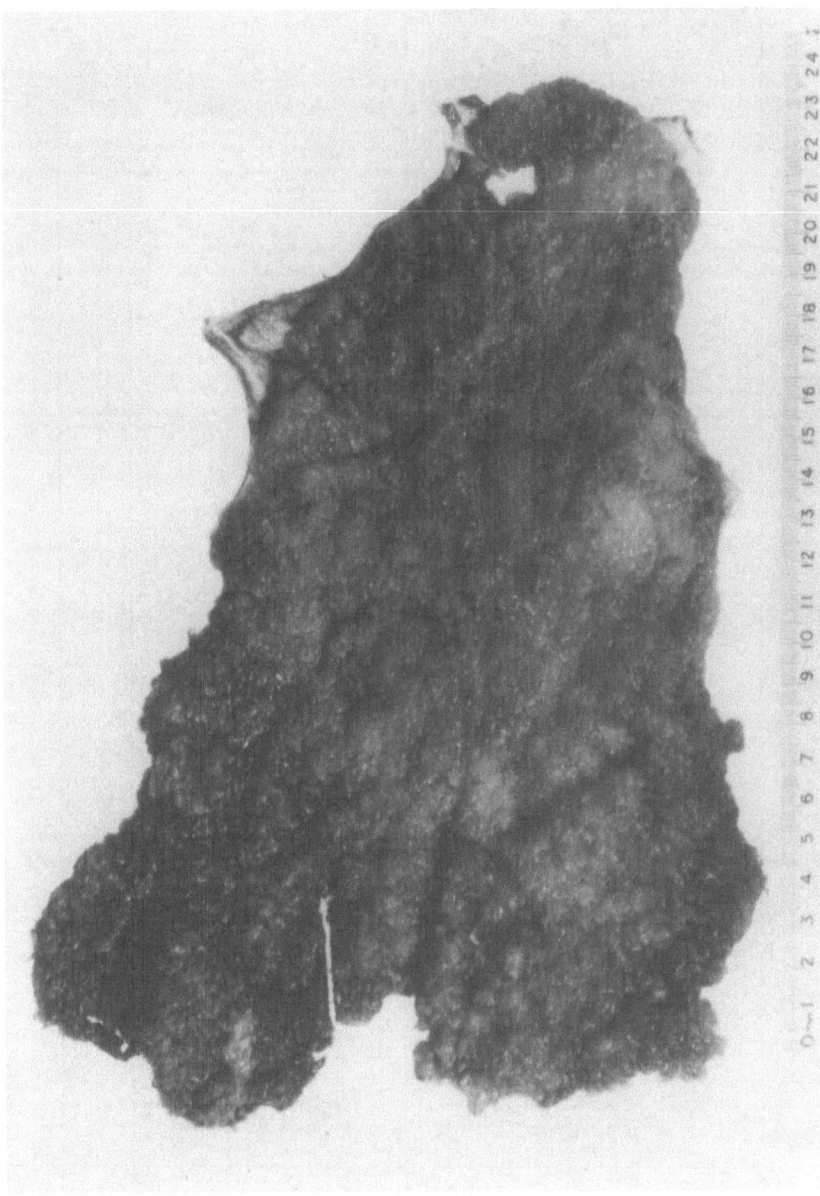

Fig. 6. A villous growth which, like the previous specimen illustrated (fig. 4) had replaced all normal rectal mucosa, confidentially assessed pre-operatively as being a benign growth, and treated by submucosal tube resection.

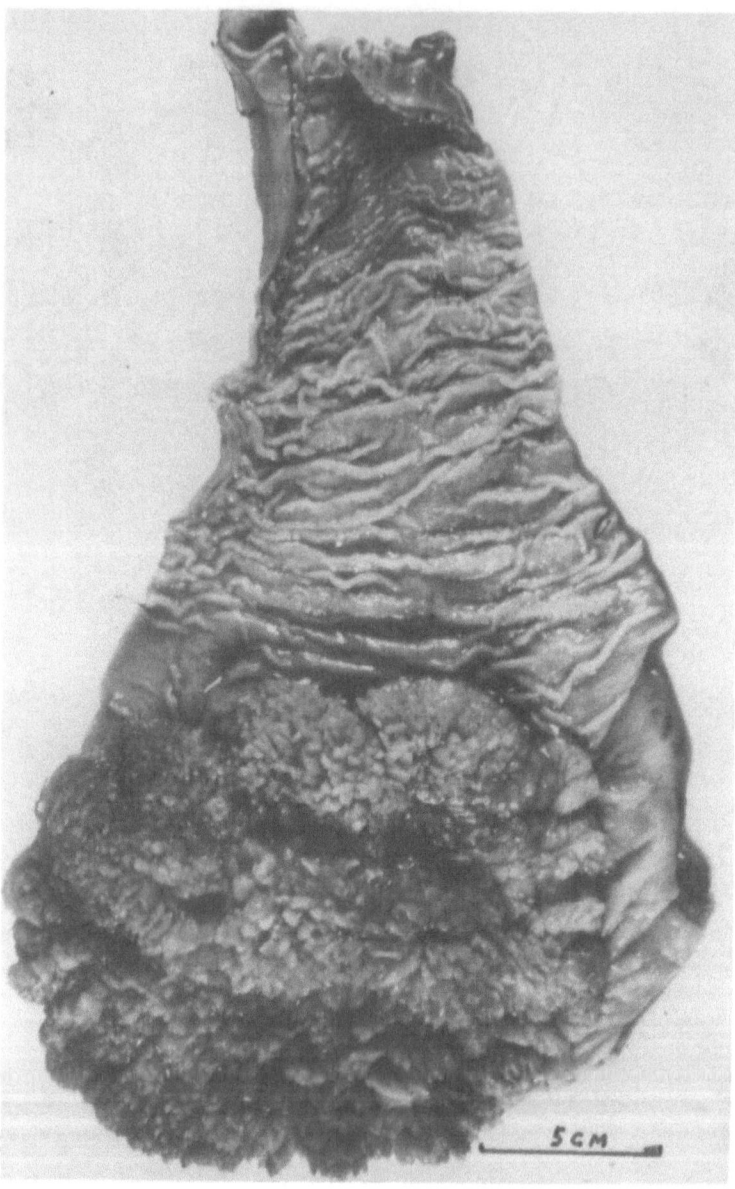

Fig. 7. A villous growth which had replaced virtually all normal rectal mucosa treated by a combined restorative procedure, with submucosal resection of the lowest 3 cm.

because the suspicious hard area was due to previous partial diathermy excision. But, more about the alternatives when I come to talk about the trans-sphincteric approach.

EXAMINATION OF THE RESECTED SPECIMEN

Complete surgical excision, by whatever operative technique, is preferable to destruction by diathermy or by electrocoagulation, because we need a specimen! And surgeons do need the collaboration of pathologist colleagues. Ideally this should be at the level of close personal contact.

Going back to the early history, it is clear that Quain recognised this need, and, although reputed to have been at times a somewhat 'difficult character', it is obvious that he did enjoy a friendly relationship with his colleague, Dr. Jenner, Professor of Pathological Anatomy. They examined the specimen together, in the fresh state, before Dr. Jenner proceeded to his microscopic examination, illustrating and describing the architecture of the villous processes. He confirmed Quain's clinical assessment, also that removal was complete (further careful search was made by Professor Quekett of the Royal College of Surgeons). This is the ideal arrangement whenever possible, but in any case it is the responsibility of the surgeon to see that the resected specimen reaches the laboratory in good condition, well set-out and correctly orientated. A photographic record is highly desirable, together with an outline drawing on which the sites are marked from which blocks of tissue have been taken for microscopic examination.

FOLLOW UP

Careful follow-up is essential because, even after the most detailed examination of resected specimens, it is not always possible to be sure that excision in depth has been complete. Depending upon the circumstances it may have been agreed that a policy of 'wait and see' was the right one. If there were microscopic foci of viable carcinoma left, then these will grow to palpable size, requiring further treatment. The 'wait and see' time must not be a long one.

Reappearance of villous growth near the site of the original lesion is not uncommon and diagnosed as 'recurrence', but this term needs to be qualified. The visible villous growth could be due to microscopic villous change which was present at the time of operation but not recognisable to the naked eye. Alternatively, it could be due to subsequent villous change in an area of mucosa which was normal, but inherently unstable at the time of resection of the first visible lesion. Unfortunately, I have seen the sad consequences of both processes going on; the surgeon has concentrated on removing benign fringe recurrences and has failed to note the ominous continuing growth of residual cancer cells deep to rectal mucosa.

I now approach all 'Villous Tumours' of the rectum with a high index of

130

suspicion; the fact that some can, over the course of many years, grow to enormous size, and still remain benign mucosal lesions, has led to an over-optimistic approach. I remember that Quain, with his interest in the subtleties of the English language, decided to call them 'Peculiar'.

REFERENCES

1. Quain Richard: Villous tumour. In: *Diseases of the rectum*, 2nd edition 1855. Walton and Maberly, London, p 295-298.
2. Quain Richard: *Illustrations of a peculiar bleeding tumour of the rectum*. Walton and Maberly, London 1855.
3. Fitzgerald MG: Extreme fluid and electrolyte loss due to villous papillomae of the rectum. *Br Med J* 1: 831-832, 1955.
4. Cooling C and Marrack D: Potassium secreting tumour of the colon. *Proc Roy Soc Med* 50: 272-274, 1957.
5. Roy AD and Ellis H: Potassium secreting tumours by the large intestine. *Lancet*, 759-760, April 11, 1959.
6. Lee RO and Keown D: Villous tumours of the rectum associated with severe fluid and electrolyte disturbance. *Br J Surg* 57: 197-201, 1970.
7. Gavis RW: Pre-renal uraemia due to papillomae of rectum. *Ann Int Med* 15: 916-926, 1941.
8. McKittrick LS and Wheelock FC(J): In: *Carcinoma of Colon*, Charl C Thomas, Springfield, Illinois, p 61-63.
9. Duthrie HL and Atwell JD: The absorption of water, sodium and potassium in the large intestine with particular reference to the effects of villous papillomas. *Gut* 4: 373-377, 1963.
10. Parks AG: A technique for excising extensive villous papillomatous change in the lower rectum. *Proc Roy Soc Med* 61: 441-443, 1968.

15. ENDOSCOPIC POLYPECTOMY

D.M. VAN DEN BOOMGAARD

Since the beginning of the seventies endoscopic polypectomy has been possible, and with the use of fiberoptic instruments polyps can be removed from the entire colon. It has proved to be a safe and easy method in the hands of an experienced endoscopist. Only a short admission to the hospital is needed.

Colon polyps are mostly found during endoscopy, while barium enema miss them in 20-50%. If a polyp is found, it has to be removed completely, even if it is a small one. A biopsy should not be taken, because it does not give enough information about the character of the polyp and a malignancy can easily be missed.

After medical evaluation on an out-patient basis, including physical examination, routine preoperative blood investigation, blood grouping, coagulation study, barium enema, diagnostic endoscopy, e.c.g. and X-thorax, the patient is admitted to the hospital on the day of the planned polypectomy. All patients spend one night in the hospital after polypectomy. No special diet or convalescent regime is recommended. The patient is informed about the procedure and the small risk that could be made in an operation.

Bowel preparation is important and should be done properly. The method depends on the location of the polyp and can range from total lavage or a two day scheme of low fibre diet with laxatives for polyps in the proximal colon to a water tap enema for polyps in the rectosigmoid. Most of the patients initiate their bowel preparation at home. Only the elderly or those living at a distance are admitted to the hospital one day early for purgation.

The type of endoscope used also depends on the location of the polyp and ranges from the colonoscope for polyps in the right colon to the flexible fiberoptic rectoscope for polyps in the rectosigmoid. Fluoroscopy is needed when the colonoscope is used.

The patient is placed in the recumbant position, close to the edge of the table, with his legs in stirups. Premedication usually is not needed. Occasionally diazepam or buscopan intravenously is used. The endoscope is introduced and passed to the known position of the polyp. If more than one polyp has to be removed in the same session, one starts with the most proximal polyp. The colon is insufflated with an inert gas (like CO_2), to avoid explosion of the gasses usually present in the colon (primarily methane).

The polyp can be removed in two ways. First by using a special polypectomy snare which is placed and closed around the base of the polyp high enough to minimize the risk of heat necrosis of the bowel wall, but low enough to include early malignant invasion into the stalk. After tightening the snare and elevating the polyp away from the bowel wall, the stalk is cut by using alternatively during short periods a coagulation current of an intermittently flowing damp sine wave form that has excellent haemostatic effects, and a cutting current of a regular sine wave form. This method is fitted for all polyps up to a diameter of 4 cm. If the patient has a polyp larger than 4 cm and at the same time too high a risk for abdominal operation, these large polyps can also be removed piecemeal or in several sessions endoscopically. Secondly polyps with a diameter up to 7 mm can be simultaneously biopsied and destroyed in a few seconds with the hot biopsy forceps. The tissue enclosed in the conductive material of the forceps is bypassed by the current and therefore not heated. So a pathological diagnosis can be made.

The removed polyps can be retrieved by suction on the tip of the endoscope. This method has the disadvantage that the distal bowel cannot be inspected. Therefore one can use a special retrieval forceps, Dormiabasket or the polypectomy snare itself making bowel inspection on withdrawal and holding more than one polyp possible.

It is important to mark the coagulation plane for the pathologist, so he can make the right judgment. Each removed polyp is put in a separate jar with formaldehyde, with the name of the patient mentioned and the place of removal.

Complications of the endoscopic polypectomy could be due to the bowel preparation in the form of hypervolaemia and dehydration, or it could be due to the premedication, if given, in the form of respiratory depression. Finally complications could occur due to the procedure itself and include haemorrhage, perforation, vagal-vagal reflex, explosion or electric burns.

Reasons for failure of polypectomy are the patient's refusal to cooperate, presence of adhesions following diverticulitis, large sessile polyps, technical difficulties or inexperience of the endoscopist.

Our own experience started in June 1975 and up to March 1979, 431 polyps were removed from 270 patients. Looking at the age and sex distribution it is clear that the incidence was greatest in the 6th and 7th decades and that the sex ratio was two females to three males. Our youngest patient was a boy of four years old, who complained of irregular stools and frequent rectal blood loss making blood transfusions necessary. A large juvenile polyp could be removed from the descending colon without complications. Afterwards he was completely without complaints. Our oldest patient was a woman 97 years old from whom a bleeding benign adenomatous polyp was removed from the proximal sigmoid.

In our series most polyps (89.1%) were found in the left colon, and therefore

Table 1. Age and sex distribution.

Age	Number of patients	Females	Males
0 - 10	2	1	1
11 - 20	3	–	3
21 - 30	6	4	2
31 - 40	18	8	10
41 - 50	33	9	24
51 - 60	69	23	46
61 - 70	73	27	46
71 - 80	52	26	26
81 - 90	11	4	7
91 - 100	3	2	1
Total	270	104	166

Table 2. Anatomical location of removed polyps.

Location	Number of polyps	Percentage
rectum	85	19.7
sigmoid	239	55.5
descending	60	13.9
transverse	32	7.4
ascending	9	2.1
cecum	6	1.4
Total	431	100.00

could be removed with simple sigmoidoscopy without the aid of fluoroscopy. During obductions a larger percentage of polyps was present in the right colon. Since we did not perform a total colonoscopy in all patients, it is certain that we missed a number of polyps present in the right colon. Therefore if possible a diagnostic total colonoscopy should be done.

In 65.2% a single polyp was removed. In 34.8% more than one polyp with a maximum of 9 polyps in one patient were removed in one session. The polyps removed with the hot biopsy forceps are not included in this study. With the hot biopsy forceps we once removed 75 polyps from the rectum of a boy of 16 years old with an ileorectal anastomosis for familial polyposis.

We saw no malignant incidence in those polyps with a diameter up to 15 mm, so it reassured us slightly regarding those polyps not retrieved. They were all of the small type. However in the literature 1% malignant degeneration is recorded in polyps smaller than 1 cm. The smallest polyp recorded that contained malignant degeneration was 3 mm.

324 polyps, that is 75.1%, were neoplastic. 295 were benign adenomas, with

Table 3. Numbers of polyps snared per patient (total 431 polyps).

No. of polyps snared	No. of patients	Percentage
more than 5	3	1.1
5	6	2.2
4	6	2.2
3	22	8.2
2	57	21.1
1	176	65.2
Total	270	100.00

Table 4. Size of removed polyps.

Size	Number	Percentage
0 - 5 mm	71	16.5
6 - 10 mm	120	27.8
11 - 15 mm	74	17.2
16 - 20 mm	49	11.4
21 - 25 mm	35	8.1
26 - 30 mm	18	4.2
31 - 40 mm	14	3.2
40 mm	5	1.2
unknown	45	10.4
Total	431	100.00

Table 5. Pathologic features of polyps removed by endoscopy.

		Number	Percentage
neoplastic polyps		324	75.2
benign adenoma	295		
villous adenoma	5		
carcinoma in situ	13		
adenocarcinoma	11		
non-neoplastic polyps		65	15.1
polyps removed but not retrieved		42	9.7
Total		431	100.00

tubular or tubulovillous adenomas with or without atypia. Five were true villous adenomas. This small number compared with other series published is due to the fact that after removing the first five villous adenomas, we stopped removing them endoscopically, because they showed malignant degeneration in pathological analysis of the removed polyp or malignancy in the remnant in the resected part of the bowel if we could not remove them completely, or showed malignant recurrence on control a few months later. 13 patients showed a carcinoma in situ and they were cured by the endoscopic polypectomy. In 11 patients there was an adenocarcinoma. In four of them the coagulation plane was free of tumor and there was no malignant invasion in the muscularis mucosae. The other seven were operated afterwards. It can be very difficult during laparotomy to find the exact place of endoscopic removal, especially if several weeks have gone by. It is a pity that we do not now have a satisfactory marker that could be used after polypectomy to mark the exact place of removal.

We saw 10 complications of polypectomy, all bleedings. No perforations or mortality were seen. Some of the bleedings could be stopped by coagulation or by adrenaline solution washings. Several times blood transfusions were necessary. Only once did the surgeon have to ligate a large bleeding vessel in the stalk of a very large rectum polyp. The recovery of the patient was uneventful.

The question of what to do after the pathological diagnosis of the polyp is known and how to control the patient afterwards is important. There are no sure rules now published. Our current methods ar the following, patients with:

A. malignant polyps with infiltration into the coagulation plane or invasion into the muscularis mucosae should have resection of the affected bowel segment as soon as possible.

B. malignant polyps with no infiltration into the coagulation plane or muscularis mucosae or a carcinoma in situ should be controlled endoscopically on a fixed scheme made arbitrarily on 6 weeks, 6 months and annually.

C. benign polyps and a not benign villous adenoma should be controlled endoscopically annually.

D. benign non-neoplastic polyps should be controlled endoscopically, if complaints recur.

E. villous adenomas should not be treated with endoscopic polypectomy, but should be referred to the surgeon for resection of the affected bowel segment.

CONCLUSIONS

Endoscopic polypectomy is a safe procedure in the hands of an experienced endoscopist and has a very low mortality and morbidity rate compared with the abdominal method.

Endoscopic polypectomy is inexpensive and only a short admission to the hospital is needed.

Endoscopic polypectomy is important in the prevention of colorectal

136

cancer if all polyps are be discovered early enough. Also those that give no symptoms and if those polyps could be removed endoscopically, the incidence of colorectal cancer would diminish dramatically.

Finally the endoscopic polypectomy is not an inconvenient procedure for the patient.

REFERENCES

1. Becker V: Polypektomie. *Allgemeinpathologische Problematik Leber, Magen, Darm* 4: 147, 1973.
2. Berci G et al.: Complications of colonoscopy and polypectomy. *Gastroent.* 67: 584, 1974.
3. Bond JH et al.: Explosion of hydrogen gas in the colon during proctosigmoidoscopy.
4 Bühler H et al.: Was bringt die kolonoskopische Polypektomie. *Schweiz med Wschr* 28: 1079, 1978.
5. Dean ACB: Problems with coloscopic polypectomy. *Endoscopy* 5: 123, 1973.
6. Dodds WJ et al.: Role of colonoscopy and roentgenology in the detection of polypoid colonic lesions. *Digestive Disease* 7: 646, 1977.
7. Frühmorgen P et al.: New aspects of therapeutic coloscopy. Endoscopy 2: 59, 1975.
8. Husen NV et al.: Zur endoskopischen Polypektomie im Magendarmkanal. Akt. Gastrologie 5: 377, 1975.
9. Knutson CO et al.: Polypoid lesions of the proximal colon. Ann Surg may, 1974.
10. Miller SF et al.: The early detection of colorectal cancer. Cancer 2: 945, 1977.
11. Ottenjahn R: Colonic Polyps and coloscopic polypectomy. *Endoscopy* 4: 212, 1973.
12. Overholt BF et al.: Colonoscopic polypectomy: silent perforation. *Gastroenterology* 70: 112, 1976.
13. Ragins H et al.: The explosive potential of colonic gas during colonoscopic electrosurgical polypectomy. Surg Gyn Obstetrics 138: 554, 1974.
14. Rogers BHG et al.: Complications of flexible fiberoptic colonoscopy and polypectomy. *Gastrointestinal endoscopy* 2: 73, 1975.
15. Rösch W: Endoscopic polypectomy – Cosmetic operation or necessity. *Acta Hepato-Gastroenteral* 21: 173, 1974.
16. Sirak MV et al.: Colonoscopic polypectomy. *Digestive Diseases* 4: 339, 1974.
17. Spencer et al.: Colonoscopic polypectomy. *Mayo Chin Proc* 1: 40, 1974.
18. Sugarbaker PH et al.: Snare polypectomy with the fiberoptic colonoscope. *Surg Gyn Obstetrics* 138: 581, 1974.
19. Williams CB et al.: Colonoscopy in the management of colonpolyps. *Br J Surg* 61: 673, 1974.
20. Wolff Shinya: Endoscopic polypectomy. *Cancer august supplement*, 1975.
21. Wolff WI Shinya H: A new approach to colonic polyps. *Annals of surgery* 3: 367, 1973.
22. Wolff WI Shinya H: Polypectomy via the fiberoptic colonoscope. *New Eng J Med* 288: 329, 1973.
23. Wyss G et al.: Resultate der Kolonoskopien und Polypektomien der Jahre 1974 und 1975 am Kantonsspital Basel. *Schweiz med Wschr* 3: 68, 1977.

16. SURGERY OF COLONIC POLYPS

MAUS W. STEARNS, JR.

The flexible colonoscope has greatly reduced the need and altered the indications for major surgical procedures in the treatment of colonic polypoid lesions. There are relatively few remaining indications for laparotomy in their treatment: 1) the pedunculated polyp that cannot be reached or visualized by the colonoscopist, 2) multiple (arbitrarily more than ten) polyps in one segment, or in a young person, especially with a familial history, when they are scattered throughout the colon, 3) sessile polyps greater than 2 cm in size and some smaller ones that cannot be removed satisfactorily via the flexible colonoscope, 4) the pedunculated polyp which after removal is found to contain clinically significant cancer.

Colonoscopists have and are acquiring great skill, not only with the passage of the instrument to the ileal-cecal valve, but also in the adeptness with which they can snare and remove polyps. However, even the best occasionally fails on repeated tries to reach a polyp demonstrated by barium enema. If the polyp is greater than a centimeter in size, unless there is a medical contra-indication, the polyp generally should be removed by laparotomy. A colotomy through a taenia after the bowel segment has been isolated and the remaining viscera protected, allows extraction of the polyp and ligation of the base with excision (fig. 1). Colonoscopy of the previous unexamined bowel for additional polyps should be performed clearing the bowel as one would do with the flexible colonoscope (fig. 2). This approach was standard procedure prior to the advent of flexible colonoscopy and it remains a very useful procedure in the occasional patient.

A relative frequent problem is where after pathologic examination of the removed polyp 'infiltrating' cancer is found by the pathologist. Close understanding between the clinician and the pathologist is all-important. Our experience in the '40s and '50s when we reoperated on a number of patients under these circumstances has been very useful in deciding who requires further operation. We extremely rarely found nodal metastases from pedunculated polyps unless: 1) the tumor was very anaplastic, 2) venous or lymphatic emboli were found in the pedicle, or 3) the cancer extended to the line of excision. These remain our indications for surgical intervention to date. Similar indications have been arrived at by others as well.

A debatable but probably valid indication is segmental resection of the

138

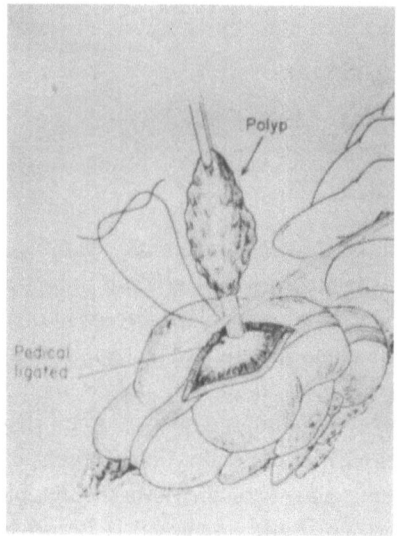

Figure 1.

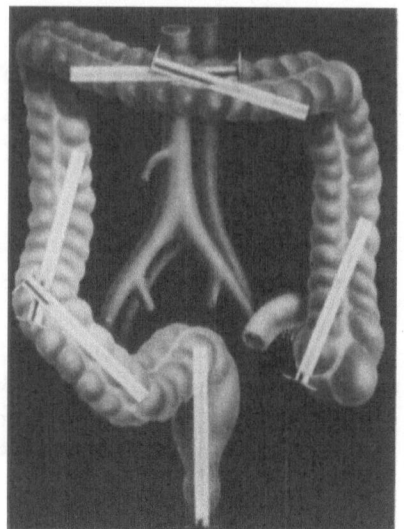

Figure 2.

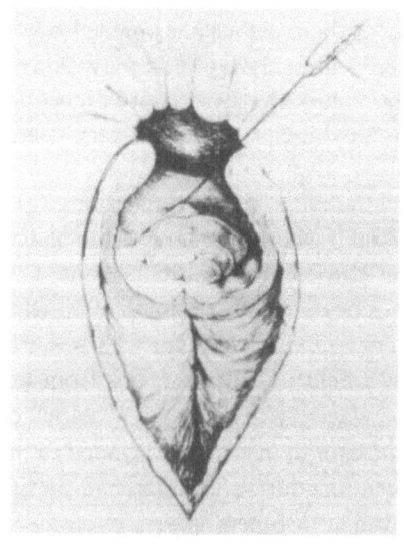

Figure 3.

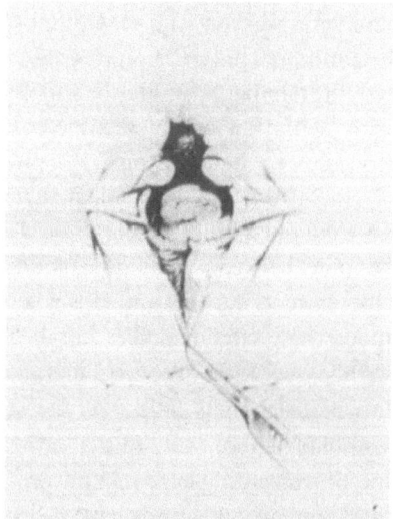

Figure 4.

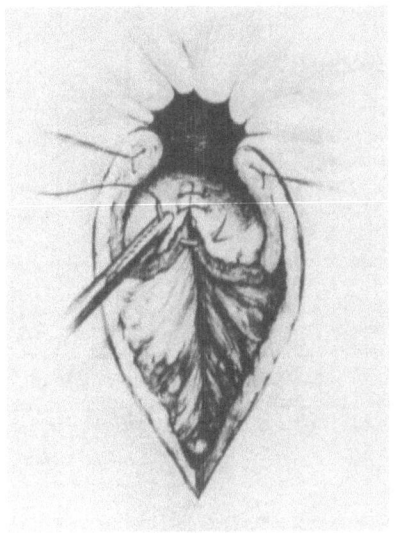

Figure 5.

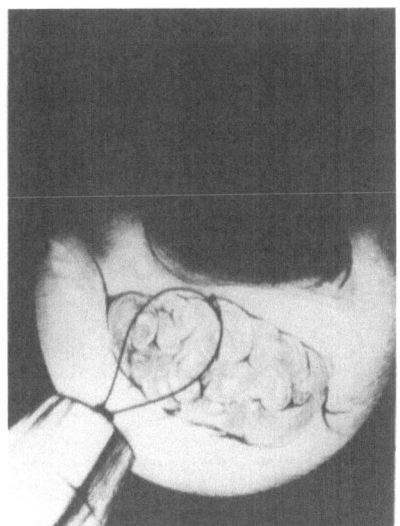

Figure 6.

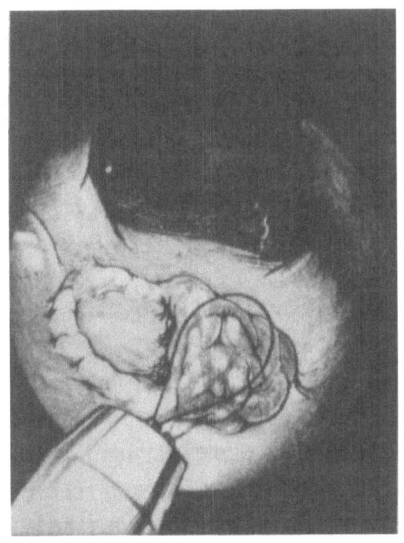

Figure 7.

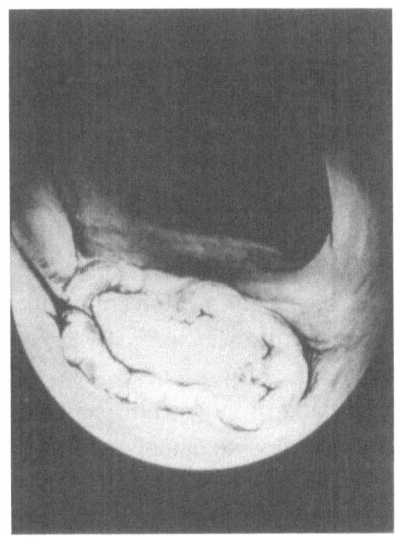

Figure 8.

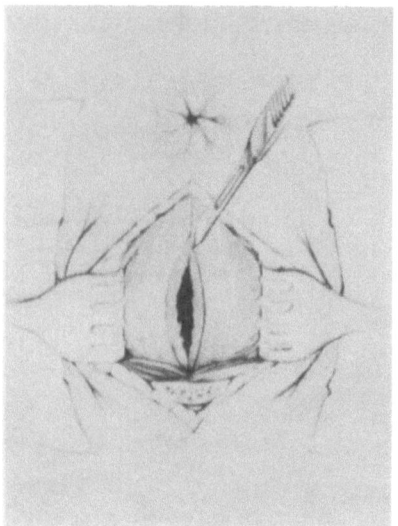 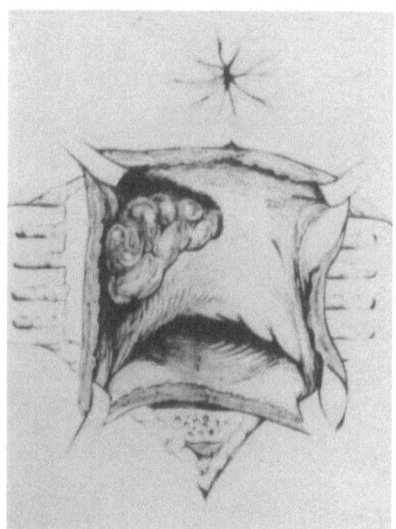

Figure 9.   *Figure 10.*

bowel segment containing a considerable number of benign neoplastic polyps, not simple mucosal hyperplasias. A generous section of the adjacent mesentery should be included on the chance that one or more will be found to have infiltrating cancer present. If this is found and the adjacent nodes do not contain metastases no additional surgery is needed. However, in the very rare event that nodal metastases are found then the patient should be operated on and an adequate cancer operation performed.

We use the same approach for the intra-colonic sessile polyp which does not have any of the clinical characteristics of malignant change, particularly ulceration and induration. We arrived at this approach as our pathologists are very unhappy with frozen sections of polyps particularly large sessile ones, as they feel the chances of over-or under reading this material are too great and much prefer careful evaluation of well prepared material. This has proved a satisfactory approach over many years.

Sessile lesions in the rectum which is a clinical entity called villous tumors has been a problem for many years. Our surgical approach to these lesions is very conservative. Unless there is clinical evidence of infiltration into the muscularis propria or the lesion is highly anaplastic a local procedure is usually done. Our management varies considerably with the local in the upper or lower rectum. In the upper rectum where sphincter-preserving types of resection can be done, and local procedures are less satisfactorily performed we prefer an anterior resection for those lesions which involve half or more of the circumference. In the lower rectum where resection involves a permanent

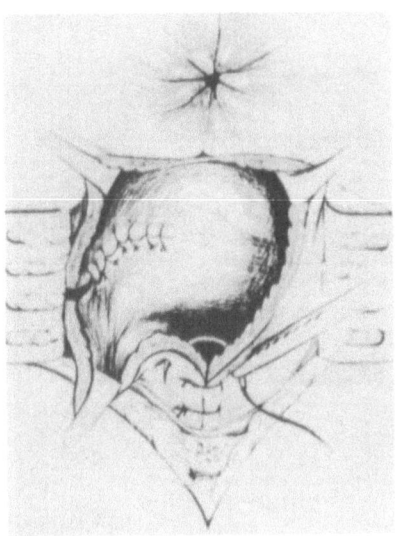

Figure 11.

colostomy and local procedures are more easily performed technically we utilize a number of local procedures. Transanal excision (figs. 3, 4 and 5) is preferred when technically possible. Staged snare removal (figs. 6, 7 and 8) is particularly useful when general anesthesia is to be avoided. Posterior procto-tomy (figs. 9, 10 and 11) is a satisfactory approach for those not used to working through the sphincter. Electrocoagulation can be used by those who prefer it. We prefer excision as it is possible to submit the entire polyp to the pathologist for his study. If there is infiltrating cancer extending deeply into the muscularis propria we then advise abdomino-perineal resection since the chance of nodal metastases increases rapidly. Occasionally we use a pull-through for annular lesions in which we are reasonably sure there is no true muscle invasion. Our results with this conservative approach is shown in table 1, which in our opinion justifies the continuation of conservativism.

Table 1. Villous adenoma (10 year study).

107 conservative procedures		
Pathology:	Benign	63
	Superficial ca	37
	Invasive ca	7
Results:	Operative mortality	0
	Died of cancer	0
	Recurrence	19 (18%)
Recurrences:	17/19 Retreated locally	
	2 APR	

PART V

TREATMENT

17. RADIOTHERAPY OF INOPERABLE OR RECURRENT CANCER OF THE RECTUM AND RECTOSIGMOID

P. THOMAS AND R.E. TJHO-HESLINGA

With an incidence rate of 20.2 per 100,000 inhabitants the annual number of patients with rectal cancer in The Netherlands amounts to 2800. About 15-25% of these patients are inoperable. The survival rate for the operable group is around 50%. At surgery liver metastases are found in 10 to 15%. It is probable that most of the other patients die of locoregional recurrence. This means that in The Netherlands each year 550 inoperable patients and 825 patients with locoregional recurrence are potential candidates for radiotherapy. With that high a percentage of local recurrences (35%) and so many inoperable patients it is necessary to explore other modalities of treatment to improve results.

The incidence of locoregional recurrence depends on the stage. The stage is determined by the extent of tumour growth through the bowel wall and by metastases in the regional lymph nodes. The original stage classification of Dukes (2) has been modified by Kirklin et al (3), by Astler and Coller (4) and lastly gy Gunderson and Sosin (5) and comprises:

group A: tumour limited to the mucosa; nodes negative.
group B: extension into but not through the muscularis propria; nodes negative.
group B2: extension through the entire bowel wall; nodes negative.
group B3: lesion adherent to or invading adjacent organs or structures; nodes negative.
group C1: tumour limited to bowel wall; nodes positive.
group C2: extension through the entire bowel wall; nodes positive.
group C3: lesion adherent to or invading adjacent organs or structures; nodes positive.
group D: lesion with distant metastases.

Table 1 summarizes the data from literature on the relationship between stage and locoregional recurrence.

INDICATIONS FOR RADIOTHERAPY

Radiotherapy plays only a modest role in the *primary treatment* of rectal cancer. Papillon (9) is famous for his local radiotherapy of small tumours of

Table 1. Stage and incidence of locoregional recurrence.

Author	Stage	Locoreg. recurr. in percentage	Number of patients
Gunderson and	B1, B2, B3	71.4	7
Sosin (5)	B2, B3	83,3	6
	C1, C2, C3	70.5	61
	C2, C3	85	40
	C1	29.4	17
Gilbert (6)	B1	16.7	35
	B2	51.4	37
	C2	78.4	37
	Dukes B	31.3	
	Dukes C	72.8	
Cass (7)	all	30	
Johnson (8)	B1	0- 5%	
	B2	20-50%	
	B3	40-80%	
	C1	20-50%	
	C2	60-85%	

the rectum. He obtained five-year survival in 78% of 133 patients. The technique is difficult, and the number of suitable patients is so small that very few radiotherapists can gain sufficient experience. None the less it is a potential method of curative radiotherapy.

More important is the radiotherapy of *inoperable rectal cancers.* In this field many radiotherapists obtain 10% five-year survival rates (10, 11), while Rider (12) even claims 29% five-year survival.

We will only deal with inoperable and recurrent rectal carcinoma.

From 1969 through 1977 107 patients with carcinoma of the rectosigmoid were treated with radiotherapy: 41 patients had recurrent growth, 46 were inoperable and 20 suffered from metastases.

RECURRENCES

The recurrent tumour was localized in the rectum in 32 out of the 41 patients and in the sigmoid in the other 9. Eighteen patients had stage B disease, six stage C (table 2). Thirty patients complained of pain, six of loss of blood and/or mucus.

The duration as well as the degree of pain alleviation resulting from irradiation can be estimated only roughly, because follow-up studies sometimes lacked depth. Pain is a subjective perception and often it is not clear whether the remaining pain is being caused by the tumour or by scar tissue.

Seventeen out of thirty-five patients showed complete remission, thirteen

Table 2. Location, operation and stage of recurrent rectosigmoidal carcinoma.

Loc.	Nr.	Operation	Nr.	Dukes B	Dukes C	Unknown
rectum	32	amputation anterior	20	11	1	8
		resection	11	4	4	3
		polypectomy	1	–	–	1
sigmoid	9	resection	9	3	1	5
Total	41			18	6	17

Table 3. Dose and its effect on pain in recurrent colorectal cancer.

Dose in rads	Complete remission	Alleviation of pain	No effect
3000 or 4000	13/28	12/28	3/28
5500 or 6000	4/ 7	1/ 7	2/ 7
	17/35	13/35	5/35

perceived alleviation of pain and only five experienced no pain relief (table 3). Five patients were irradiated twice. Insofar as these numbers permit any conclusion, a high dose does not seen to improve the results. Of six patients with loss of blood, mucus or tumour discharge, one was irradiated twice. The effect of irradiation was excellent; in all six cases the symptoms disappeared completely. This palliation lasted from 3 to 18 months. All the patients who had a recurrence of the tumour have since died.

INOPERABLE CANCERS

Inoperability was the indication for radiotherapy 46 times. The tumour was inoperable because of invasion of surrounding organs in 29 out of 46 patients, distant metastases with or without invasion of surrounding organs in 12 patients, age in 3 cases and twice the patients (80 and 84 years old) refused surgery (table 4).

Twenty patients suffered pain, thirty patients lost blood, mucus and tumour discharge and fifteen suffered bowel dysfunction.

The effect of irradiation on pain was very satisfactory in most patients, only two out of twenty-one patients reported no effects following irradiation, where as eight were in complete remission and nine experienced appreciable pain reduction (table 5). In two patients the effect of radiotherapy could not be judged. One patient was irradiated twice. The numbers are too small to

Table 4. Causes of inoperability.

	Nr. of patients
Invasion of surrounding organs	29
Distant metastases (liver)	6
Invasion and distant metastases (liver 5 ×, omentum 1 ×)	6
Age	3
Refused surgery	2
Total	46

Table 5. Dose and its effect on pain in inoperable colorectal cancer.

Dose in rads	Complete remission	Alleviation of pain	No effect	Cannot be judged
3000 or 4000	4/13	6/13	2/13	1/13
5500 or 6000	4/ 8	3/ 8	–	1/ 8
	8/21	9/21	2/21	2/21

warrant any conclusion about the relationship between dose and its effect on pain. The results are in accordance with those in literature. Williams (11) has the highest percentage (86%) of favourable results followed by Urdaneta Lafee (13) 80% and Rousseau (14) 75%.

Of thirty patients irradiated for *loss of blood, mucus* and *tumour discharge* three could not be followed . All patients showed a favourable reaction to irradiation, more than half even experienced complete remission (table 6). The remission lasted from 2 to 24 months. Here too the numbers are too small to warrant a conclusion about the relationship between dose and effect.

The effect of irradiation on bowel dysfunction was satisfactory (table 7). Of 15 patients with inoperable rectal cancer, only one had to undergo a colostomy $1\frac{1}{2}$ years after irradiation. These results are confirmed by Johnson (8), Williams (11) and Tierie (15).

The question must be raised as to whether irradiation is not a better palliative treatment for inoperable carcinoma of the rectosigmoid than a colostomy.

Of all 46 inoperable patients 3 are alive without evidence of disease after 27, 28 and 89 months, resp., and one is alive without local recurrence but with liver metastases after 30 months.

Table 6. Effect of irradiation on the loss of blood, mucus and tumour discharge.

Dose in rads	Complete remission	Alleviation of symptoms	No reaction	Unknown
3000 or 4000	9/14	4/14	–	1/14
5500 or 6000	10/16	4/16	–	2/16
	19/30	8/30		3/30

Table 7. Effect of irradiation on impairment of defecation.

Dose in rads	Complete remission	Alleviation of symptoms	No reaction	Unknown
3000 or 4000	3/ 5	1/ 5	–	1/ 5
5000 or 6000	6/10	3/10	–	1/10
	9/15	4/15		2/15

METASTASES

Irradiation of distant meatastases generally gives satisfactory results, but obviously survival is usually too short to warrant any conclusions about the long-term effect. Irradiation of liver metastases is seldom indicated. In selected cases of (peripheral) lung metastases high dose irradiation may be beneficial.

RADIO-RESISTANCE OF CARCINOMA OF THE RECTUM AND SIGMOID

Rectal cancer is a classical example of supposed radio-resistance. The results obtained by interstitial implantation or external megavoltage therapy indicate that radio-resistance or radio-sensitivity is the result of a combination of the inherent qualities of the tumour and external circumstances.

Histology is a poor determinant – we all know of adenocarcinomas cured by radiotherapy and small laryngeal carcinomas that happen to be radio-resistant. Stage and volume of the tumour are important factors, and probably volume stands for vascularisation. Necrotic tumours are poorly vascularized, this means anoxic or poorly oxygenated tumour cells and therefore diminished radio-sensitivity.

Improved radiotherapy requires improved technology, i.e. megavoltage therapy, but also a better ratio between the radiation load at the normal surrounding tissue and that at the tumour, greater knowledge of radiobiology and improvement in the detection of the extent of the tumour (CT scan).

Bulk resection might change a necrotizing, radio-resistent tumour into a residual tumour that may be cured by radiotherapy. It is conceivable that some of the local recurrences after radical surgery might be prevented by postoperative radiotherapy.

IRRADIATION VARIABLES

The most important variables in radiotherapy of rectal cancers are *dose* and *volume*. These variables are interdependent: a large volume excludes a high dose and vice versa.

Dose

A palliative dose should be chosen such that the side-effects are small, while the desired effect is attained and lasts as long as possible. Table 8 shows the wide range in doses used by different authors. Sometimes it is possible to obtain good palliation with small doses, e.g. 2000 rad. The duration of the response may depend on the dose (10, 18) but the significant correlation between dose and response postulated by Hindo (18) only applies for doses of less than 2500 rads, fractionated into 1000 rads per week, 200 rads per dose.

In our series of 108 patients, 60 (55%) reached complete remission, 53% after a moderate dose, 59% after a high dose. For the 'partial remission' group (34 of 108, i.e. 31%), there was no significant difference between the moderate and high dose groups (table 9).

Although the effect does not seem to be dose-dependent in the dose range used, the duration of remission might differ. With out series this cannot be proven, nor can it be excluded.

Volume

Although it has not been proven that a substantial number of patients die of tumours arising in para-aortic lymph nodes, a number of radiotherapists have extended the irradiation volume to include para-aortic fields up to the second lumbar vertebra. Only Tierie (15) clearly states the dose for these extended fields, i.e. 3500 rads, but he does not give data that support the desirability of the use of extended fields. In view of the significance of distant metastases and locoregional recurrence in the cause of death of these patients the benefit cannot be great.

Table 8. Rectosigmoidal cancer. Dose and indication.

Author	Dose in rads for inoperable cancer	Dose in rads for recurrence
Henry, Goffin (16)	7000-8000 (split course)	5000-7000
Tierie (15)	3500 + 1500 + 1400	–
Urdaneta Lafee (13)	3000	–
Wang, Schulz (10)	2000-5000	2000-5000
Whiteley (17)	2000-2500	2000-5000

Table 9. Dose-effect relationship for the effect of irradiation on pain, loss of blood, mucus and tumour discharge and bowel dysfunction.

Dose in rads	Complete remission	%	Partial remission	%	No effect	%	Unknown
3000/4000	35/66	53	23/66	35	5/66	7.5	3/66
5500/6000	25/42	59	11/42	26	2/42	4.5	4/42
Total	60/108	55	34/108	31	7/108	6.5	7/108

DISCUSSION AND PROSPECTS

For palliation of complaints from recurrent or inoperable cancer of the rectum and sigmoid, radiotherapy is a very valuable tool. A dose of 3000 rads/3 weeks gives a high percentage of complete or incomplete remission. It is worthwhile to investigate whether a dose higher than 3000 rads will give a substantially longer remission or is better than two courses of 3000 rads. In the palliative treatment of recurrent or inoperable rectosigmoidal cancer the benefit of an extension of the treatment volume to include the para-aortic lymph nodes has not been proven.

As hypoxia probably plays a major role in the unsatisfactory reaction to irradiation, the inoperable rectosigmoidal cancer lends itself very well for trials with agents that are independent of oxygenation, e.g. neutrons (19), or that improve sensitivity to radiation, i.e. radiosensitizers. The results of these trials will determine whether the role of these agents should be extended to the study of the combination of radiosensitizers and radiotherapy or the role of neutrons in pre- and postoperative radiotherapy. The results of radiotherapy in the palliative treatment of rectosigmoidal cancers, the prospects of the above-mentioned new developments in radiotherapy and the lack of improvement in surgical results require a very close cooperation between gastroenterologists, surgeons and radiotherapists. The number of patients is large

152

enough to draw conclusions within relatively few years. The limiting factor
will be manpower rather than patient numbers.

It must be considered unethical to start trials on the efficacy of chemotherapeutic agents as a subsitute of radiotherapy as long as the results, as
shown by Moertel, (20) are so poor.

For all three modalities it is imperative that every effort to improve the
results of therapy should be governed by well defined and well designed
prospective controlled clinical trials.

REFERENCES

1. de Waard F and van Zonneveld RJ: Epidemiologie van kanker. In: *Oncologie*, Zwaveling A, van Zonneveld RJ and Schaberg A (eds), Stafleu, Leiden 1978 (2nd ed.), p 19-27.
2. Dukes CE: Classification of cancer of rectum. *J Path Bact* 35: 323-332, 1932.
3. Kirklin JW, Dockerty MB and Waugh JM: The role of the peritoneal reflection in the prognosis of carcinoma of the rectum and sigmoid colon. *Surg Gynec Obst* 88: 326-331, 1949.
4. Astler VB and Coller FA: The prognostic significance of direct extension of carcinoma of the colon and rectum. *Ann Surg* 139: 846-851, 1954.
5. Gunderson LL and Sosin H: Areas of failure found at re-operation (second or symptomatic look) following 'curative surgery' for adenocarcinoma of the rectum. *Cancer* 34: 1278-1292, 1974.
6. Gilbert SG: Symptomatic local tumor failure following abdominal-perineal resection. *Int J Rad Oncol Biol Phys* 4: 801-807, 1978.
7. Cass AW, Million RR and Phaff WW: Patterns of recurrence following surgery alone for adenocarcinoma of the colon and rectum. *Cancer* 37: 2861-2865, 1976.
8. Johnson RJ: Gastro-intestinal cancer – colon (surgery/radiotherapy). The role of radiation therapy in the management of rectosigmoid cancer. *Cancer* 40 (1 suppl.): 595-603, 1977.
9. Papillon J: Intracavitary irradiation of early rectal cancer for cure. *Am J Proctol* 26: 37-41, 1975.
10. Wang CC and Schulz MD: The role of radiation therapy in the management of carcinoma of the sigmoid, rectosigmoid and rectum. *Radiology* 79: 1-5, 1962.
11. Williams JG: Radiotherapy of carcinoma of the rectum. In: *Cancer of the rectum*, Dukes C, London, E.S. Livingstone Ltd, 1960.
12. Rider WD: Is the Miles operation really necessary? *J Canad Ass Radiol* 26: 167-175, 1975.
13. Urdaneta Lafee N, Kligerman MM and Knowlton AH: Evaluation of palliative irradiation in rectal carcinoma. *Radiology*, 104: 673-677, 1972.
14. Rouseau J, Cuzin J, Debertrand Ph, Mathieu G and Fenton J: La cobaltthérapie dans le cancer du rectum. *Arch Fr Mal App Dig* 58: 9 bis 49, 1969.
15. Tierie AH: Radiotherapy of marginal resectable and non-resectable rectum cancer. *Radiologia Clin* 47: 222-227, 1978.
16. Henry J and Goffin JC: La place de l'irradiation par betatron dans le traitement des cancers du rectum. *J Radiol Electrol* 55: 491-494, 1974.
17. Whiteley HW, Stearns MW, Leaning RH and Debbish MR: Palliative radiation therapy in patients with cancer of the colon and rectum. *Cancer* 25: 343-346, 1970.
18. Hindo WA, Soleimani PK, Miller WA and Henrickson FR: Patterns of recurrent and metastatic carcinoma of the colon and rectum treated with radiation. *Dis Col Rect* 15: 436-440, 1972.
19. Catterall M: Clinical experience with fast neutrons. *Proc Roy Soc Med* 65: 839-843, 1972.
20. Moertel CG: Chemotherapy of gastro-intestinal cancer. *N Eng J Med* 299: 1049-1052, 1978.

18. PRE- OR POSTOPERATIVE RADIATION IN RESECTABLE TUMORS

MAUS W. STEARNS JR.

PREOPERATIVE RADIATION THERAPY

Our interest at Memorial Sloan-Kettering Cancer Center in preoperative radiation dates back to the late thirties and early forties where the accepted practice under the late Dr. George Binkley was to give patients with cancer of the rectum preoperative radiation therapy three to four weeks prior to operation. In the late forties and early fifties the emphasis was on the surgical approach and the routine preoperative radiation therapy was abandoned, except for questionably operably lesions. When it became apparent that the extended surgical approach alone did not improve survival we reviewed the early experience with preoperative radiation from 1939-1951. This experience is summarized in tables 1, 2 and 3, where it seems apparent that the patients with the poorest prognosis, that is the Dukes' C lesions those with nodal metastases benefited materially from preoperative radiation (2). Thus in 1957 we resumed preoperative radiation therapy for patients with any but the most superficial cancers of the rectum. In 1960 we began to randomize patients. Because these were almost all patients seen in private offices and it was in the days before informed consent we randomized patients purely on the basis of an odd or even birth date. This allowed us to discuss with the patient his treatment program immediately without having to wait for an outside randomization. We continued this program through 1967. In 1972 we evaluated our results, which are shown in tables 4, 5 and 6, which indicated there was no difference in survival with or without preoperative radiation therapy (3).

This experience has been criticized because of the method of randomization. This defect is to some extent compensated by the fact that all of the surgery was performed or closely supervised by six surgeons who limited their practice to colon cancer, that the patient population was uniform, that the radiation therapy was given by two radiotherapists, that the pathology was all reviewed by two or three pathologists, that the survival in all parameters was almost identical, that the location of the tumors was the same and that the incidence of nodal metastases were the same, that is 37% in the control series and 35% in the treated series. Our conclusion was that in our practice routine preoperative X-ray therapy had not influenced survival in our patients. However, as demonstrated in table 7 the proportion of failures due to

K. Welvaart et al. (eds.), Colorectal Cancer, 153-159. All rights reserved.
Copyright © 1980 by Martinus Nijhoff Publishers, The Hague/Boston/London.

Table 1. Five-year survival.

	Total patients	Five-year survivors	Five-year survival rate
Total series	1786	505	28.5%
Operated patients	1276	479	37.4%
No X-ray	549	225	41.0%
With X-ray	727	254	35.0%
Resected patients	971	479	49.0%
No X-ray	473	225	47.5%
With X-ray	498	254	51.0%

Table 2. Effect of preoperative X-ray therapy on cancer of rectum.

	No. of patients	Incidence in series %	Overall 5-year survivors %	Determinate 5-year survivors %
Dukes A				
s̄ X-ray	74	23	74	82
c̄ X-ray	101	23	73	86
Dukes B				
s̄ X-ray	108	33	66	77
c̄ X-ray	158	35	65	70
Dukes C				
s̄ X-ray	141	44	23	25
c̄ X-ray	188	42	37	39
Totals	770		53%	58%

Table 3. Effect of preoperative X-ray therapy on cancer of rectum.

	No. of patients	Incidence of series %	Overall 10-year survival %	Determinate 10-year survival %
Dukes A				
s̄ X-ray	74	23	58	70
c̄ X-ray	101	23	53	68
Dukes B				
s̄ X-ray	108	33	45	56
c̄ X-ray	158	35	47	56
Dukes C				
s̄ X-ray	141	44	10	11
c̄ X-ray	188	42	27	30
Totals	770		38%	43%

Table 4. Preop X-ray.

	Overall	
	No. X-ray	Plus X-ray
Total number patients	414	376
Indeterminate	44	57
5-year survivors	242	215
5-year survival		
Overall	58%	57%
Determinate	65%	67%

Table 5. Preop X-ray regional metastases.

	No metastases		Pos. metastases	
	No X-ray	Plus X-ray	No X-ray	Plus X-ray
Determinate patients	231	209	139	110
5-year survivors	182	164	63	49
Determinate				
5-year survival	79%	78%	45%	45%

Table 6. Preop X-ray location.

	No X-ray	Plus X-ray
Below 6 cm		
Determinate patients	62	70
5-year survival	62%	56%
6-10 cm		
Determinate patients	114	170
5-year survival	59%	66%
11-16 cm		
Determinate patients	184	76
5-year survival	70%	68%

Table 7. Preop X-ray site of failure.

	Positive nodes	
Total patients	79	107
Failures		
Local	30%	16%
Liver	11%	10%
Other	14%	29%

pelvic recurrence had been lowered, but the proportion due to distant metastases had increased.

Opposed to this experience was that of the Veterans' Administration which has been so ably reported by Dr. George Higgins (1). The course of pre-operative therapy of approximately 2000 rads given over a period of two to three weeks was essentially the same as we had used. The results of that study are shown in tables 8 and 9. It seemed apparent that their significant improvement in survival was for those patients who had abdomino-perineal resection. Table 10 shows the results in our patients having abdomino-perineal resection with and without radiation therapy. It is obvious that our patients did not have the same beneficial effect from radiation. Since the Veterans' Administration patients were almost entirely males, we also looked at any difference according to sex shown in table 11. It is interesting to note that in the patients who did not have X-ray therapy the survival in men was considerably poorer than in women, which is the usual finding in colon and rectal cancer. However, when preoperative radiation had been given the survival in men approached that of women. Another discrepancy between our series was the finding in the Veterans' Administration series that there was a significantly lower incidence of nodal metastases in those treated preoperatively (table 12). This lower incidence has been attributed to the effect of radiation in sterilizing lymph nodes. Using the same amount of radiation this effect was not observed in either our early series where there was a 44% incidence of Dukes' C lesion in the untreated and 42% in those having radiation, or in our later series where the incidence was 37% in the untreated and 35% in the treated group. In passing it would appear that the difference in incidence of nodal metastases in the controlled series and in the treated series of the Veterans' Administration was about the same difference as the survival. The real significance of these observations remains to be determined.

Most other completed studies of preoperative X-ray are of relatively small numbers of patients or they lack control arm and have been well summarized by Higgins (1). The dosage of radiation in these reports varied from that by Ryder of a single dose of 500 rads to the pelvis immediately preoperative to 5000 rads over a five to eight week period as given by Fletcher, Allan Dunphey and Stephens. A report from Leningrad of a series of some 242 patients in whom patients having surgery alone were compared with those having 3000 rads five to ten days prior to surgery. The six-year survival of combined treatment was 52.5% and 40% for those with surgery alone.

There are a number of on-going studies of preoperative X-ray whose final report should provide additional significant information. The British Medical Research Council have entered a substantial number of patients in three-arm study: surgery alone; 500 rads immediately prior to surgery; 2000 rads over 12 to 15 days preoperatively. The European Organization for Research

Table 8. Overall 5-year survival.

	No of patients	5-year survival
Control	353	28.9%
Treated	347	35.2%

(Higgings 1979)

Table 9. Survival curative abdominoperineal resection.

	No of patients	5-year survival
Control	143	34.3%
Treated	162	46.9%

(Higgins 1979)

Table 10. APR.

	No X-ray	Plus X-ray
Total	90	139
(POD	0	6)
Indeterminate-total	10	22
5-year survivors	45	70
Ca after 5 years	3	8
5-year survival		
Overall	50%	50%
Determinate	55%	60%
NEC	53%	53%

Table 11. Preop X-ray sex.

	No X-ray		Plus X-ray	
	Men	Women	Men	Women
Determinate patients	192	178	186	133
5-year survivors	114	128	126	87
Determinate				
5-year survival	59%	72%	68%	65%

Table 12. Incidence nodal metastases.

	Control	Preop XRT
Positive nodes	32.1%	21.8%

(Higgins 1979)

in The Treatment of Cancer also has a three-arm study: surgery alone; 3450 rads over 19 days; 5'Fluouracil during the first week of radiation therapy.

POSTOPERATIVE RADIATION THERAPY

Postoperative radiation has one outstanding theoretical advantage in that only those patients with the greatest chance of local recurrence need be treated. There are also theoretical disadvantages. Cancer cells that are disseminated by the trauma of surgery will not have received an attenuating course of X-ray and may implant and grow more readily. The tissues in the pelvis will have relative deprivation of blood supply and hence less effective oxygenation which may make the cells more resistent to radiation. Moreover, after surgery in the pelvis loops of small bowel are almost always found adherent by scar tissue. Fixed small bowel is much more easily damaged by radiation then when it is freely movable and the same segment is not always in the field of therapy.

Reports of the results of postoperative radiation therapy are of small numbers of patients. Dose levels have been used from 4600-5100 rads. These levels raise concern about the induction of radiation enteritis and at least one death from this complication was reported in a series of 40 patients with a substantial early complication rate in others. These reports, however, suggest that there may be some decrease in the number of intra-pelvic recurrences.

There are a number of on-going studies such as the Gasrointestinal Study Group including an arm with no additional treatment comparing postoperative radiation 4500-5100 rads, chemotherapy and combined radiation and chemotherapy. These studies will be of great interest.

PRE- AND POSTOPERATIVE RADIATION THERAPY

If I were to be asked to design a protocol for study of the role of radiation therapy as an adjunct to surgery, I would employ the 'sandwich' technique, a modest course of 2000-3000 rads preoperatively for those with low-lying rectal cancer, followed by a similar postoperative course for those having Dukes' C lesions or extensive B lesions where the lateral margins were suspect. This has very distinct advantages with few disadvantages. If cancer cells are attenuated by radiation preoperative treatment is essential. The Veterans' Administration study demonstrates that at least in their patients preoperative X-ray therapy has improved the survival of those having abdomino-perineal resection. This low dose is well tolerated and creates no surgical problems. After surgery those who have the greatest potential for pelvic recurrence can be selected for additional treatment, which at these lower levels should not cause complications of radiation enteristis. It has the distinct advantage of being a simple two-arm study in which clear cut results should be readily apparent.

REFERENCES

1. Higgins GA and Roswit B: The role of radiotherapy in the surgical treatment of large bowel cancer. In: *Progress in clinical cancer*. Vol VII. Irving M Ariel (ed), 1978, Grune and Stratton, Inc.
2. Stearns MW Jr, Deddish MR and Quan SHQ: Preoperative roentgen therapy for cancer of the rectum. *Surg Gynecol Obs* 109: 225-229, 1959.
3. Stearns MW Jr, Deddish MR, Wuan SHO and Leaming RH: Preoperative roentgen therapy for cancer of the rectum and rectosigmoid. *Surg Gynecol Obs* 138: 584-586, 1974.

19. CRYOTHERAPY IN RECTAL CARCINOMA

G. FEIFEL AND H. LETZEL

INTRODUCTION

Resection is undoubtedly the only cure for rectal carcinoma (2, 4, 23). However, depending on the extent of the tumor and on the general condition of the patient resection is not always feasible.

Alternative or palliative methods are local excision, electrocoagulation, radiotherapy or colostomy (16, 25, 28). Only circumscribed tumors with limited invasion of the rectal wall may be cured by local surgery or electrocoagulation. The indications for electrofulguration as a palliative measure are limited (3). Sufficient experience with radiotherapy for inoperable rectal carcinoma is presently not available. A simple colostomy is unavoidable when a high stenosis is present. Unfortunately it is the method which most significantly alters the patient's quality of life. Moreover, the lethality is considerable, particularly for patients with advanced growth (1, 2, 9, 15, 26).

In view of this background therapeutic alternatives have to meet at least three requirements: a low risk, a marked reduction of the tumor and preservation of the natural bowel function. First reports concerning cryotherapy for tumors have been encouraging (6, 10, 14, 22, 24), and as a result we undertook a study to determine the extent to which this method fulfills these criteria.

MECHANISM OF THE CRYOGENIC LESION

The biological application of cryogenic temperatures has apparently paradoxical aims:
1. The preservation of biological material; and
2. the selective destruction of tissues by means of freezing them. The survival or death of living tissues is determined by several factors, the most important being the rates of cooling and warming (9, 12, 19, 20, 21). Depending on these rates phenomena develop which are deleterious to the cells (table 1). In a tissue, temperatures below $-22\,°C$ lead to capillary stasis followed by thrombosis. This is probably the most important factor for the origin of a necrosis. A cooling rate of more than $200\,°C$ per min has proven adequate

162

Table 1. Types of freezing injury.

Cell compression
Loss of water
Damage to cell protein
Membrane rupture
Ischaemic necrosis

---

for clinical application. Fast freezing followed by slow thawing is the most suitable approach for destruction of living tissues. However, because of various factors which influence the destruction of tissues, the extent of destruction cannot be predicted precisely in an individual case (8, 13).
Fig. 1 shows an example: Within an area of necrosis caused by preoperative cryotherapy remnants of a carcinoma are still to be seen. Probably the vascularity in this area had a protective effect.

According to Fraser (9) the size of the cryolesion is not only related to the probe size, its temperature, the duration of freezing and the vascularity but also to the thermal conductivity of tissues previously stressed by freezing injury. Therefore, the volume of frozen tissue increases with each successive freezing. There are two consequences for the application of cryotherapy to large tumors which can be derived from Fraser's findings: the optimum size of the cryolesion is obtained by choosing a low probe temperature and

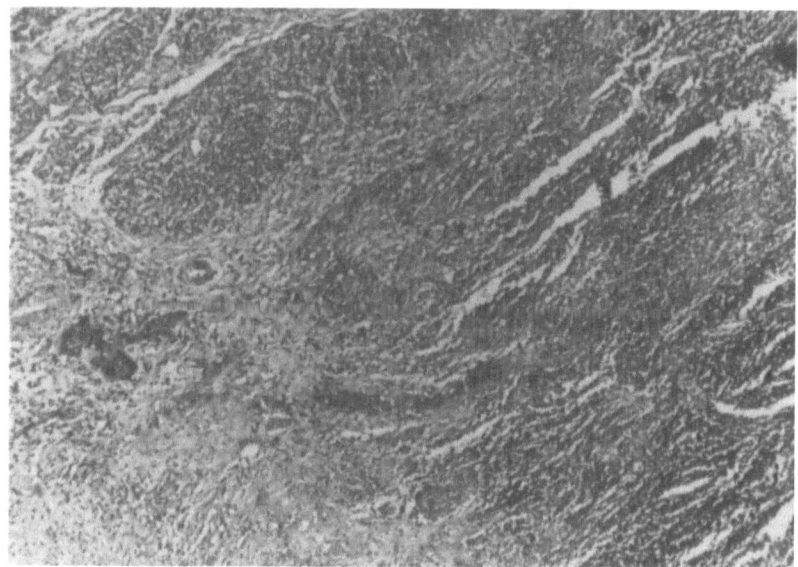

Fig. 1. Histological appearance of a cryolesion 4 weeks after freezing in a patient with squamous cell carcinoma of the anus. On the left (dark) remnants of the carcinoma are still to be seen.

repetitive freeze-thaw cycles. Unfortunately, the extent of the final necrosis cannot be predicted precisely, although the amount of frozen tissue can be exactly controlled by the surgeon. Obviously malignant growths have a lower thermal conductivity. Therefore, when cryotherapy is considered as a method of curing cancer, there is reason to be cautious (11, 27, 30).

Cryotherapy is not associated with immediate tissue destruction. Relatively slow tissue destruction seems to lead to the release of antigenic substances (6, 22). More significance has yet to be accorded this phenomenon in conjunction with cryotherapy.

INSTRUMENTS AND METHODS

Since the fundamental investigations of Smith, Cooper and others a variety of instruments has become available. I only mention the two most important ones (5, 17).

1. Instruments which are *cooled by expansion of gas*. The tip of the probe is cooled according to Joule-Thompson's principle. N_2O under high pressure is released through a jet and absorbs warmth from the outside. Warm gas is removed via another tube. Using N_2O a temperature down to $-70\,°C$ can be reached.

2. Instruments which are *cooled by change of state*. Cooling is achieved by the absorption of heat upon changing the refrigerant from a liquid state to vapor. For the freezing of large tumors liquid nitrogen is to be recommended because the tip of the probe can be cooled down to $-190\,°C$. This requires, however, more complicated equipment which is more expensive.

In Munich, we use the latter system, i.e. the cryosurgical unit CE_2A (Union Carbide) with liquid nitrogen. It is a closed circuit system with a flexible vacuum-insulated probe. Probe tips of various shapes and sizes are used: round tips are, for instance, preferred for contact freezing, sharp probes are suitable for penetrating the tumor. The probe diameter ranges from 7 to 10 mm, the freezing tip is 2.5 cm long. The tip contains a temperature sensor by means of which a preset temperature is electronically controlled. A heating system allows immediate removal of the probe after freezing is finished.

In fig. 2 the course of the temperature during freezing and thawing is illustrated in a patient with rectal carcinoma. The temperature drops down to $-160\,°C$ within 30 sec. That means a cooling rate of $400\,°C$ per min. The temperature is more or less precisely kept at the present level until freezing is interrupted by switching on the heating.

The *preparation of the patient* is easy. After an enema he simply empties his bowels before he is brought to the rectoscopy-room. Cryotherapy is usually performed without anesthetics. The patient can leave the hospital a few hours

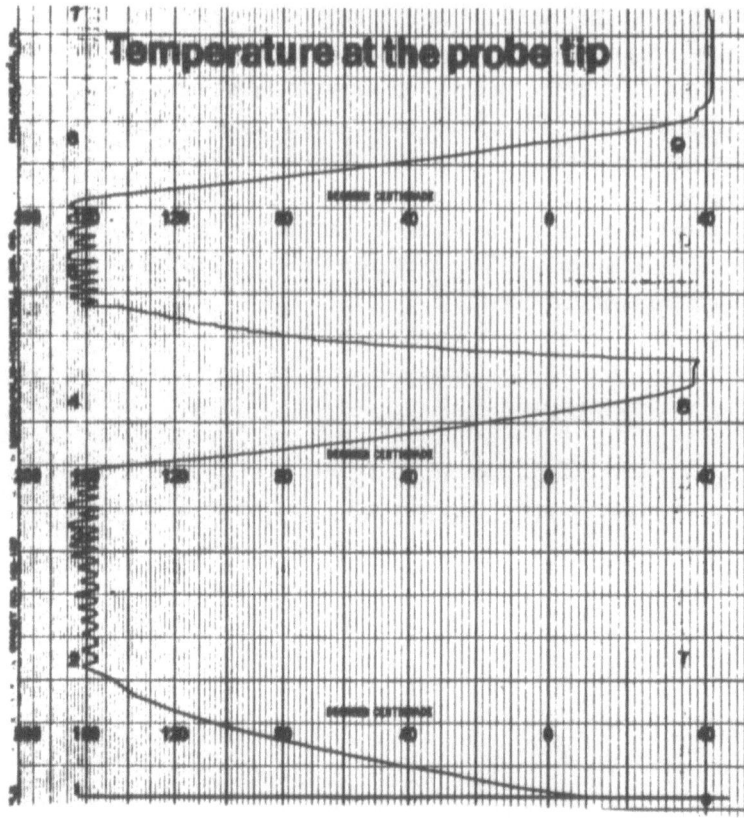

Fig. 2. Temperature measurements recorded at the probe tip during freezing and thawing of a rectal carcinoma.

later. Only in the case of large or high rectal tumors is general anesthesia recommended. This allows the use of a surgical rectoscope which provides a good view of these tumors. Essentially the freezing has to be restricted to areas which are fully visible to the surgeon. Only then is it guaranteed that the amount of frozen tissue can be exactly controlled and the risk of perforation or damage to normal tissue can be minimized.

PATIENTS

In our clinic cryotherapy has been used since 1976. Only 3 surgeons took part in the study; thus the procedure may be regarded as fairly standardized. Between May 1976 and May 1979, the proportion of patients receiving cryotherapy amounted to about 30%. The results presented in this paper will refer to the upper two groups in fig. 3.

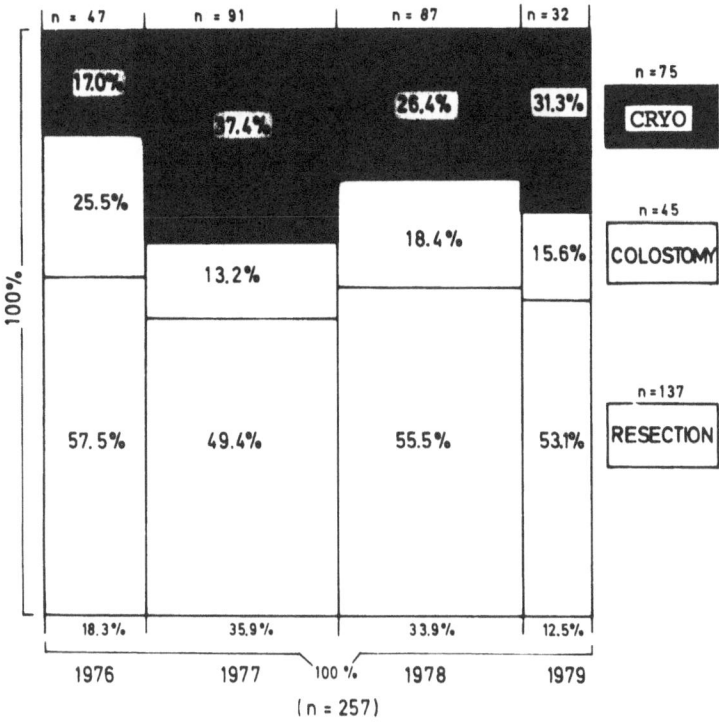

Fig. 3. Treatment of 257 patients with rectal carcinoma (1976-79).

To evaluate our results we divided our patients into three groups:

Group A: patients who only received cryotherapy (n = 61)

Group B: patients primarily treated with palliative colostomy followed by cryotherapy (n = 13)

Group C: a control group of patients who only underwent palliative colostomy (n = 26).

Whereas the course of the patients in groups A and B could be followed completely, this could be achieved in only 56% of group C.

The *indication for local treatment* with cryotherapy was exclusively restricted to patients who were either generally or locally or transiently inoperable or who had refused surgery. It should be emphasized that all patients of group A had one or more concomitant diseases. The causes of inoperability were for instance second tumors, blindness, paralysis, general metastases and in particular cardiac and/or respiratory failure.

The basic aim of cryotherapy was reduction of the tumor, elimination of a stenosis and palliation of symptoms like bleeding, tenesmus or pain. Our most important aim, however, was to avoid colostomy. The success or failure of cryotherapy depended on whether we could achieve these aims or not.

Partial success means that one of several aims could be achieved or that the severity of symptoms could be reduced. The local results were controlled by rectoscopy, including a biopsy at least every 4 months. For patients in whom a laparotomy could not be performed, the search for metastases included a liver sonogram, an X-ray of the lungs and, since 1977, CEA determinations (7).

To evaluate the results of cryotherapy in this retrospective, non-randomized study we tried to answer 4 questions:

1. Are there differences between groups A, B and C with respect to age, site and extention of the tumor, clinical stage and metastases?
2. What are the factors influencing success or failure, or survival, after cryotherapy?
3. In what percentage of our patients could the aims of cryotherapy be achieved?
4. What kind of complications are to be expected during or after cryotherapy?

RESULTS

Fig. 4 shows cumulative age distribution for our 3 groups. Group A and group C have a similar tendency with a steep rise above 70 years of age. The patients of group B on the other hand were younger on average. This becomes particularly apparent when looking at the medians and their confidence intervals. Half of our patients on cryotherapy as the only treatment were more than 76 years old (fig. 5).

Moreover, there is a marked difference in the proportion of patients with clinically proven metastases on entering the study. Of the patients in group A 27.1% had metastases versus 48% in group C. But one will agree that the certainty of diagnosing existing metastases should be higher in patients who have undergone laparotomy (fig. 6).

For staging we used the system of clinical staging described by Mason. Here too, there is a marked difference between the groups. Only 44.1% of the patients primarily treated with cryotherapy were judged as having stage 4 disease in contrast to over 80% in each of the other two groups (fig. 7).

In fig. 8 the upper and lower limits of the tumors are drawn as they were determined endoscopically. Site and extention of the tumors seem to be similarly distributed in all 3 groups – the peak lying between 4 and 12 cm from the anal verge in patients' upper end of the tumor could be defined. For anatomical reasons freezing should be restricted to this zone to avoid the neighborhood of the peritoneal reflection or the anal sphincter, respectively.

As to the factors influencing success or failure or cryotherapy, semi-circumferential tumors had a better prognosis than circumferential or constricting tumors, the percentage of failure being 5-fold higher for the latter

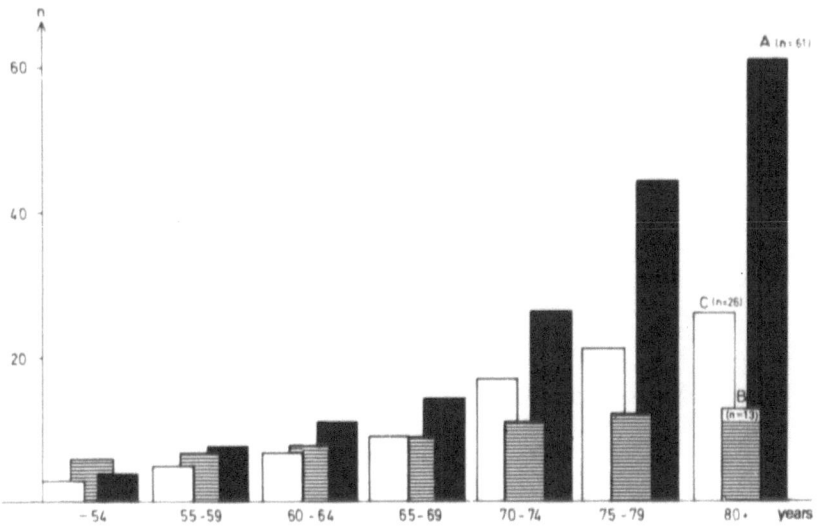

Fig. 4. Cumulative age distribution. A cryotherapy, B cryotherapy after colostomy, C colostomy.

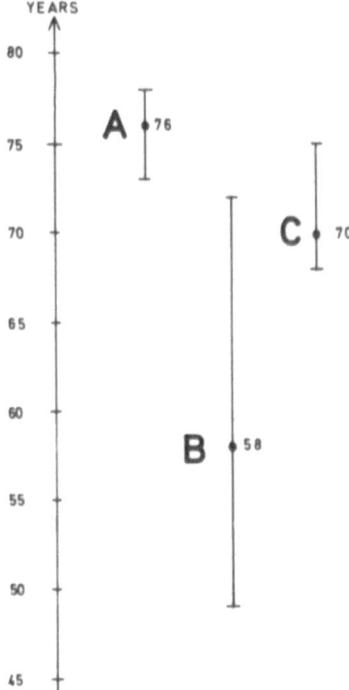

Fig. 5. Age: Median 95% – confidence interval. A cryotherapy, B cryotherapy after colostomy, C colostomy.

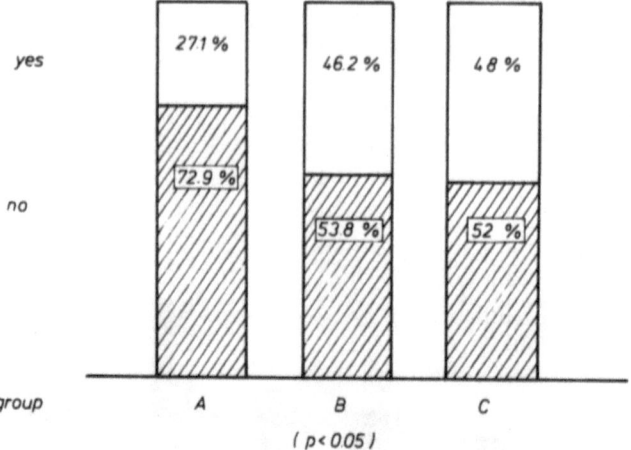

Fig. 6. Metastases in patients of groups A, B and C.

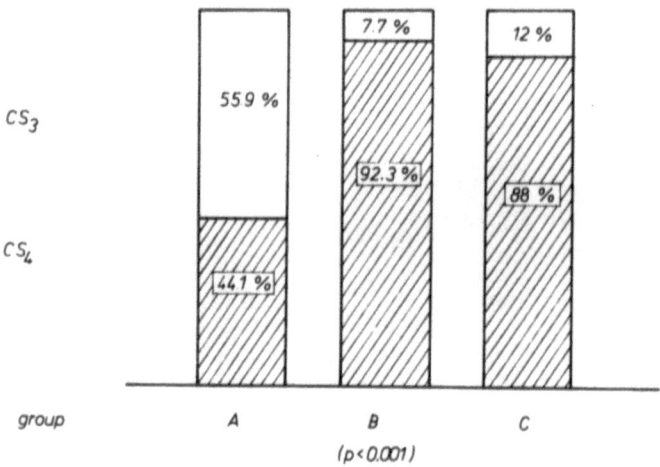

Fig. 7. Clinical staging (CS) according to Mason.

(fig. 9). The success of cryotherapy was apparently more obvious in polypous tumors than in ulcerating ones. Age was not a decisive factor in the final outcome; stage and secondary spread, however, were all the more so. Therefore it is not surprising that patients of group A with more tumors in stage 3 and fewer metastases showed the lowest overall mortality.

Nevertheless the duration of survival after cryotherapy was remarkably long for these seriously ill patients. The median survival time was found to be 20 months in contrast to 6 and 8 months for the other two groups (fig. 10). The difference in survival is striking but must be interpreted with care since it may

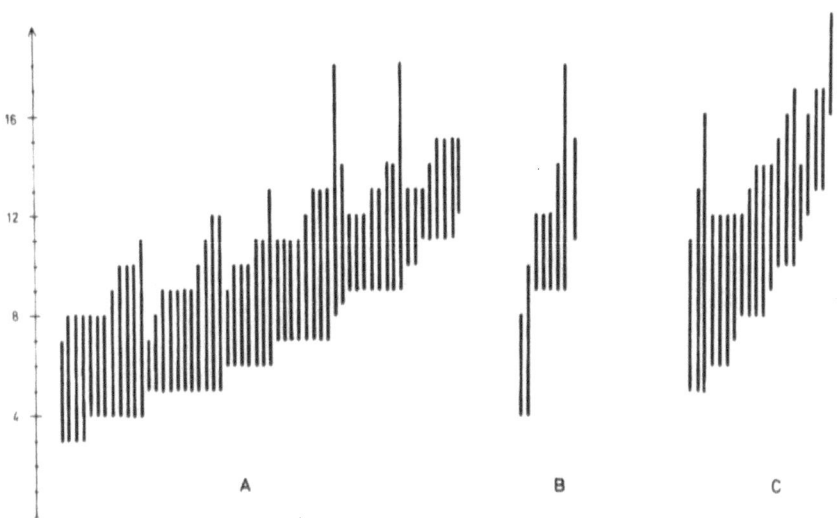

Fig. 8. Extent (cm) of tumor in patients receiving cryotherapy and controls. See text.

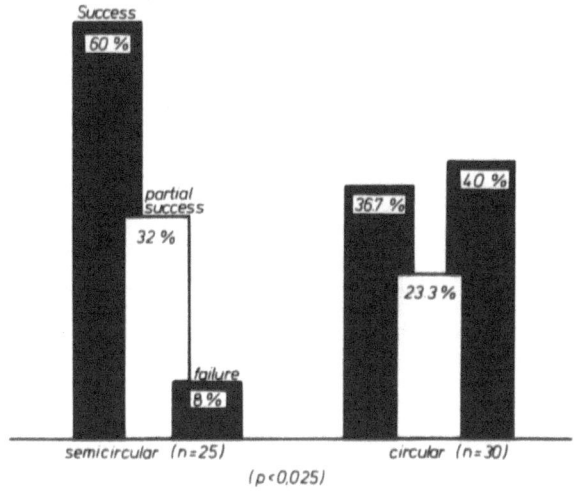

Fig. 9. Success and failure of cryotherapy and type of growth (group A).

be influenced by some of the differences between the groups. Another observation deserves notice: no patient in the cryo-group died during hospitalization, whereas 4 patients in group C died postoperatively. Summarizing this point, circumferential spread, stage and especially metastases influence success and survival after cryotherapy. Cryotherapy itself however did not cause immediate fatality.

In comparing the aims of cryotherapy with the local results it is obvious that this form of local treatment can only partially solve the problems of

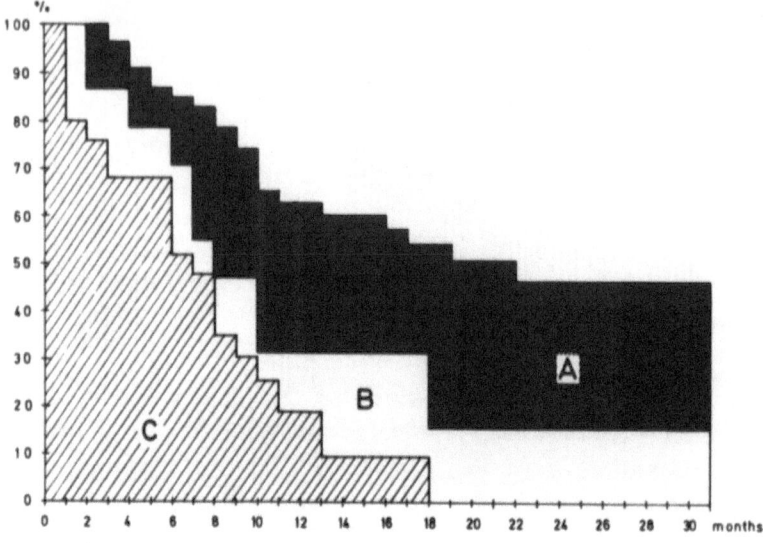

Fig. 10. Survival time for patients with and without cryotherapy (log. Rank test: p < 0.001).

patients with inoperable rectal carcinoma. In only 4 of our patients was all known growth destroyed with a negative biopsy during a follow-up of two years. In the others the tumor was reduced or even removed but recurrent growth developed.

The most encouraging result is the fact that in 65% the tumor could be reduced and a stenosis prevented. Accordingly a colostomy could be prevented in 65% of the patients (table 2). One could ask whether a more aggressive approach, for instance prolongation of the freezing time, could improve the results. In fact the therapeutic range for the freezing time is rather small. Therefore one has to fear a higher rate of complications, especially the increased danger of injuring adjacent organs or normal mucosa.

In the present series there were few major complications. Bleeding, although the most frequent unpleasant side-effect after cryotherapy, could be stopped by local means in each case. In contrast, incontinency, fibrotic stenosis or perforation of the rectum occasionally required surgical intervention with drainage and colostomy (table 3).

Table 2. Local results of cryotherapy.

Aims	Success	
	yes	no
Abolition of stenosis	59.1%	40.9%
Reduction of tumor and prevention of stenosis	65.0%	35.0%
Control of bleeding or discharge	55.6%	44.4%

Table 3. Complications in 74 patients during and after cryotherapy.

	Minor	Major
Bleeding	9.3%	—
Incontinency	2.7%	4.0%
Fibrotic stenosis	4.0%	1.3%
Perforation/infection	1.3%	4.0%
		26.6%

With regard to monitoring the treatment it should be mentioned that the control of CEA levels has proven to be a reliable parameter. The tumor-reducing effect of cryotherapy is reflected in a concomitant drop in the CEA levels a few days after cryotherapy. A discrepancy between good local results and unchanged or even rising CEA levels points to secondary growth.

CONCLUSIONS

As yet cryotherapy as a nonsurgical treatment does not appear to be acceptable as an alternative to excision or resection, not even in the early stages of rectal carcinoma. In our view the indication for cryotherapy should be restricted to patients who are inoperable because of either their general state of health or local conditions. The evaluation of these conditions is difficult but can be revised during the course of treatment, as was the case with 2 of our patients. In such cases cryotherapy serves by providing preoperative devitalisation, as is recommended by Langer (18).

The improvement in the quality of life after cryotherapy in patients with inoperable rectal carcinoma seems so obvious that a randomized clinical trial comparing cryotherapy versus palliative colostomy does not appear to be justified. The question does arise, however, as to whether a randomized trial comparing cryotherapy and radiation could throw some light on the issue of the best nonsurgical method for the treatment of inoperable rectal carcinoma.

SUMMARY

During the past 3 years 74 patients with either generally or locally inoperable rectal carcinoma were treated with cryotherapy. The use of a liquid nitrogen system allowing temperatures down to $-180\,°C$ proved adequate, especially for large tumors. Cryotherapy is most suitable for tumors in the middle third of the rectum. The best results of this non-surgical treatment are achieved in semicircular and polypous tumors. As compared to patients of a control group undergoing only palliative colostomy, the survival time turned out to be remarkably longer for patients receiving cryotherapy. However, there were differences between these groups in clinical stage and the presence of metastases. Nevertheless the risk of the method is low, colostomy can often be avoided and satisfying local results can be achieved in more than 50% of the cases.

REFERENCES

1. Adam YG, Calabrese C and Volk H: Colorectal cancer in patients over 80 years of age. *Surg Clin North Amer* 52: 883-889, 1972.
2. Baden H and Andersen B: Survival of patients with untreated liver metastases from colorectal cancer. *Scand J Gastroent* 10: 221-223, 1975.
3. Beahrs AH: Status of fulguration and cryosurgery in the management of colonic and rectal cancer and polyps. *Cancer* 34: 965-968, 1974.
4. Bussey HJR: The survival rate patients with advanced rectal cancer. *Proc Roy Soc Med* 62: 29-34, 1969.
5. Cooper IS: Cryobiology as viewed by the surgeon. *Cryobiology* 1: 44-51, 1964.
6. Cooper, I.S: Cryogenic surgery. *Surg Ann* 2, 239-264. 1970.
7. Feifel G, Beutel V and Lamerz R: Cryotherapy for palliation in rectal carcinoma. *Front gastrointest Res* 5: 195-201, 1979.
8. Fraser J and Gill W: Observations on ultra-frozen tissue. *Br J Surg* 54: 770-776, 1967.
9. Fraser J: Cryosurgery. *Prog Surg* 14: 136-159, 1975.
10. Gage AA: Cryotherapy for inoperable rectal cancer. *Dis Colon Rectum* 11: 36-44, 1968.
11. Gage AA: Cryosurgery for cancer. *Cryobiology* 5: 241-249, 1969.
12. Gill W, Fraser J and Carter DC: Repeated freeze-thaw cycles in cryosurgery. *Nature* 219:410-413, 1968.
13. Gill W, Fraser J, da Costa J and Beazley R: The cryosurgical lesion. *Amer Surgeon* 437-445, 1970.
14. Gill W, Long W, Fraser J and Lee P: Cryosurgery for neoplasia. *Br J Surg* 57: 494-502, 1970.
15. Godwin JD and Brown ChC: Some prognostic factors in survival of patients with cancer of the colon and rectum. *J Chron Dis* 28: 441-454, 1975.
16. Goligher JC: Current trends in the radical management of carcinoma of the rectum. In: *Recent advances in surgery*. Taylor S (ed), 1977, p 1-32.
17. Holden HD and Saunders SL. Cryosurgery. Its scientific basis and clinical application. *Practitioner* 210: 543-550, 1973.
18. Langer S and Buss H: Der Mastdarmkrebs. Klinik und Morphologie der lokalen Kryotherapie. *Dtsch med Wschr* 104: 768-771, 1979.
19. Mazur P: Theoretical and experimental effects of cooling and warming velocity on the survival of frozen and thawed cells. *Cryobiology* 2: 181-192, 1966.
20. Meryman HT: Mechanics of freezing in living cells and tissues. *Science* 124: 515-521, 1956.
21. Meryman HT: The interpretation of freezing rates in biological materials. *Cryobiology* 2: 165-170, 1966.
22. Moore FT, Blackwood J, Sanzenbacher L and Pace WG: Cryotherapy for malignant tumors: immunologic response. *Arch Surg* 96: 527-529, 1968.
23. Newman HK and Stearns MW: Re-exploration for 'unresectable' colonic cancer. *Dis Col Rect* 18: 576-580, 1975.
24. Osborne DR, Higgins AF and Hobbs KEF: Cryosurgery in the management of rectal tumours. *Br J Surg* 65: 859-861, 1978.

25. Papillon J: Endocavitary irradiation in the curative treatment of early rectal cancers. *Dis Col Rect* 17: 172-180, 1974.
26. Pestana C, Reitemeier RJ, Moertel ChG, Judd ES and Dockerty MB: The natural history of carcinoma of the colon and rectum. *Am J Surg* 108: 826-829, 1964.
27. Rella W, Schandalik R, Walzel C, Wrba H, Holzner JH and Pantucek F: Investigation of cell-vitality in tumor specimen after cryosurgical operations. *Österr Ztsch Onkologie* 2: 47-48.
28. Stearns MW: Limitations of local treatment of carcinoma of the rectum. In: *Controversy in Surgery*. Varca RL (ed), 1976, 401-406.
29. Winkler R and Rauchenberger B: Das inkurable kolorektale Karzinom. *Münch med Wschr* 119: 997-1002, 1977.
30. Whittaker DK: Ice crystals formed in tissues during cryosurgery. *Cryobiology* 11: 192-201, 1974.
31. Whittaker M and Goligher JC: The prognosis after surgical treatment for carcinoma of the rectum. *Br J Surg* 63: 384-388, 1976.

20. ELECTROFULGURATION FOR RECTAL CANCER

E.A. VAN SLOOTEN AND O.A. VAN DOBBENBURGH

Purely local treatment for a malignant disease which has a tendency to metastasize to regional nodes would seem to be oncological heresy, all the more so when the regional nodes are not easily accessible for routine examination and when these nodes are often the first and temporarily the sole localization of metastatic spread.

Orthodox treatment for cancer of the distal rectum, the Quénu-Miles operation, entails a permanent colostomy and still carries a relatively high postoperative mortality and morbidity, so that any procedure which would be less onerous for the patient would be very welcome. In some areas (head and neck, extremities) the primary tumour and the regional lymph nodes can be approached individually as separate procedures, thereby reducing operative trauma and mutilation. Furthermore the two areas need not be treated simultaneously and different therapeutic modalities, e.g. radiotherapy and surgery, may be applied; the risk for elderly and/or debilitated patients can thus be minimized.

Although in some cases of locally treated cancer of the rectum this has been attempted, excision of regional retrorectal and sigmoidal nodes is not a satisfactory procedure. The area is difficult to define anatomically and is not easily accessible; furthermore an attempt at truly radical excision is liable to jeopardize the blood supply to the rectum. Moreover the operation can only be carried out through a laparotomy with wide exposure of the pelvic contents.

It is evident that a two-step treatment of distal carcinoma of the rectum, removal of the primary tumour followed by node excision, is not a practical proposition.

Pathological studies have shown that metastatic spread to lymph nodes mainly depends on the invasive properties of the primary tumour. When malignant growth is limited to mucosa and submucosa, nodal metastasis is very rare. Only poorly differentiated tumours will occasionally metastasize to nodes even when local invasion is still limited to the submucosa.

Differentiated tumours invading the muscular wall without penetrating into the perirectal tissues have a distinctly higher rate of nodal metastasis. This, however, is to some extent dependent on the size of the primary tumour. When only one-third of the circumference is involved, metastases are found in less than 15% of the cases.

K. Welvaart et al. (eds.), Colorectal Cancer, 175-180. All rights reserved.
Copyright © 1980 by Martinus Nijhoff Publishers, The Hague/Boston/London.

As soon as invasive growth has reached the perirectal tissues, the incidence of nodal metastasis becomes very high, around 60% with some slight variation due to tumour size. It follows from these figures that there is a small category of patients with rectal carcinoma, consisting of those with superficial tumours of all sizes and those with small tumours invading but not breaking through the muscular wall, in whom local treatment of the rectal tumour would appear to be warranted.

For curative local treatment of sessile infiltrating tumours several modalities have been developed and each has its enthusiastic advocate(s):
1. contact intracavitary radiotherapy (1, 2);
2. local excision (3);
3. electrocoagulation (4, 5, 6, 7);
4. Laser destruction (8);
5. cryosurgery (9);
6. transanal diathermy loop resection (10).
The main factors which influence the results are selection of the cases and experience with the method.

By means of selection the number of cases in which nodal metastasis becomes apparent after treatment of the primary tumour can be limited. Experience, patience and accuracy are needed to prevent local recurrence.

Although the appearance of nodal metastasis in the presacral space after successful local treatment of the primary tumour is disappointing, its influence on the eventual prognosis is – at least theoretically – not very great for those patients in Dukes' C category for the following reasons:
1. The 5-year survival for Dukes'C disease treated by orthodox surgery is 30% at best; of the other 70% most deaths are due to distant metastatic spread.
2. More than half of the patients with secondary nodal metastasis can be cured locally by orthodox surgery. As a rule these will fall under the favourable 30% of Dukes' C category.

If it is assumed that in 15% of the patients nodal metastasis will become apparent after 'curative' local treatment, one may calculate that about 2 or 3% of all the patients treated originally will actually die as a consequence of the 'limited' approach. If adominoperineal excision has been performed in the same group, surgical mortality would have reached a similar figure.

At the Netherlands Cancer Institute electrocoagulation-fulguration has for many years been the method of choice for the treatment of sessile rectal cancer suitable for local treatment, whether the aim be cure or palliation. Surgical excision has not been performed for several reasons, the assumed risk of implantation being the strongest, and local intracavitary radiotherapy has not yet been applied although it is a very appealing method because patients do not have to be hospitalized and the inconvenience is very slight.

A small number of cases with involvement of the anus were treated by radioactive implant in the hope of preserving the sphincter mechanism. This, however, proved to be a mistake since in most of these cases radio necrosis and/or ulceration led to a permanent colostomy with or without excision of the rectum. The newer techniques of cryosurgery and laser excision have not been used chiefly because the procedures are more time-consuming and can only be applied in a few selected cases. Maybe the new Nd-Yag laser will prove to be a satisfactory tool.

The fulguration apparatus is relatively simple and consists of a 15 cm bevelended non-conductive tube, 3 cm in diameter, with built-in suction and an adaptable handle. The energy source is a high frequency (300,000 Hz) electrosurgical unit supplying 2.5 A at a voltage of 100-1000 V. The current is adjusted so that short sparks develop which heat the tissue to such a degree that evaporation of all the elements occurs without any charring. With this technique it is possible to recognize all the structures in the treated area: mucosa, submucosa, circular and longitudinal muscle, perirectal fat, tumour strands and blood vessels. The depth of infiltration can be quite accurately defined. Depending on the blood supply, which acts as a cooling system, a 2-3 mm layer of surrounding tissue reaches a temperature that leads to necrosis.

It is advisable to start destruction in the normal surrounding mucosa, 5 mm from the edge of the tumour and to proceed towards the centre. This ensures a sufficiently wide safety margin. In the centre where invasion is deepest, fulguration should be continued until all tumour strands have disappeared and only normal-looking tissue remains.

In some cases, notwithstanding conscientious preoperative assessment of the depth of infiltration, it appears during the procedure that tumour strands penetrate into the outer longitudinal muscular layer or the perirectal tissues. If the patient's general condition permits an abdomino-perineal excision, the procedure should be stopped and the Miles operation should be performed a few weeks later.

The necrotic tissue is sloughed off within 15 days. When arteries more than ± 1 mm in diameter have been exposed at the demarcation zone, haemorrhage may occur between the 8th and 15th day after treatment. This can always be stopped by electrocoagulation (not fulguration) using the same apparatus.

During healing of the burn retraction occurs, chiefly when the muscular wall has been destroyed (Dukes'B cases). If the burn covers less than one-half the circumference of the bowel a distinct stricture will develop. This, however, usually causes very little trouble. When scarring takes place over a larger part of the circumference, problems are likely to arise.

When an adenocarcinoma which has its point of origin in the rectal mucosa grows down into the anal canal and encroaches upon the squamous cell epithelium or involves the sphincter, this is a sign that it has such invasive properties that local treatment should not be tried. Moreover at this level destruction of one-half of the circumference and the ensuing scar formation will cause much greater functional problems than destruction of a similar proportion of the rectal wall at a somewhat higher level. On the basis of these data and considerations the following rules for the selection of cases suitable for 'curative' electrofulguration can be formulated:

1. Limited invasion of rectal wall, no deeper than the inner (circular) muscular layer.
2. Tumour involves no more than 1/3 of the circumference.
3. No invasion of the anal canal.
4. Upper limit below the assumed level of the peritoneal reflection.
5. No suspect nodes in the presacral space.

The composition of the group of patients with respect to criteria 2 and 3 is shown in tables 1 and 2.

In a number of cases one or more of these rules were not followed. Reasons for transgression were:

1. Old age and poor general condition precluding abdomino-perineal excision.
2. Patient's firm decision not to have a colostomy.
3. Surgeon's reluctance to make a permanent colostomy in a young patient.

When judging the results of electrofulguration in 60 cases, it is essential to divide the series into two groups: 43 cases in which the rules for selection were followed and 17 in which there was a transgression of these rules. It should be noted that when there is no evidence of disease 2 years after the first treatment, it is very unusual for a recurrence to develop at a later date. Although the tumour did not quite satisfy the criteria, a number of patients were selected for local treatment because they were old or generally unfit; as a result the number of loco-regional recurrences needing treatment was rather high.

Table 1. Cancer of the rectum. Curative Electrofulguration. Distance between lower tumour margin and dentate line; 60 patients.

cm	0-1	2-3	4-5	6-7	8-9	10-11	12-13
Number	7	20	18	6	4	4	1

Table 2. Cancer of the rectum. Curative Electrofulguration. Part of the circumference involved.

Involved	$\frac{1}{12}$	$\frac{2}{12}$	$\frac{3}{12}$	$\frac{4}{12}$	$\frac{5}{12}$	$\frac{6}{12}$	$\frac{12}{12}$	not recorded
Number	3	11	16	11	6	5	2	6

This means an additional burden, which by the way was never regarded as being so great that no further treatment could be given, but resulted in eventual cure in 3 of the 11 cases. The results are given in table 3.

One may conclude from the figures that with electrofulguration ± 65% of the selected patients with rectal carcinoma survived without evidence of disease and that out of a group of 11 patients (± 20%) with local recurrence only 4 could not be cured locally after secondary treatment. These results are comparable to those of local intracavitary radiotherapy. Complications occurred in 16 out of 60 patients and consisted mainly of haemorrhage during the second post-treatment week (Table 4). Whenever possible recurrence should be treated by abdomino-perineal excision. A second course of fulgura-

Table 3. Cancer of the rectum. Curative Electrofulguration. Results 2 years after first treatment.

		N.E.D. 5 yrs.	Local residual tumour	Distant spread and other causes of death
Selection rules followed 43	No loco-regional recurrence	31	25	6
	Local recurrence	6 treated	2	1	3
	Presacral nodes involved	6 treated	4		2
Rules not followed 17	No local recurrence	8 treated	6		2
	Local recurrence	5 treated	1	3	1
	Pre-sacral nodes involved	0			
	Treatment modified 4 →Radical surgery	2		2
60			40	4	16

Table 4. Cancer of the rectum. Curative Electrofulguration. Complications.

	Bleeding	Stenosis	Incontinence	Miscellaneous	Death
Selection rules followed 43	12	1	–	1	–
Rules not followed 17	2	2	–	2	–

tion may have some temporary palliative effect but will rarely lead to a local cure. Electrofulguration for palliation only is a completely different aspect which should not be discussed in this context.

Suffice it to list the three main indications:

1. Local (cicatricial) recurrence in the perineum after abdomino-perineal excision.
2. Prevention of symptoms and complaints caused by a local tumour in patients with incurable disseminated disease; often combined with radio-therapy.
3. Destruction of a sufficiently large portion of a locally inoperable obstruc-ting tumour to allow passage of faeces in an attempt to avoid a colostomy.

REFERENCES

1. Papillon J: Place de la Radiothérapie intracavitaire à visée curative dans le traitement du cancer du rectum. *Nouv Presse Méd* 6, 250, 1977.
2. Papillon J: Intracavitary irradiation of early rectal cancer for cure. *Cancer* 36: 696, 1975.
3. Mason AY: Transsphincteric approach to rectal lesions. *Surg Annu* 9: 171, 1977.
4. Strauss AA: Immunologic resistance to carcinoma produced by electrocoagulation. Based on fifty-seven years of experimental and clinical results. C.C. Thomas, Springfield 1969.
5. Wassink WF: The curative treatment of carcinoma recti by means of electrocoagulation and radium. *Arch Chir Neerl.* 8: 313, 1956.
6. Klok PAA: Onderzoek van de waarde van electrocoagulatie als behandeling van het adeno-carcinoma recti. Acad proefschrift Amsterdam 1963.
7. Crile Jr G, Turnbull Jr RB: The role of electrocoagulation in the treatment of carcinoma of the rectum. *Surg Gynecol Obstet* 135: 391, 1972.
8. Verschueren RJ. Koudstaal J and Oldhoff J: Surgery with the CO_2 laser. *Panminerva Med* 17: 241, 1975.
9. Kratzer GL and Onsanit T: Fulguration of selected cancers of the rectum. *Diss;ses Colon Rectum* 14: 431, 1972.
10. Crile G and Turnbull Jr RB: The role of electrocoagulation in the treatment of carcinoma of the rectum. *Surg Gynecol Obstet* 135: 391, 1972.
11. Wilson E: Local treatment of cancer of the rectum. *Diseases Colon Rectum* 16: 194, 1973.
12. Lacour J. Prade M. Lasser P and Apelbaum H: La place de l'électrocoagulation dans le traitement de cancers du rectum. *Bull Cancer* 63: 191, 1976.
13. Lock MR et al : The treatment of early colorectal cancer by local excision. *Brit J Surg* 65, 346, 1978.
14. Zinkin LD, Katz LD, Rosin JD: A method of palliation for obstructive carcinoma of the rectum. *Surg Gyn Obst* 148, 427, 1979.
15. Sischy B. Remington JH and Sobel SH: Treatment of rectal carcinomas by means of endocavity irradiation. *Cancer* 42, 1073, 1978.
16. Lamarque R and Gros C: La Radiothérapie de contact des cancers du rectum. *J Radiol Electrol* 27, 333, 1946.
17. Ager P, Samala E, Bosworth J, Rubin M and Ghosseris NA: The conservative management of anorectal cancer by radiotherapy. *Am J Surg* 137-338, 1979.

21. THE EXTENT OF THE RESECTION

K. WELVAART

INTRODUCTION

The first surgical treatment of an obstructing carcinoma of the rectum was described by Pillore in 1776; therapy consisted of a caecostomy. The patient survived one month (Amussat, 1839). In 1826 Lisfranc performed a resection of the rectum, leaving the patient with a perineal colostomy. Primary resection and anastomosis of the colon was reported by Reybard in 1833; his patient survived 1 year (8). One of the first large series of patients with a colon tumor was recorded in 1892 by Oscar Block (2), a Danish surgeon. He reported 138 cases of carcinoma of the colon. Only 30 of these tumors were treated by local excision and anastomosis. Mortality was as high as 50%. Unfortunately survival rates are unknown.

Primary *resection* of the colon was accompanied by high morbidity and mortality, until in the early 1900's the aseptic technique of anastomosis was developed. Better support of blood volume, use of intestinal intubation, preoperative mechanical cleansing of the bowel and antibiotic therapy have further reduced surgical mortality to the present-day levels. However, chances of survival remained poor.

Improvement of survival rates is related to an understanding of the biology of a malignant tumor, with particular reference to the potency of dissemination, local spread and recurrence. Based on these characteristics, the principles of the surgical technique have been developed.

These principles demand that cancer of the colon and rectum should be treated by a *wide* resection of the tumor, including predictable areas of vascular and lymphatic drainage. Reconstruction and restoration of normal colonic function is integral to the surgical procedure.

Over the past two decades the cure rate has not altered significantly. Many reports, from many institutes, describing retrospective analyses of their patients yield essentially the same figures for survival. Therapy as a rule consisted of en-bloc removal of the tumor in a segment of the colon with its mesentery containing possibly affected lymph nodes. Even super-radical and extended types of resection with removal of adjacent organs as a routine procedure, such as removal of the spleen and tail of the pancreas for left colon carcinomas (5, 6), or total colectomy for any tumor located in the splenic flexure (4) did not significantly improve the results (fig. 1).

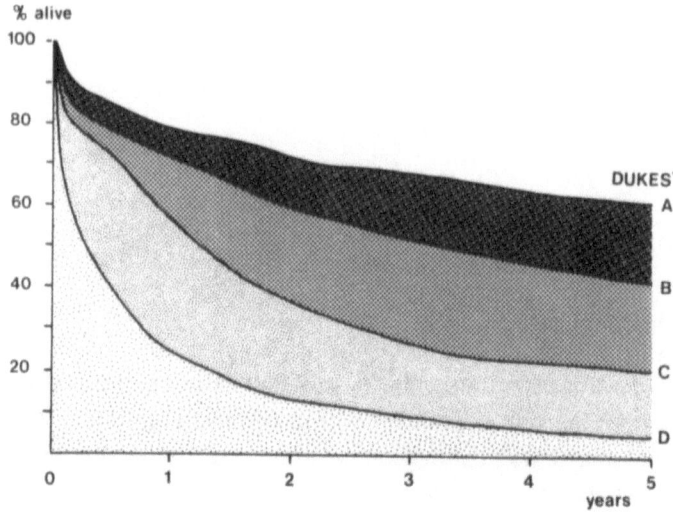

Fig. 1. Five-year survival based on Dukes classification.

THE EXTENT OF THE RESECTION

When I discuss the extent of the resection, I want to try to determine the *optimum* amount of tissue to be removed, based on scientific grouds and taking into account the biology of the cancerous process. The tumor spreads lymphogenically as well as haematogenically; haematogenic dissemination is directed towards the portal vein; lymphogenic spread follows the course of the main arteries (fig. 2a) and occurs in the lymph nodes situated in the segment of the affected colon (9).

The *paracolic* group of lymph nodes along the marginal vascular arcades are by far the most important and numerous filters. Collecting lymphatic trunks extend from these nodes to the *intermediate* group of nodes, situated in the mid-portion of the mesentery near the colic vessels.

Each intermediate node receives several collecting trunks from the *regional group of paracolic nodes.*

The intermediate nodes drain into the *central or principal* nodes at the base of the mesentery (fig. 2). Although this pattern of lymph node metastases usually progresses in an orderly fashion, metastases sometimes skip the para-colic or intermediate nodes and directly involve the central nodes. This is estimated to occur in about 12% of the cases, mainly when the tumor is located in the lower left colon.

Fig. 3 is reproduced from Haagensen's book *The Lymphatics in Cancer.* It shows the actual distribution of lymph node metastases from colorectal

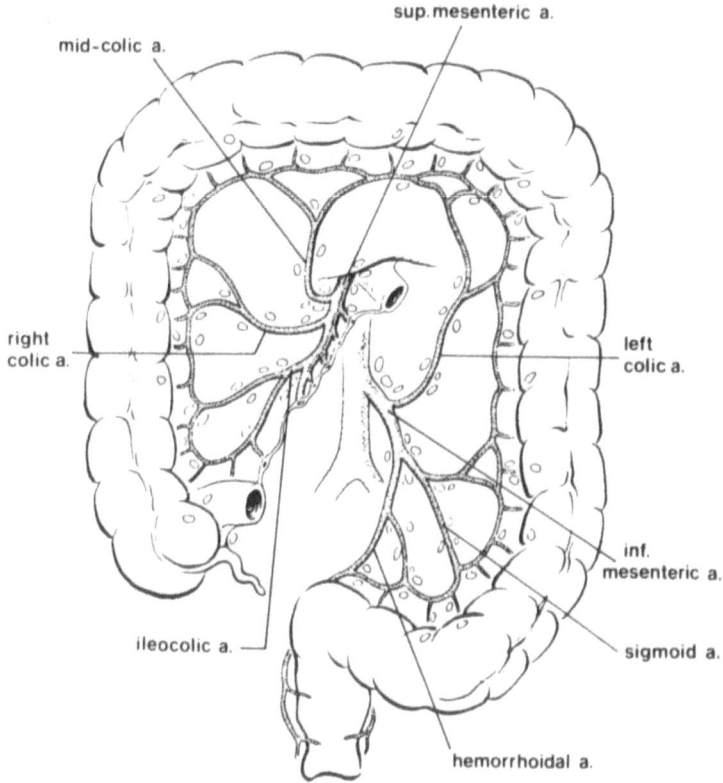

Fig. 2a. Arterial blood supply to colon and rectum.

cancer, according to the localisation of the tumor. When we define the extent of the resection, we assume that the rationale of our definition is the probability that tumor cells have only involved *specific* lymph nodes.

Thus the extent should be calculated to the limitations of the mesentery, noticing that enough healthy bowel on either side of the tumor will be removed automatically.

The extent of the resection for tumors located in the *caecum and ascending colon* is shown in fig. 4. The part of the mesentery to be resected should contain the ileocolic artery, right colic artery and right branch of the midcolic artery.

According to Haagensen's table (fig. 3), which shows that no lymph node metastases will be found around the mid-colic artery, one wonders why one still has to include the right branch of this artery in the resection. The reason is that there may be an anatomical variation in the arterial blood supply to the right colon; the mid-colic branch is absent in 12% of the cases. Therefore, in order to stay on the safe side, it is advisable to include the hepatic flexure in the

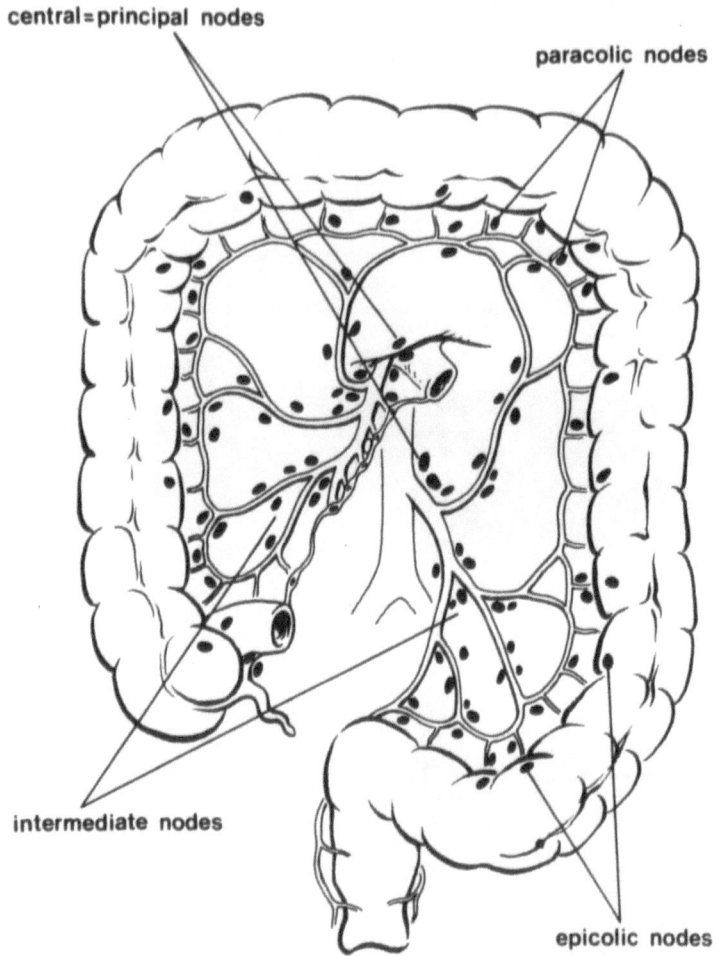

central=principal nodes

paracolic nodes

intermediate nodes

epicolic nodes

Fig. 2b. The lymph nodes of the large intestine.

resection. There is no argument for minimizing the resection; the anastomosis between the ileum and the remaining transverse colon is a relatively simple operation and the loss of the ascending colon has no influence on the patient's bowel function.

Tumors located in the *hepatic flexure* (fig. 5) tend to send cells to lymph nodes along the mid-colic, right colic and ileocolic artery. For this reason *all* three vessels should be included in the resected mesentery; continuity is subsequently restored by an end-to-end anastomosis between the ileum and the remaining transverse colon.

For any tumor in the *transverse colon* (fig. 6) the specimen should contain the mid-colic and left colic artery. As you may observe in Haagensen's table

Site of primary carcinoma	Regional lymphatic system	Per cent of metastases in node groups		
		paracolic	intermediate	central
Cecum and ascending colon	Right colic	10%	10%	5%
	Ileocolic	70%	40%	25%
Hepatic flexure and proximal transverse colon	Mid colic	70%	-	-
	Right colic	20%	5%	20%
	Ileocolic	15%	-	5%
Mid and distal transverse colon	Mid colic	79%	32%	21%
	Left colic	11%	5,3%	-
Splenic flexure	Mid colic	56%	19%	6%
	Left colic	31%	19%	-
Descending colon	Mid colic	10%	5%	-
	Left colic	100%	25%	5%

		para-colic or para-rectal	intermediate		
			distal	proximal	central
Sigmoid colon	Inferior mesenteric	94%	32%	9,1%	7,8%
Rectosigmoid and rectum	Inferior mesenteric	96%	35%	19%	7,8%

Fig. 3. Distribution of lymph node metastases according to region. Cleared specimens.

(fig. 3), the central nodes located at the base of the left colic artery are *never* involved. Thus ligation of this artery with preservation of the inferior mesenteric artery is fully justified in a curative resection. Of course, the greater omentum with the gastroepiploic nodes should also be included in the resection.

Tumors in the *splenic flexure* are not always removed in the same fashion. Fig. 7 shows sacrifice of both branches of the mid-colic artery; the inferior mesenteric artery is saved and only the left colic artery is ligated at its origin. In fig. 8 the right branch of the mid-colic artery is spared. The left colic artery is handled in the same way as in the previous picture.

The decision to either sacrifice or save the right branch of the mid-colic artery depends mainly on appreciation of the localisation of the tumor: is it closer to the transverse side or to the side of the descending colon?

In fig. 9, the extent of the resection is increased by sacrificing the inferior mesenteric artery. Subsequently the entire left colon must be removed.

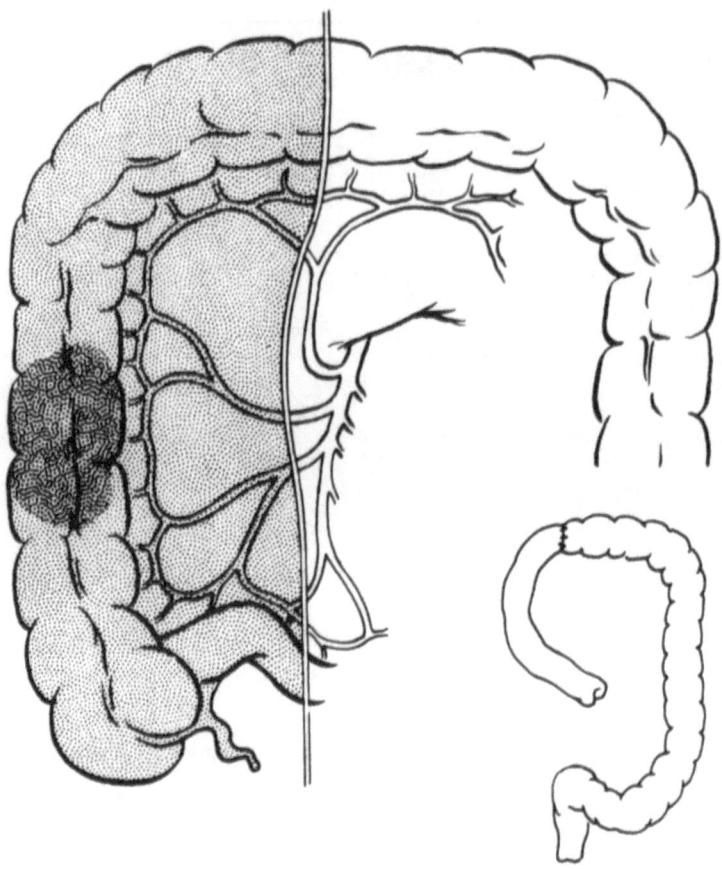

Fig. 4. The extent of the resection for tumors in the caecum and ascending colon. The mesentery includes the ileocolic, right colic and right branch of the mid-colic artery.

Many reports in literature indicate a preference for ligation of the inferior mesenteric artery at its origin in the treatment of tumors in the splenic flexure. However, in Haagensen's table (fig. 3), you can see that the central nodes are never involved and thus sacrifice of the inferior mesenteric artery is, in my opinion, unnecessary.

Tumors in the *descending colon* (fig. 10) spread almost exclusively along the left colic artery. However when central blockage of lymph occurs, retrograde dissemination may occur as far as the left branch of the mid-colic artery. Therefore, the left branch of the mid-colic artery must be included in the resection. In 5% of cases the central nodes around the inferior mesenteric artery are involved. This fact explains the rationale for sacrifice of the inferior mesenteric artery by ligation at the base above the aorta.

In spite of this theoretical rationale I disagree with this procedure. True,

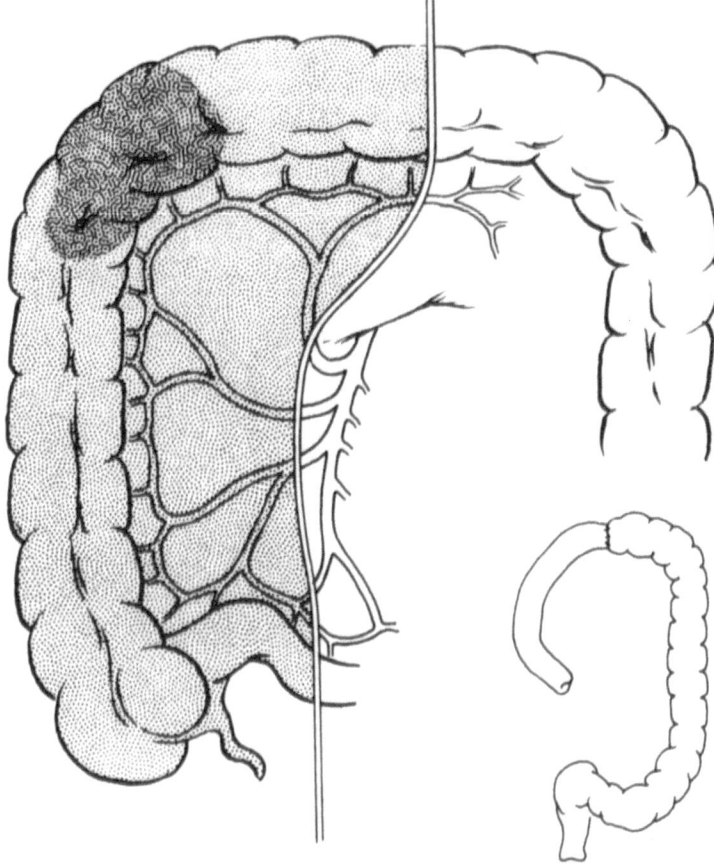

Fig. 5. The extent of the resection for tumors in the hepatic flexure. The mesentery includes the ileocolic, right colic and mid-colic arteries.

there is a 5% chance of nodal involvement, but I doubt very much whether an attempt to remove these central nodes provides an increase in survival. In spite of an adequate resection, survival for patients with Dukes C tumors usually does not exceed 30%. We must keep the biology of the tumor in mind: the greater the increase in lymphogenic dissemination, the greater the likelihood of haematogenic dessemination. If venous involvement at the site of the primary growth becomes a fact, more than 90% of the patients die within 5 years. I consider removal of the central nodes in an effort to prolong the patient's life to be comparable to an extended radical mastectomy in an effort to cure breast cancer already metastasized to the apical nodes. We know from several trials in the past that this procedure does not lead to better therapeutic results. When a tumor which is capable of *both* lymphogenic and haematogenic dissemination has spread to the apical nodes then haematogenic dis-

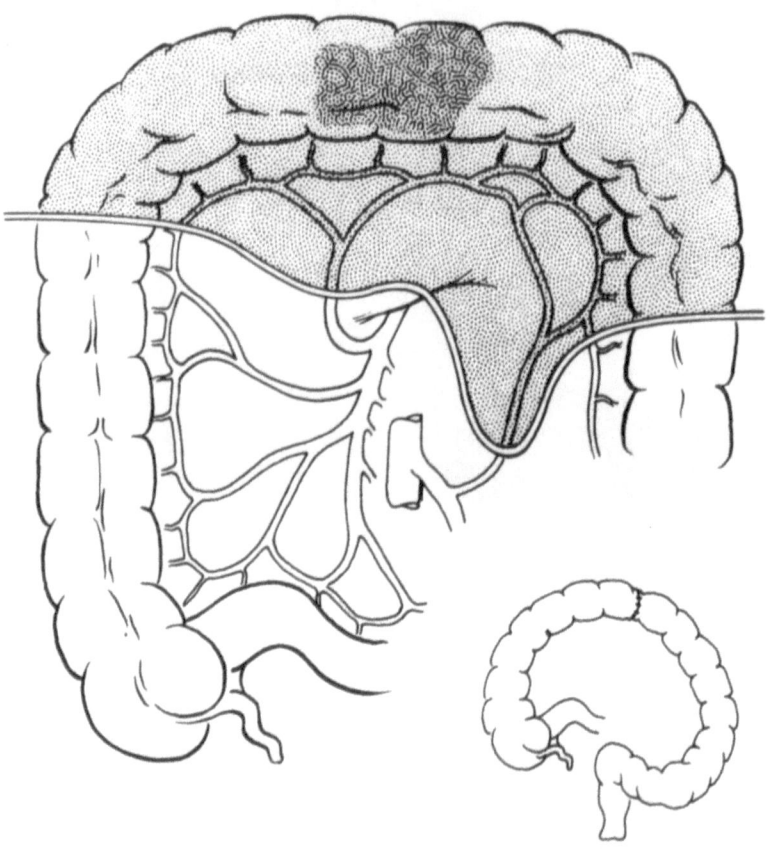

Fig. 6. The extent of the resection for tumors in the transverse colon. The mesentery includes the mid colic and left colic arteries.

semination must have already taken place, resulting in a very poor chance of survival. Comparable tumors with a very poor prognosis when extensive lymphogenic dissemination has become a fact are, as I already have mentioned, breast cancer but also malignant melanoma, oesophageal cancer, pancreatic cancer and many other malignances. The assumption that in colorectal cancer the biological behavior of the tumor would differ from that of these other tumors and that removal of the apex (the central nodes) therefore makes sense is in my opinion self-deception.

   Why do I make such a fuss about it? Removal of the entire left colon demands a more extensive operation with the chance of a difficult anastomosis, the need for a temporary colostomy and, especially in the elderly patient, an increased risk of mortality and morbidity due, for instance, to a leaking anastomosis. Occasionally, the primary anastomosis cannot even be performed because of an inadequate colonic length. Consequently anasto-

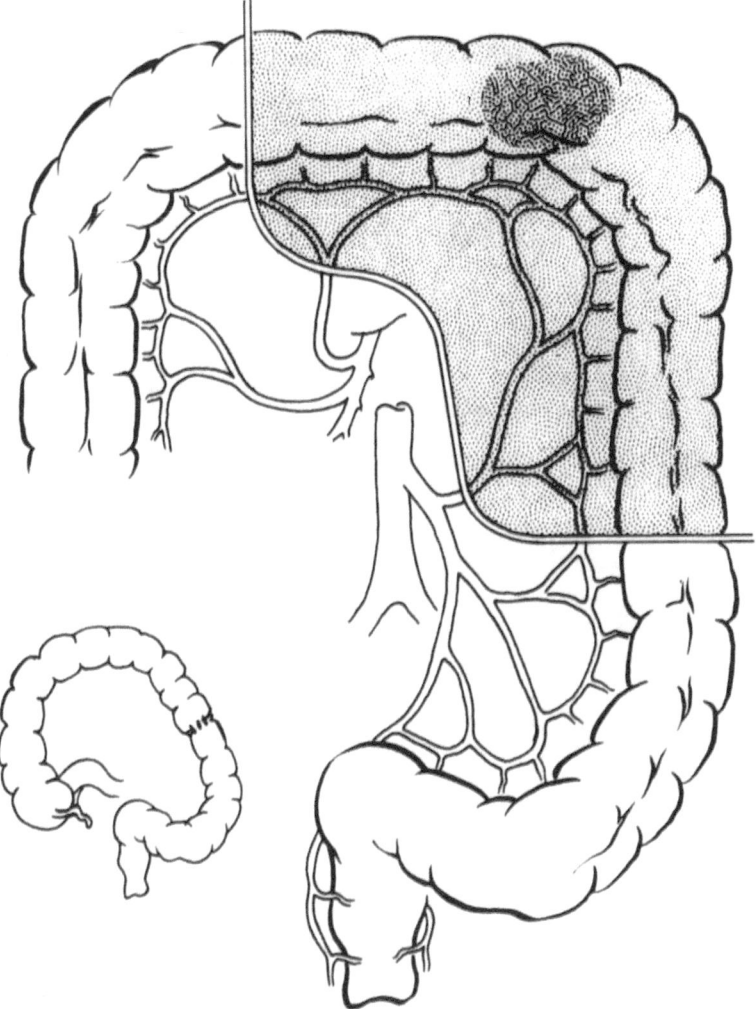

Fig. 7. The extent of the resection for tumors in the splenic flexure. Sacrifice of both branches of the mid-colic artery.

motic tension prompts the decision for a colonic stoma. Finally one should realize that loss of the left colon affects the consistency and frequency of the normal stool. For this reason, I like to treat tumors located in the proximal part of the left colon in the same manner as tumors in the splenic flexure to save the inferior mesenteric artery.

Tumors in *the sigmoid* (fig. 11) spread to the central nodes along the inferior mesenteric artery in 7.8% of the cases. Retrograde spread towards the proximal part of the left colon along the left colic artery, or along the marginal artery, does not occur and removal of the left colic artery is not indicated in sigmoidal

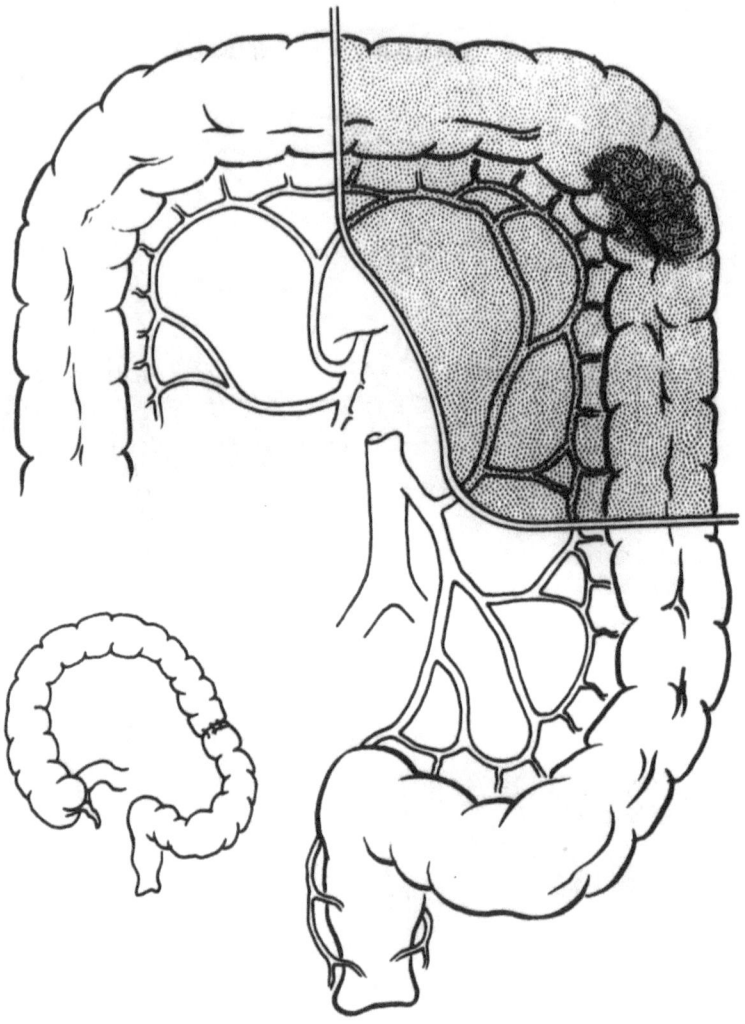

Fig. 8. The extent of the resection for tumors in the splenic flexure; the right branch of the mid-colic artery is spared.

cancer. For the same reason as I explained before, we preserve the inferior mesenteric artery and ligate the artery *below* the origin of the left colic artery. This type of resection is essentially the same when we deal with tumors in the rectosigmoid and an anterior resection is feasible with preservation of the anus.

When an *abdomino-perineal resection* (fig. 12) is carried out, the abdominal part of the resection implies removal of a segment of the large bowel after ligation of the inferior mesenteric artery below the orgin of the left colic artery. A permanent colostomy is created in the left lower quadrant of the

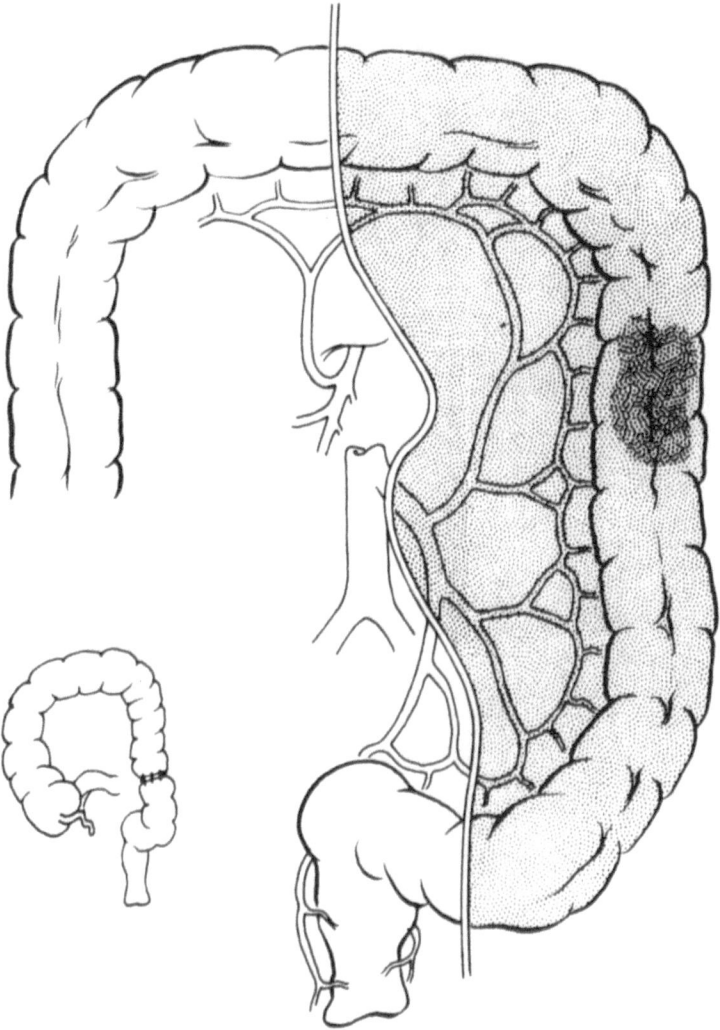

Fig. 9. The extent of the resection for tumors in the splenic flexure when the inferior mesenteric artery is ligated at its origin.

abdomen. The abdominal part of the resection as you will observe does not differ essentially from a sigmoid resection.

CONCLUSIONS

I have tried to outline the extent of the resection for colorectal cancers in different localisations of the large bowel. Lesser procedures are insufficient

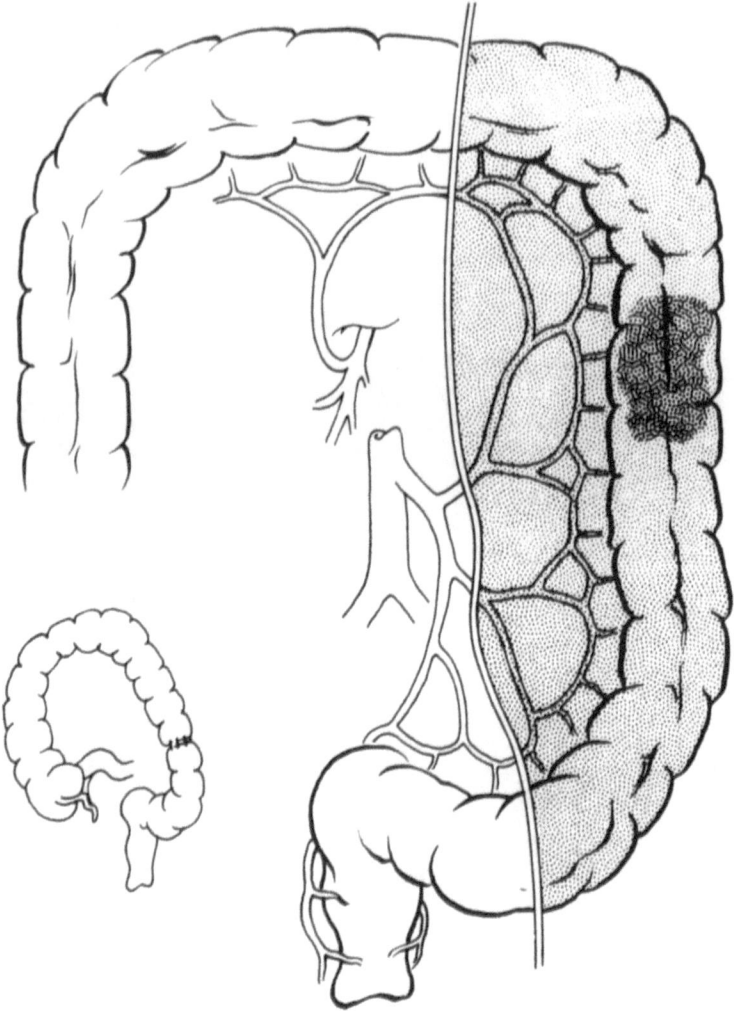

Fig. 10. The extent of the resection for tumors in the left colon with preservation of the inferior mesenteric artery.

efforts to control the disease and should not be considered acceptable in curative cancer surgery. Increasing the extent of the resection does not lead to better results and therefore should not be advocated. We must realize that, like many other cancers, colorectal carcinoma in many cases is not a localised disease that can be treated with local treatment. The significance of micrometastases in other organs is well understood. They are responsible for our final results. Therefore probably in the future others, rather than surgeons, will have to improve the survival rate for colorectal cancer.

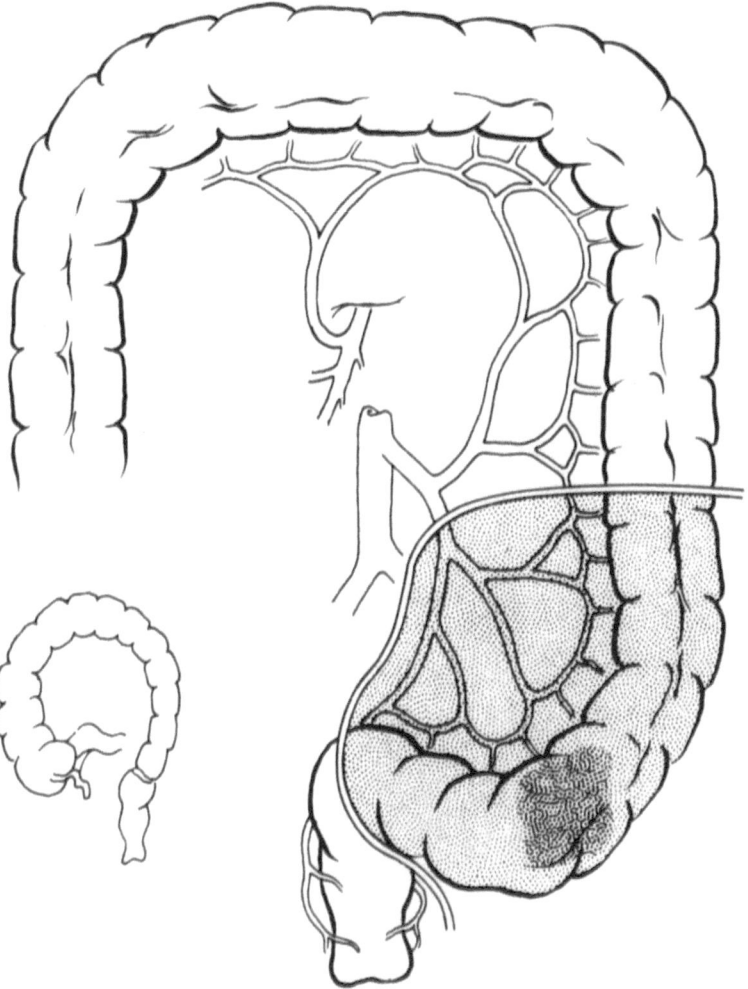

Fig. 11. The extent of the resection for sigmoid cancer. The mesentery includes the sigmoid arteries; both the inferior mesenteric artery and left colic artery are spared.

REFERENCES

1. Amussat JZ: Mémoire sur la possibilité d'établir un anus artificiel dans la région lombaire sans pénétrer dans le peritoine. Paris 1839.
2. Block O: Om extra-abdominal Behandlung vor cancer intestinales (rectum derfra und taget). *Nordiskt Medicinskt Arkiv*, N.F. 2, No. 1 and 2, 1892.
3. Haagensen CD, Feind CR, Herter FP, Slanetz CA and Weinberg JA: *The lymphatics in cancer*, W.B. Saunders Company, Philadelphia, 1972.
4. Husemann B, Löw R, Panhans W, Schellerer W and Schweiger M: Überlebenszeit und Lebensqualität beim operierten Dickdarm Karzinom. *Zbl Chirurgie*, 102, 1977.

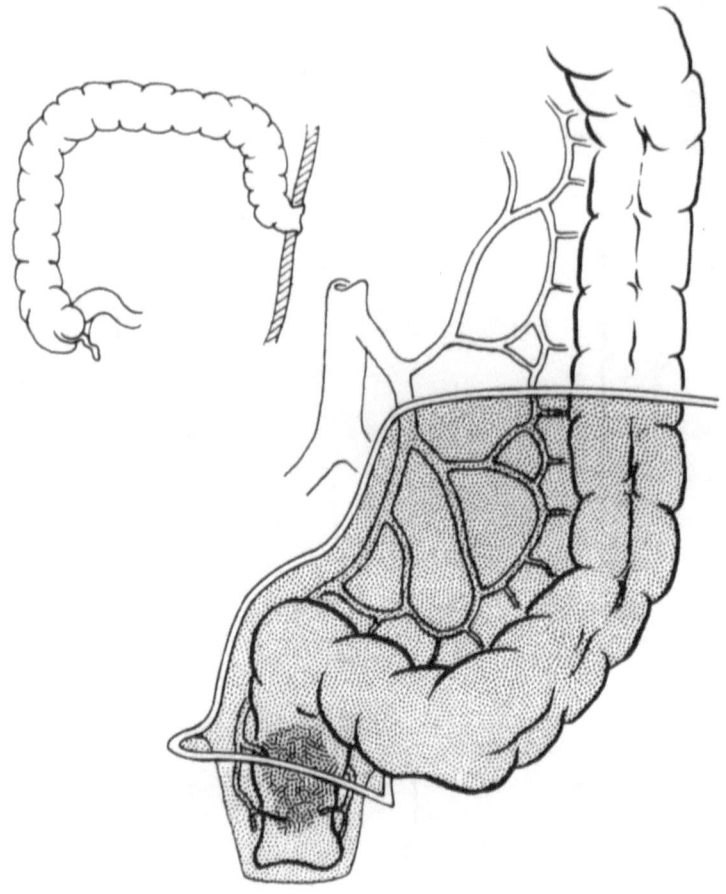

Fig. 12. Carcinoma of the lower rectum demanding an abdominoperineal resection. Ligation of the inferior mesenteric artery below the left colic artery; removal of the rectum; permanent colostomy.

5. Jünemann A, Sailer R and Derra E: Probleme der ein- oder mehrzeitigen Operationsverfahren am linken Colonabschnitt beim Dickdarm Karzinom. *Langenbecks Arch Chir* 340, 1975.
6. Khafagy MM and Stearns MW: Carcinoma of the splenic flexure. *Dis Colon Rect* 16: 504, 1973.
7. Lisfranc: Quoted in Kelsey, CB: *Diseases of rectum and anus.* Wood, New York 1882.
8. Reybard TF: Mémoire sur une tumeur cancéreuse affectant l'os iliaque du colon: ablation de la tumeur et de l'intestine; réunion directe et immédiate de deux bouts de cet organe; guérison. *Bull Acad Roy Méd* 9: 1031, 1943.
9. Rouviere H: *Anatomy of the human lymphatic system.* Edwards Brothers, Inc., Ann Arbor, Mich. 1938.

22. CANCER OF THE COLON [+] [*]

The Five- and Ten- Year Survival Rates following Resection utilizing the Isolation Technique

RUPERT B. TURNBULL

Like all surgeons I feel a certain kinship to Lord Moynihan, through our late chief of surgery, Doctor Robert Dinsmore of The Cleveland Clinic Foundation. Dr. Dinsmore visited him at Leeds many years ago and came away with a wealth of knowledge and with a surgical philosophy that he passed on to us.

The title of my presentation would suggest that something new in cancer surgery has been brought forward. In truth, the idea that cancer could be spread by surgical manipulation is now more than 55 years old. What is new, is the presentation of clinical evidence that operative handling of a cancer-bearing organ (colon) may explain the continuing had constantly poor survival rates following resection.

HISTORICAL ASPECTS

In 1913 Tyzzer (1), working in the laboratory of the Cancer Commission at Harvard University, suggested that local trauma to cancers resulted in metastases. As an experimental model, he used Japanese waltzing mice and a spontaneously occurring cancer in that strain. The tumour was implanted in the chest wall. Digital trauma of these growing tumours produced extensive metastases as compared with control animals. Tyzzer concluded:

Do the procedures followed in the course of physical examinations or surgical operations increase or diminish the incidence of metastases?... every physician should realize the irreparable harm which may result from the manipulation of malignant tumours... I have repeatedly observed the palpation of the mass in question in repeated physical examinations, the violent scrubbing often employed in preparing the field of operation. It is almost identical with that which I have employed for the experimental production of metastases. It would be of advantage to the patient if each questionable tumour of the breast, for example, could be regarded as highly explosive, the least manipulation of which should be absolutely avoided both prior to and during the operation. It is not improbable that by this means metastasis and extension beyond the field of operation could be prevented and the percentage of cases cured by operation increased.

In 1952 Barnes (2) described a 'physiologic' method for resecting the right side of the colon for cancer. He advocated ligation of the vascular pedicles and

[+] Moynihan Lecture delivered at the Royal College of surgeons on 23rd June 1969.

[*] Reprinted from *Annals of the Royal College of Surgeons of England* 46: 243-250, May 1970.

196

division of the bowel before handling the cancer-bearing sergment to prevent traumatic spread of cancer through the veins and lymphatics.

In 1954 Cole, Packard and Southwick reported finding cancer cells in the portal venous blood of a perfused resected cancer-bearing segment of human colon. This observation gave rise to their suggestion that the mesenteric veins draining the cancer-bearing sergment should be ligated before significant operative manipulation.

In 1955 Dr. Edwin Fisher and I (4) reported cancer cells in the portal venous blood of 8 of 25 resected segments (for cancer) of colon, and suggested that the cells had been scattered by operative manipulation. We had previously been so interested in this problem and its possible significance that in 1953 I altered my standard method of resection of the colon to one wherein the cancer-bearing segment was not manipulated or handled in any manner until after the lymphovascular pedicles were ligated and the colon divided at the elected sites for resection (Fig. 1). To emphasize the objectives of this method of resection, the name *No-Touch Isolation* was adopted. It was now found necessary to change time-honoured practices. For instance, a palpable abdominal mass discovered pre-operatively was immediately labelled with adhesive tape, DO NOT PALPATE, and the radiologist was asked to avoid manual (lead glove) manipulation during diagnostic barium enema. In the operating room, under anaesthesia, the skin of the abdomen was superficially lavaged, rather than prepared by 'scrubbing', and when the abdomen was opened members of the operating team were not allowed to palpate the tumour. The question of resectability was settled by determining whether or not the pancreas or duodenum was directly invaded ty tumour. Cancers of the right side of the colon deserve special mention since most of the locally incurable tumours occupy this segment. The method of resection of the right colon has been described elsewhere (5). The small intestine is delivered from

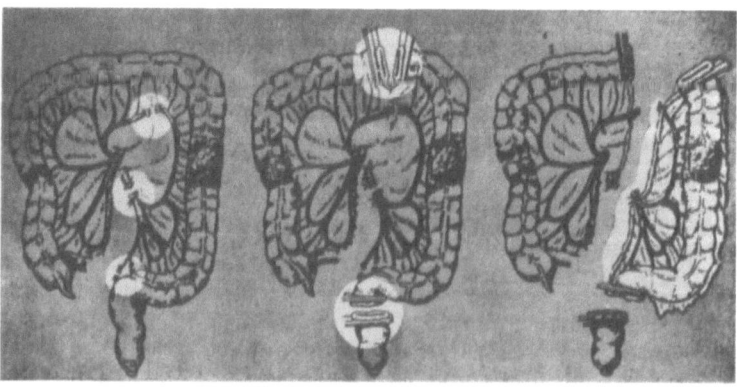

Fig. 1. No-touch isolation technique. Reproduced by permission from *Ann Surg* 166: 420, 1967.

the abdomen (wrapped in silastic drapes) to expose the duodeno-jejunal flexure (fig. 2a). The peritoneum over the terminal duodenum is devided and a finger inserted along the lateral duodenal border from the third portion to the pylorus of the stomach (fig. 2b). Any medial extension or fixation of tumour to the duodenum or pancreas is immediately discovered. At the same time the ileo-colic, right colic, and hepatic flexure mid-colic lymphovascular pedicles are ready for division and ligation as the first step in isolating the cancer-bearing segment (fig. 3).

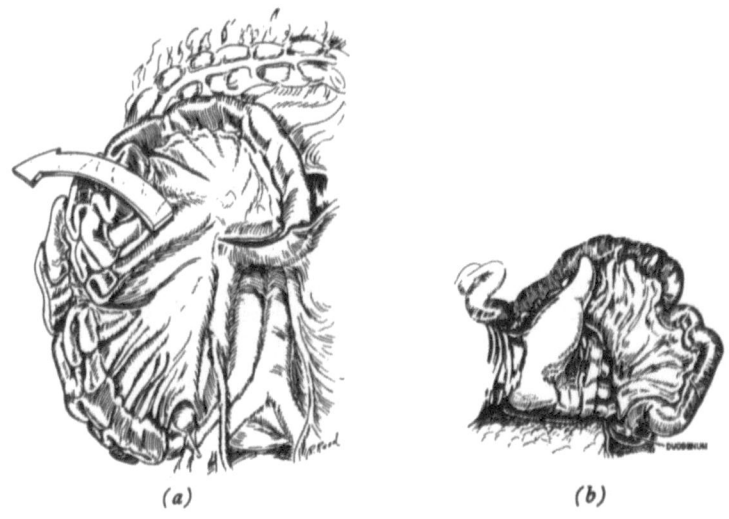

(a)   *(b)*

Fig. 2. (a) Right colectomy: isolation method. The small intestine is delivered out of the abdomen to expose the retroperitoneal duodenum. The overlying peritoneum is incised. (b) the lateral duodenal border is followed by the fingers of the surgeon who stands on the left side of the patient. (Figure reproduced from Maingot, R. (1969) *Abdominal Operation,* by permission of Appleton-Century-Crofts. Publishers)

Cancers of the left side of the colon present fewer problems in determining resectability. Any attached or invaded organ can be sacrificed with hope for cure as long as the inferior mesenteric artery, the inferior mesenteric vein at the ligament of Treitz and the splenic flexure division of the mid-colic artery are not directly invaded or fixed by tumour.

This report is based on a computer analysis of the results of the surgical treatment of 676 consecutive patients with cancer of the colon, admitted exclusively to the Colon and Rectal Surgery Department from 1950 to 1964. The number is increased by 12 over our original report (6) because of the inclusion of cases of a new departmental surgeon. The final survival rates are increased also because all rates previously reported (6) are here corrected for age. I am indebted to Mr. Kenneth Kyle (6) of Glasgow who, as a cancer

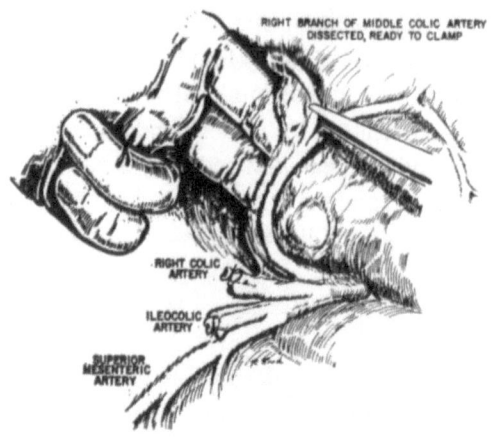

Fig. 3. The lymphovascular bundles are selectively ligated and divided. The small intestine has been returned to the abdomen for this manoevre. (Figure reproduced from Maingot, R (1969) *Abdominal Operation*, by permission of Appleton-Century-Crofts, publishers)

scholar in 1966, reviewed the records of and traced 2,225 patients with cancer of the colon and rectum seen at The Cleveland Clinic during those years. The statistical analysis of our data has been expertly handled by Dr. Frank R. Watson (6) and Dr. John Spratt (6) of the University of Missouri. Without my co-workers, this report would have been impossible.

Because this report is based on survival rates among patients with cancer of the colon treated exclusively at The Cleveland Clinic, the following patients were excluded from the study: patients with cancer in a polyp, with carcinoid tumours of the colon, malignancy other than adenocarcinoma, patients operated upon first at other hospitals, and patients not presenting themselves for treatment at The Cleveland Clinic Hospital. Of these, some were seen in consultation at other hospitals. A few declined to undergo surgical treatment or were operated on elsewhere.

Patients with cancer of the rectum and anus were excluded from the analysis because we have so far not been able to devise a method of rectal resection utilizing a *No-Touch Isolation* technique.

Cancers of the colon were defined as those tumours located at or above a point 14 cm above the anus, as recorded at the time of proctosigmoidoscopic examination.

PATHOLOGY

Adenocarcinoma of the colon was divided into four clinico-pathological stages or classes.

Stage A – tumour confined to the colon and its coats.

Stage B – tumour extension into pericolic fat. No metastses to lymph nodes or distant spread.

Stage C – tumour metastases to regional lymph nodes but no clinical or radiological evidence of distant spread.

Stage D – tumour metastases to liver, lung, bone, peritoneal seeding to tumour; irremovable because of parietal invasion; adjacent organ invasion.

The histological grade of each tumour was recorded but was not included in the clinico-pathological staging of this report.

Most of the tumours were reported as Grade 3 or moderately undifferentiated. After operation, the pathological specimens were immediately fixed in alcohol-formalin and later were opened through the base of the tumour, and the depth of fat invasion measured and recorded. The mesenteric fat was cut into 3-mm slices and the lymph nodes were dissected out and sectioned. No attempt was made to record the location of metastatic nodes in relation to the tumour.

The pathological reporting of specimens was consistently performed by the same three pathologists over the 15 years of this study, and I am indebted to John B. Hazard, M.D., Lawrence J. McCormack, M.D., and to William Hawk, M.D., for their diagnoses of the operative material.

CALCULATION OF SURVIVAL RATES

Survival rates were calculated by the actuarial method, and life tables were prepared to show correction for age. The median ages are recorded on each life table for each stage of tumour. The age-corrected survival rates were calculated in the usual manner utilizing the life tables (7) State of 'Ohio' white males 1959 through 1961.

RESULTS

Six-hundred-and-seventy-six consecutive patients with cancer of the colon were operated utilizing the *No-Touch Isolation* method when resection was indicated. The proportions of stages of cancer were as follows:

Stage of tumour	No. of patients	Percentage of patients
A	103	15.2
B	212	31.4
C	156	23.1
D	205	30.3
Total	676	

All of the patients in Classes A, B and C underwent resection with intent to cure the tumour but, in Class D, only half the patients had resection. The operability rate was 96%. The operative mortality was 2.2%. It is to be noted that almost one-third of the patients operated upon belonged to the incurable category. Of the 676 patients, 21 were lost to follow-up observation and were presumed to be dead of their disease.

CRUDE SURVIVAL RATES – OVERVIEW

The life table for Stages A, B, C and D cancers of the colon is shown in Figure 4 (a). The cumulative five-year survival rate (corrected for age) for the 676 patients was 61.3%. Of the total, 205 patients, or 30.4%, were judged to belong to Stage D. Nevertheless half of these underwent resection. I have already noted that all of the Stage A, B and C cancers were resected with intent to cure. The median age was 62 years.

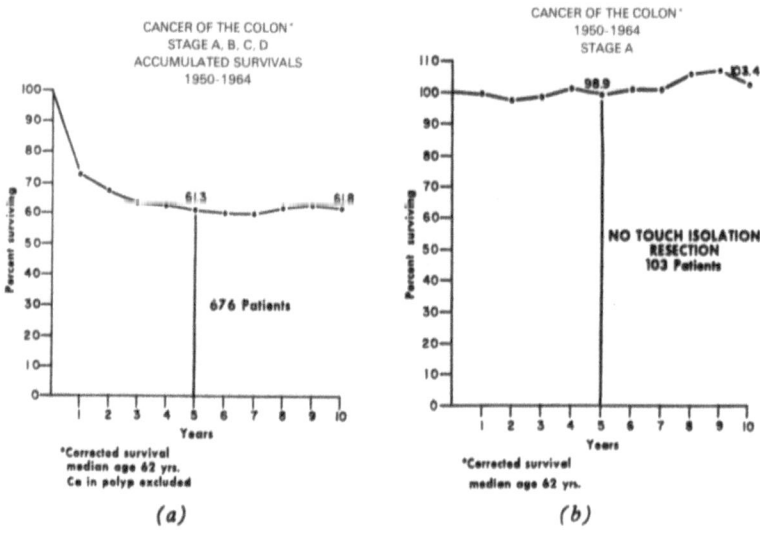

Figure 4.

SUVIVALS ACCORDING TO CLINICO-PATHOLOGICAL STAGES OF
CANCER

There were 103 patients with cancer of the colon who were judged to have Stage (Class) A cancers. All were resected with intent to cure. The age-corrected five-year survival rate was 98.9% (fig. 4b). The life table shows a false rise in the ten-year survival rate. This is due to the influence of correction for age on the diminishing number of patients after the fifth year. The median age was 62 years.

The life table for Stage (Class) B cancers of the colon is shown in fig. 5 (a). The five-year survival rate for 212 patients was 84.9%. The cancers invaded the pericolic fat for a distance of $\frac{1}{2}$ cm or less in 133 patients and over $\frac{1}{2}$ cm in depth in 79 patients. The median age was 63 years.

The life table for Stage (Class) C cancers of the colon is shown in fig. 5 (b). There were 156 patients who had one or more lymph nodes in the mesentery containing metastatic cancer. The five-year survival rate was 67.3%. The median age was 60 years.

It is in Stage C cancers of the colon that we have most improved our survival rates by the *No-Touch Isolation* method of resection (5). One might expect that cancers that have invaded the pericolic fat and spread to the regional lymph nodes are more easily spread through the veins and lymphatics by surgical manipulation than those tumours that are well localized.

The life table for Stage (Class) D cancers of the colon is shown in fig. 6 (a).

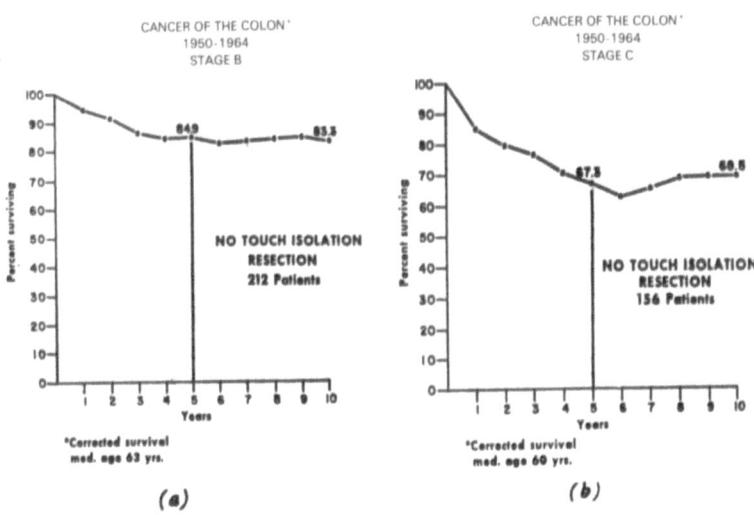

(a) *(b)*

Figure 5.

202

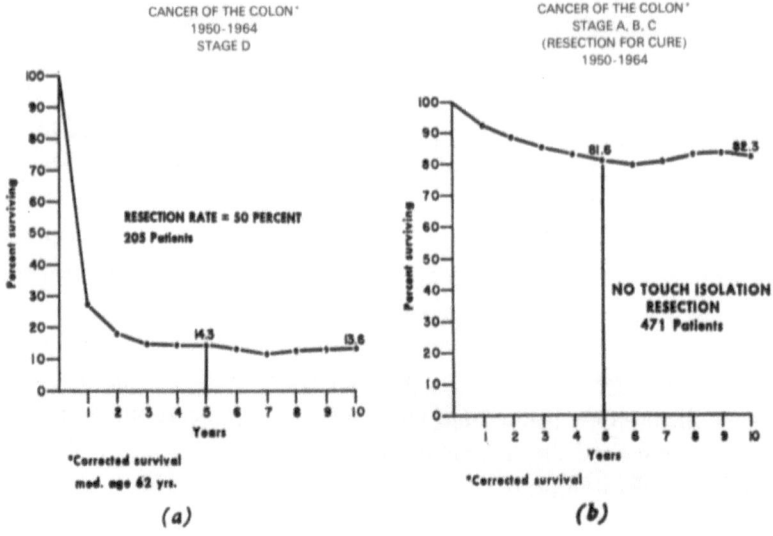

Figure 6.

There were 205 patients or 30.4% of the total number of patients that comprise this report. Half of these patients had resection on a palliative basis or with intent to cure whenever an adjacent organ was invaded by the tumour. The five-year survival was 14.3%. The median age was 62 years.

RESECTION FOR CURE

Fig. 6 (*b*) shows the five- and ten-year survival rates for 471 patients having resection for Stage A, B and C cancers of the colon. In each instance, a *No-Touch Isolation* method of resection was used. The five-year survival rate was 81.6%.

SUMMARY

It has been suggested that operative manipulation of a cancer-bearing segment of colon will increase the incidence of fatal metastasis. Since 1953, I have carefully avoided manipulation until the lymphovascular pedicles have been defined, ligated and divided, and the colon divided at the elected sites of resection.

We have modified the old pathological classification of cancer of the colon to include clinical components having to do with survival – thus a *clinico-pathological* classification: A, B, C and D.

The five- and ten-year survival rates following resection of colon cancer utilizing a *No-Touch Isolation* method are considerably increased (boubled), particularly Stage C cancers of the colon.

The *No-Touch Isolation* method of resection was utilized in patients with Stage A, B and C cancers of the colon from 1953 to 1964, with an age-corrected survival rate of 81.6%. The evidence presented in this retrospective analysis suggests that the greatly improved survival rates, particularly in Stage C cancers, are due to the *non-manipulative* method of resection. It is suggested that the heretofore conventional *manipulative* resection techniques for cancer of the colon be abandoned.

REFERENCES

1. Tyzzer EE: *J Med Res* 28: 309, 1913.
2. Barnes JP: *Surg Gynec Obstet* 94: 723, 1952.
3. Cole WH, Packard D and Southwick HW: *J Amer Med Ass* 155: 1549, 1954.
4. Fisher ER and Turnbull RB Jr: *Surg Gynecol Obstet* 100: 102, 1955.
5. Maingot R: *Abdominal operations* 2, pp 1660-1674, 1969. Appleton-Century-Crofts, Meredith Corporation, New York. Also Seventh edition, vol. 2, p 2165.
6. Turnbull RB Jr, Kyle K, Watson FR and Spratt J: *Ann Surg* 166: 420, 1967.
7. *Life Table for Ohio White Males* 1959-1961 No. 1252, vol. 2, no. 36, p. 500. U.S. Dept. of Health, Education and Welfare.

23. THE CURRENT STATUS OF THE PULL-THROUGH PROCEDURE FOR RECTAL CANCER

VICTOR W. FAZIO

For carcinomas located in the middle one-third of the rectum, i.e., from 7.0 to 12.0 cm from the anal verge, the surgeon may choose a variety of procedures to deal with the condition. These procedures include anterior resection of the rectum and sigmoid, in the case of sphincter-saving procedures, with a variety of anastomotic techniques; end-to-end; side to-end (Baker); abdomino-trans-sacral; transsphincteric (York Mason); end-to-end stapled anastomoses and pull-through colorectal and coloanal anastomoses. The Miles' abdominope-rineal resection and the extended Hartmann's operation with permanent colostomy also are used by surgeons for these med-rectal cancers in certain circumstances. While no single factor always influences the surgeon to pre-serve anorectal sphincters, factors which incline the surgeon to do so include in the patient, lack of obesity; a wide pelvis (females); no history of pelvic irradiation; 'reasonable' general good health (i.e. freedom from attendant serious cardiovascular disease); patients under the age of 70; good preopera-tive sphincter tone. Factors in the tumor itself favoring sphincter preservation include well-differentiated lesions histologically; mobile or slightly tethered lesions (lack of fixation); absence of distant metastases or peritoneal seeding. Finally, the surgeon's own experience and training will be a major factor not only in deciding whether or not to perform a sphincter-saving operation, but also in choosing which *type* of these operations to do.

Despite the wide variation in surgical procedures available for mid-rectal cancers, the differences occur in the techniques of restoring colonic continuity and the construction of the colostomy. For curative surgery, an 'adequate' cancer resection involves resection of the cancerbearing rectal segment with its adjacent fat, blood vessels, nerves and lymph nodes, including a margin of normal rectum of 5 cm or more below the level of the lesion, as measured in the freshly resected specimen. In addition, the colonic and rectal mesentery with its contained blood vessels and lymph nodes are resected en bloc. In the case of mid-rectal cancers, this involves resection of the rectum and *all* of the sigmoid colon with its mesentery, utilizing high ligation of the inferior mesen-teric artery and vein.

This paper deals with the Cleveland Clinic experience of anterior procto-sigmoidectomy with the pull-through method of anastomosis as described by Turnbull, Jr. and Cuthbertson (1) and, Cutait and Figlioni (2) in 1961. This experience was reviewed in 1978 by Kirwan et al. (3). Certain variations in the technique have been made by the author which are outlined below. In addition, comment is made on the status of the pull-through procedure in the light of the recent advances with end-to-end anastomotic stapling.

PATIENT MATERIAL AND METHODS

I. Technique of resection

A. Abdominal phase. A long midline incision is used. The sigmoid and descending colon are mobilized out of the left colic gutter and a retroperitoneal approach is made medially to the origin of the inferior mesenteric artery where it and its accompanying inferior mesenteric vein are doubly ligated and divided. The left ureter and gonadal veins are identified and preserved. The splenic flexure is mobilized off the pre-renal fascia and the omentum is detached from the left transverse colon and the superior aspect of the transverse mesocolon. The left colic artery is ligated and divided, preserving the arcade between the ascending and descending branch of the left colic artery (fig. 1). Further mobilization of the left colon is obtained by ligating the inferior mesenteric vein once again at the lower border of the pancreas. The colon is transected* at the junction of the descending colon and sigmoid, transecting the left colon mesentery inferior to the descending branch of the left colic artery. The distal colon is then irrigated with 150 cm^3 of 40% ethyl alcohol, this being collected into a plastic bag connected to a indwelling rectal catheter. Mobilization of the rectum is carried out to the level of the coccyx, superior surface of the levators and to the lower border of the prostate gland anteriorly. One then assesses if a sufficient distal margin of clearance from the cancer has been obtained, and if so, one proceeds with the pull-through operation. A heavy tape is tied below the cancer. The lower rectal segment is then irrigated with 10% providoneiodine (Betadine). The bowel is then transected 5 cm below the rectal cancer, and the specimen is examined. A tape is then tied around the end of the divided descending colon and attached to a metal ring which is then placed into the now empty presacral space, care being taken not to twist the colon.

B. Perineal phase. The patient has been previously placed in a semi-lithotomy position with head down tilt, using Lloyd-Davies stirrups. The rectal tube is

* With the Turnbull-Cutait procedure, the colon is not transected at this time, but is marked with a silk suture.

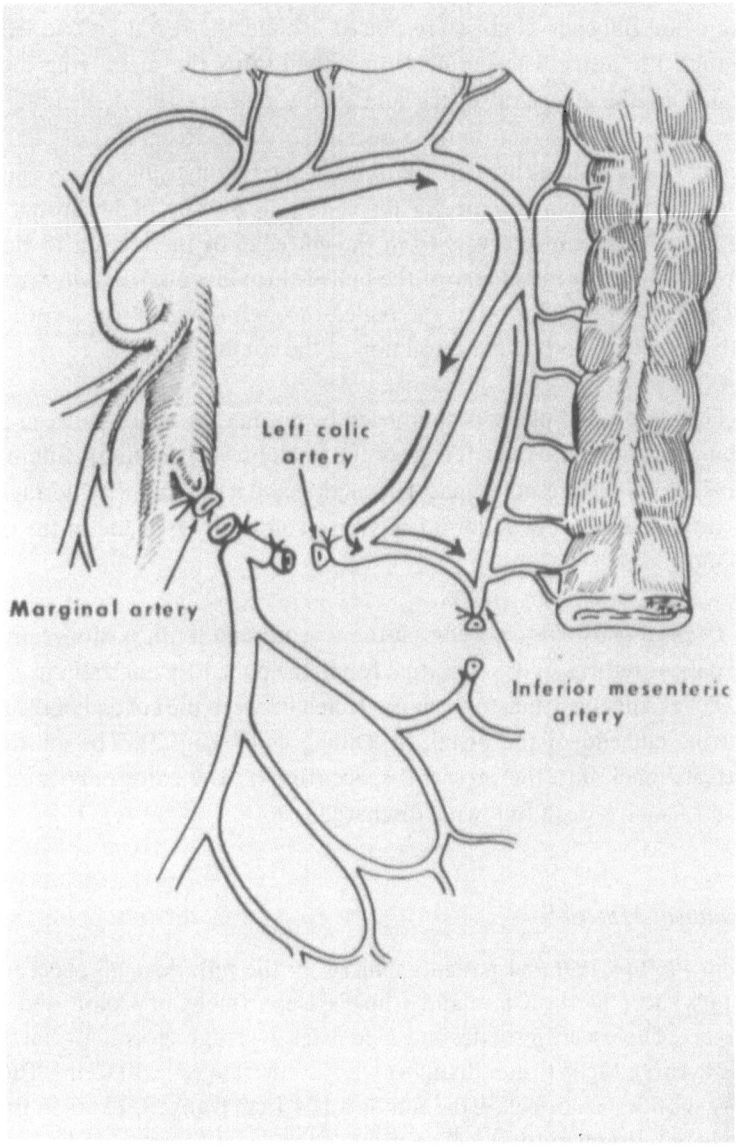

Fig. 1. Preservation of the arcade between ascending and descending branches of the left colic artery, and removal of all sigmoid colon ensures a good blood supply to the 'pulled-through' descending colon.

removed and the perineum is prepared and draped. Anorectal dilatation is done. The rectal cuff is mobilized digitally if complete mobilization has not been effected from the abdominal phase. The cut edge is seen more clearly with four large Allis clamps placed on the perianal skin for retraction. Stay sutures or Babcock clamps are placed around the rectal cuff to deliver it through the anus. The perineal operator grasps the metal ring and tape located in the presacral space and gently delivers the descending colon through the everted rectum for a distance of 10 to 15 cm (fig. 2). The blood supply of the pulled-through colon is checked by incising an appendix epiploica, and observing for arterial type bleeding. Sutures of 30 chromic catgut are placed at 1 cm intervals from the cut edge of the rectum to the seromuscular layer or mesentery of the pulled-through colon. A two inch gauge roll is then wrapped around the pulled-through segment and kept in place with rectal clips to prevent retraction of the colon.

C. The abdominal phase is completed by closing the space between the left colon mesentery and the left edge of the small bowel mesentery. Sump drains are placed in the presacral space for suction and irrigation with normal saline for a five-day period. A loop transverse colostomy is made in the midline wound.

D. *Delayed anastomosis.* Between the seventh and tenth postoperative day, the patient returns to the operating room, the pulled-through stump is amputated and a delayed anastomosis is effected between the cut end of the rectum and the cut end of the distal descending colon (fig. 3). The anastomosis 'retreats' back into the presacral space (fig. 4). The colostomy is closed at eight to twelve week following discharge.

II. Patient Material

From 1960 to 1976, 84 patients underwent the pull-through procedure for rectal cancer at the Cleveland Clinic's Department of Colon and Rectal Surgery. There were 59 males and 25 females. Average age was 57 years (range 35-74 years). Mean tumor diameter was 4.5 cm (range 1.3-10.0 cm). The mean margin of clearance below the tumor was 4.1 cm (range 1-12 cm in the fixed specimen). Preoperative measurement of the distance between the anal margin and the lower border of the cancer was 7.6 cm (range 5-12.5 cm). The staging of the tumors is outlined in table 1. All lesions save one were moderately well-differentiated.

RESULTS

Mortality. One patient is the series (1.2%) died, of a pulmonary embolus on the ninth postoperative day.

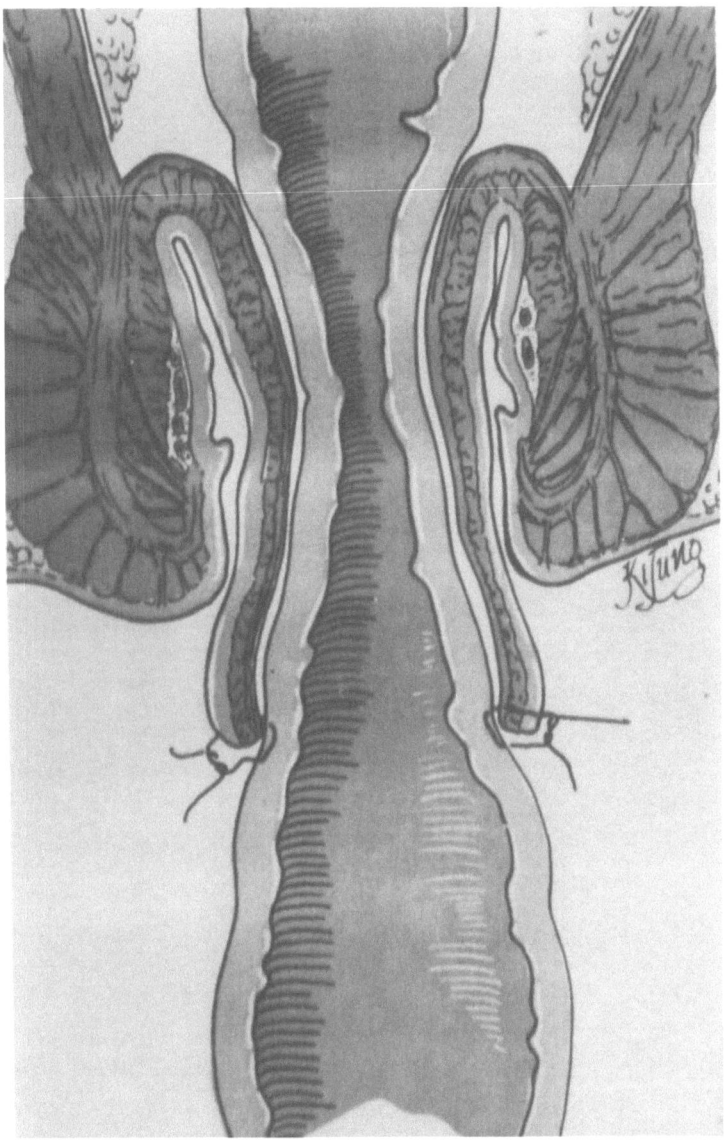

Fig. 2. The rectal cuff is everted through the anus and the descending colon is pulled through this everted cuff. Seromuscular 30 chromic sutures are placed between the rectal cuff and serosa of the pulled-through colon.

Morbididy. Table 2 lists the morbidity. The one patient who developed ischemic necrosis of the pulled-through segment had had a previous abdominal aortic graft replacement at which procedure, the inferior mesenteric artery had been ligated. Of the six patients with evidence of pelvic sepsis, all

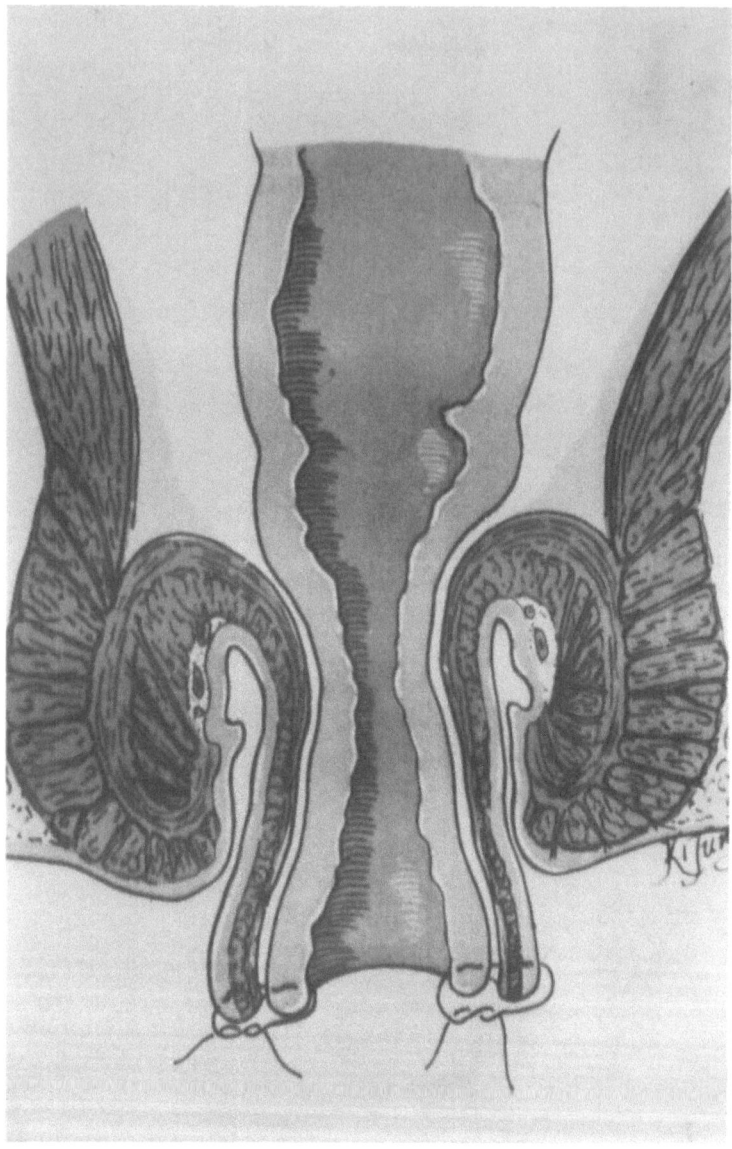

Fig. 3. The pulled-through stump is amputated between day 7 and day 10. The anastomosis is completed.

cases were minor requiring drainage in only two and no patient required a permanent colostomy on that score. Six of 59 male patients (10%) required transurethral prostatectomy for urinary retention.

Survival. All patients were followed up. Forty-seven patients had had their

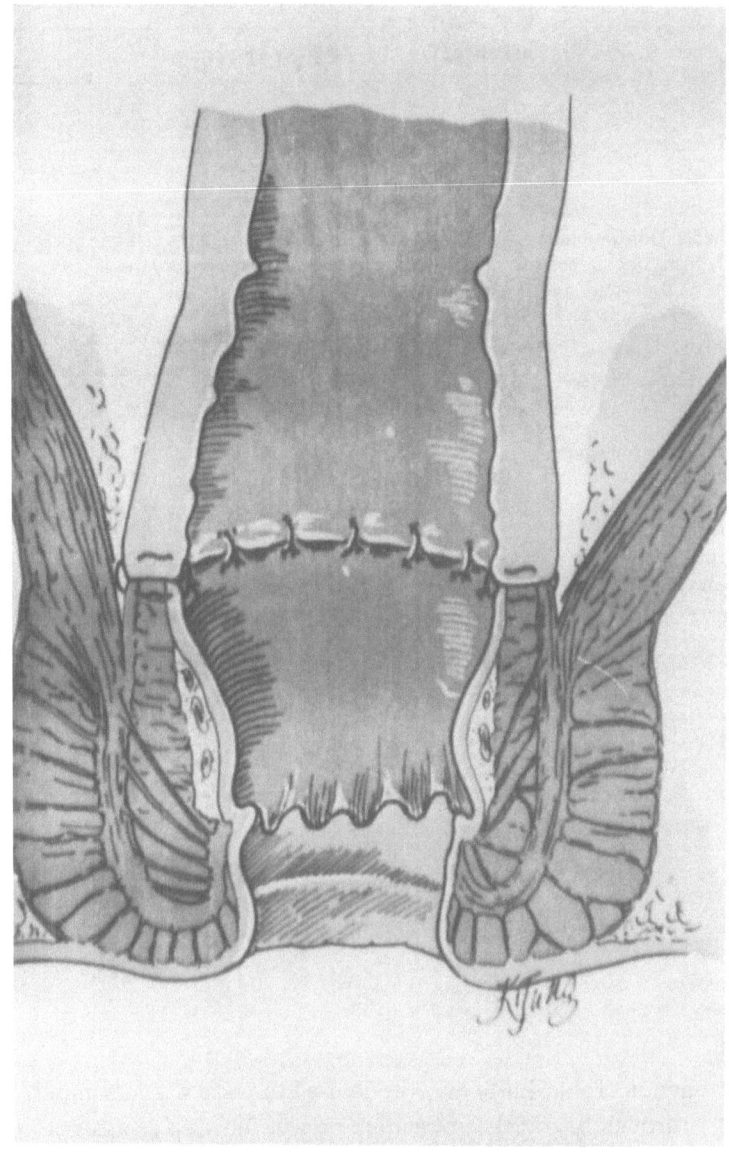

Fig. 4. The completed anastomosis 'retreats' back into the pelvis at the completion of this second stage.

operation five years or more before review. Table 3 lists survivorship. Five patients, in the entire group of 84, developed pelvic recurrences. Four of the five tumors were Dukes' Stage C and one was Dukes' B.

Bowel function. All surviving patients were assessed by interview concerning

212

Table 1. Dukes' staging of 84 rectal cancers resected using the pull-through technique.

Dukes' stage	Number	Percent
A	17	20.2
B	33	39.3
C	32	38.1
'D' [a]	2	2.4

[a] A modified Dukes' staging was used where Stage D refers to a tumor which has spread to distal or local organs or adjacent viscera, or where peritoneal implants are observed.

Table 2. Complications following pull-through procedure in 84 patients.

Complications	Number	(%)
Ischemic necrosis of colon	1	(1.2%)
Pelvic sepsis	6	(7.1%)
Urinary tract infection	11	(13.0%)
Urinary retention	6	(10.0%)
Myocardial infarct	1	(1.2%)
Small bowel obstruction	1	(1.2%)
Pulmonary embolus	2	(2.4%)

[a] Six of 59 male patients with retention required transurethral resection.

Table 3. Five-year survivorship in 47 patients undergoing pull-through procedure for rectal cancer – relationship to Dukes' staging.

Dukes' stage	No.	No. 5-year survivors	%
A	9	9	100
B	21	12	57
C	17	9	53
A, B and C	47	30	63.8

bowel function. Table 4 lists the criteria used to place patients in particular grades 1 through 5, grade 1 representing perfect function as assessed by the patient, grade 5 representing a need for making a permanent colostomy due to poor bowel function.

Sexual function in male patients. Twenty-seven patients were eligible for evaluation. Five (18.5%) were totally impotent. Partial dysfunction, that is, inability to sustain an erection or retrograde ejaculation was present in eight patients (30%).

Discussion. When discussing sphincter-saving procedures for rectal cancer,

Table 4. Assessment of Bowel function in 39 patients alive more than one year postoperatively.

Grade 1	Grade 2	Grade 3	Grade 4	Grade 5
Perfect	Occasional enema or cannot hold gas	Uses drugs or regular enemas or wears pad or occasional minor leak	Major soiling	Colostomy
10 (25.6%)	14 (35.9%)	15 (38.5%)	0	0

the two major issues that arise are first, is it as effective as the Miles' resection for cancer cure and, secondly, is the resulting bowel function preferable to having a colostomy? The first issue is an objective one that can be rapidly settled. The second issue is subjective but nonetheless answerable on the basis that patients have experienced a temporary colostomy and have a yardstick by which they can make a judgment. A third issue, that must be stated for completeness, is that the morbidity and mortality rate should be acceptably low. Finally having rated the pull-through procedure against the Miles' resection, one nowadays must compare it against other sphincter-saving alternatives, in particular, the stapled end-to-end anastomosis.

Cancer cure. The overall crude five-year survival rate in the group presented here was 63%. This compares favorably with other series where survivals of 53% (3) and 52.7% (4) (excluding operative deaths) were reported for pull-through operations. Grage (6) reported a 49% overall five-year survival for surgically treated cancer of the rectum. The low rate (6%) of pelvic recurrence in the Cleveland Clinic series also serves as an indication that the pull-through procedure is an adequate cancer operation in that wide local clearance is possible.

Bowel function. The concern of most surgeons who do not use the pull-through procedure, is that one is creating for the patient a perineal colostomy. By dilating the anus and everting the anorectum, sphincter trauma undoubtedly occurs and contributes significantly to the 'indifferent' function that occurs ab initio in patients where no temporary colostomy is used, or for a time following closure of the temporary colostomy. However, this 'indifferent' function is temporary and, as seen from the above results, an excellent to reasonable functional result can be achieved in almost all patients. The charge that the pull-through operation gives the patient a perineal colostomy is rejected. The difference lies in the fact that the pull-through patients are capable of holding a quart tap water enema, should they require it. All

214

patients in this series who used enemas regularly (and they were mostly those having a coloanal anastomosis) expressed a preference to do this over having a colostomy.

Morbidity and mortality. Only one patient in this series died in the post-operative period. The particular complication of the pull-through operation has been the occurrence of ischemic necrosis of the pulled-through segment, extending up into the pelvis. This occurred in one patient in this series where evidence for mesenteric ischemia and general atherosclerosis existed, factors promoting the likelihood of this complication. The key to this problem is prevention by not relying upon the sigmoid colon as part of the pulled-through segment. All the sigmoid colon is resected and prior to pulling the proximal colon down into the pelvis, its blood supply is assessed by incising an appendix epiloica and observing arterial-type bleeding.

Overview of the pull-through procedure. This operation has provided an excellent alternative to the abdominoperineal resection of the rectum with permanent colostomy. The more rectum that is removed implies, in general, a less favorable than usual type of continence and a longer period of time that it takes for continence to be obtained. However, even with colo-anal anastomosis, reasonable function can usually be attained. The advantage of not having a colostomy is self evident. A further advantage with the delayed anastomosis is the freedom from anastomotic leakage, and fecal fistula, a problem that is occasionally seen with the abdomino-transsacral procedure.

The stapled end-to-end anastomosis. The current status of the pull-through procedure should be considered with respect to the stapler (E.E.A.). With respect to technique of rectal resection, lines of clearance, amount of bowel resected and assessment of blood supply, the procedure is the same. The difference lies in the technique of anastomosis and in the problems that may occur with the techniques. Those associated with the pull-through have already been outlined. Those problems associated with the E.E.A. are listed in table 5. Our experience with the E.E.A. stapler over the past two years has been a favorable one to the effect that most patients who would have previously qualified for a pull-through anastomosis, have in fact had a stapled anastomosis performed. While initially the time-saving features of a stapled versus a hand-sewn anastomosis for a conventional anterior resection were perhaps comparable, with further experience it is our belief that the E.E.A. provides a faster and better anastomosis than the hand-sewn one. When compared to the pull-through procedure, the time taken for each procedure is comparable. The major advantage of the E.E.A. is that a temporary colostomy is rarely necessary except in the case of finding incomplete rings or

Table 5. Pitfalls in the use of the E.E.A. stapler.

Pitfalls:
 1. Cartridege fires during loading.
 2. If loading guide used, firing on withdrawal.
 3. Knurled knob not secured – (leaves gap).
 4. Purse string suture incomplete or pick up opposing wall.
 5. Suture fails to 'run' – use prolene or wax.
 6. Suture breaks on tying.
 7. Difficulty advancing instrument thru rectum (usually short rectal mesentery).
 8. Bowel wall too thick.
 9. Incomplete cutting of mucosa – difficulty in extraction.
10. Incomplete donuts – leak.
11. Bleeding
12. Stricture

donuts of tissue. It is probable that in comparing the procedures by level of anastomosis, that continence will prove to be superior with the E.E.A. One of the earlier problems identified when the E.E.A. was used for low anastomosis at or just above the level of the levator muscles, was the difficulty in placing a purse string suture in the cut edge of the rectal cuff, a site which is poorly seen in the narrow male pelvis. Furthermore, using the E.E.A. in the conventional way, occasionally leads to difficulty in tying the purse string with both the proximal and distal ties. Since 1978, Lavery and Fazio have used the technique of placing the distal purse string in position by the transanal route utilizing a Hill-Ferguson retractor. The closed instrument is then advanced through the rectal cuff up to the pelvic brim before opening the instrument. The proximal colon is then placed over the anvil and the purse string is tied. The instrument is withdrawn until the cartridge appears at the anus at which point the distal rectal purse string is tied under direct vision from the anal aspect. The two ends of bowel are then approximated by turning the wing nut and the instrument is fired.

Notwithstanding the excellence of the completed stapled anastomosis, leaks may occur, although this is unusual. Since this is more likely to occur in radiated bowel, as when significant doses of preoperative irradiation have been used for rectal cancers, it is probable that the pull-through procedure will still have a place in this circumstance. Similarly, if a sphincter-saving procedure is being considered for patients with radiation stricture of the rectum or rectovaginal fistula, then the pull-through procedure may prove to be a more secure anastomosis than the E.E.A.

For the majority of patients, however, the E.E.A. will, I believe, prove to be superior to the pull-through method of anastomosis.

216

ACKNOWLEDGEMENT

The author wishes to acknowledge the contribution of Ms. Kathleen Jung, Department of Medical Illustration, in preparing the diagrams for this section. Dr. W.O. Kirwan, Department of Surgery, St. Finbarr's Hospital, Cork, Ireland, extracted the chart data on patients undergoing the Pull Through operation and interviewed patients with respect to functional results.

REFERENCES

1. Turnbull RB Jr and Cuthbertson AM: Abdomino-rectal pull-through resection for cancer and Hirschsprung's disease. *Cleveland Clinic Quarterly* 28: 109, 1961.
2. Cutait DE and Figlioni FJ: A new method of colorectal anastomosis in abdomino-perineal resection. *Dis Colon Rect* 6: 415, 1961.
3. Kirwan WO, Turnbull RB Jr, Fazio VW and Weakley FL: Pull through Operation with Delayed Anastomosisis for Rectal Cancer, *Br J Surg* 65: 695-699, 1978.
4. Black BM and Botham RJ: Combined Abdomino-endorectal Resections for Lesions of the Mid and Upper Parts of the Rectum, *Arch Surg* 76: 688, 1958.
5. Waugh JM and Turner JC Jr: Abdomino-perineal Resection with Preservation of the Anal Sphincter for Carcinoma of the Mid-rectum, *S G & O* 107: 777, 1958.
6. Grage TB: preoperative radiation in rectal surgery. In: Varco AL and Delaney WB (eds), p 417-433, Saunders, Philadelphia, 1976.

24. THE TRANSSPHINCTERIC APPROACH

A. YORK MASON

This surgical access to the rectum was first presented to an International Conference on Proctology at the Royal Society of Medicine in June 1969. For this record of the Boerhaave International Course on Colorectal Cancer, held almost exactly ten years later, I feel that it would be appropriate to begin by reproducing a few of my original illustrations (1 and 2), to remind you of the basic technique of exposure and closure.

EXPOSURE

Fig. 1. The incision extends from a point just to the left of the sacro-coccygeal junction, downwards to the anal verge in the midline posteriorly. Two muscular landmarks can be recognised at this stage, the lower fibres of the gluteus maximus at the upper end, and the superficial fibres of the external sphincter at the lower end of the wound. Between these two there is a considerable depth of fat, because the ano-rectal junction is angulated forward by the puborectalis sling.

Fig. 2. This is a composite picture, drawn from photographs taken from different angles, in order to illustrate the concept of three tubes, simplifying

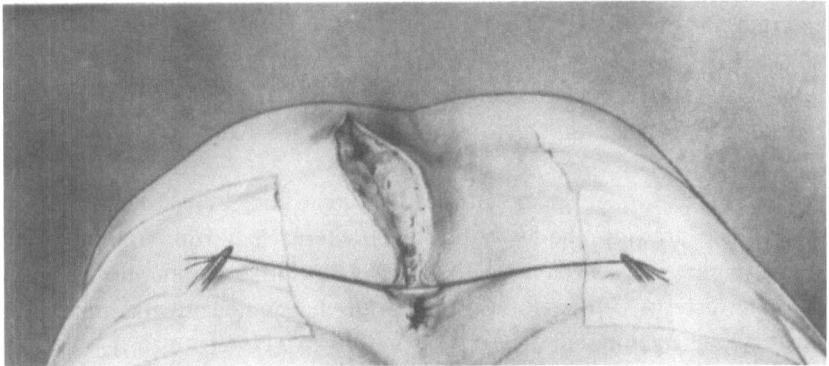

Fig. 1. The line of the incision.

K. Welvaart et al. (eds.), Colorectal Cancer, 217-234. All rights reserved.
Copyright © 1980 by Martinus Nijhoff Publishers, The Hague/Boston/London.

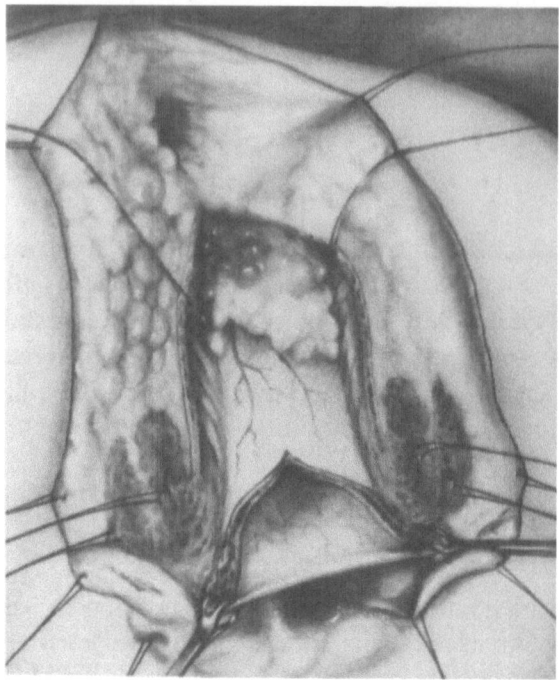

Fig. 2. The anatomy of the exposure.

an anatomy which may appear very complicated. The outer tube, a muscle complex, made up of the levator-ani, the puborectalis and the various rather artificial subdivisions of the external sphincter, is shown opened up completely. This reveals the posterior para-rectal space, filled with fat, containing lymph nodes, in its upper half, but becoming narrower at the anal end where external and internal sphincters are closely adjacent and linked by their muscle fibres. Below the fat, the whiteness of the fascia propria is characteristic, and superior haemorrhoidal vessels can be recognised. It is through this para-rectal space that a closed tube of rectum, together with peri-rectal fat and lymph nodes, can be dissected out.

The musculature of the rectum and anal canal constitute the middle tube, and, in this drawing, the lower part, characteristically white muscle of internal sphincter, has been divided to reveal the third and innermost, mainly mucosal, tube, which has only a small muscle component, the muscularis mucosae. The sub-mucosal plexus of vessels can be seen clearly, and it is through this submucosal plane that a tube of rectal mucosa with its muscularis mucosae, can be dissected out. Division of this mucosal tube (here shown stratched out by Babcock's forceps) exposes the interior of the rectum and anal canal, and permits transluminal surgery under direct vision.

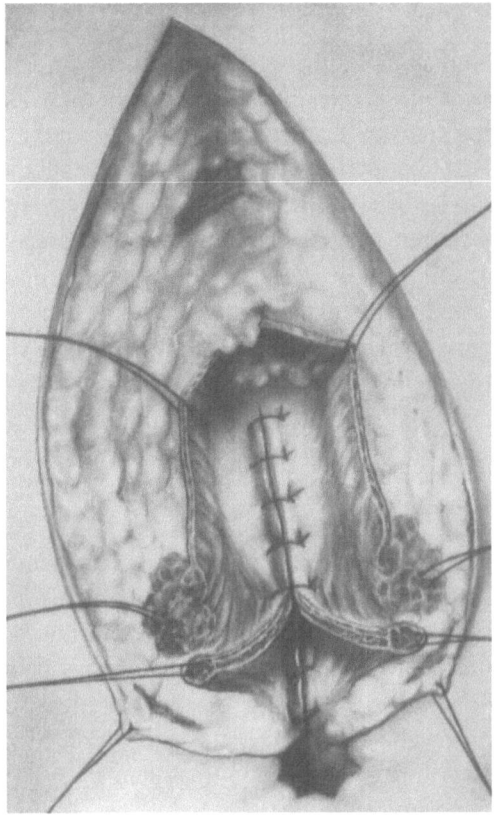

Fig. 3. The method of closure in layers.

CLOSURE

Fig. 3. Illustrates the method of closure in layers, a continuous fine chromic catgut suture for the mucosa, stronger interrupted chromic catgut sutures are used for the muscle coat of rectum and anal canal and for the outer somatic muscle tube.

INDICATIONS

There are many other indications, but my present purpose is to outline the potential value of a transsphincteric approach in the selective treatment of one group of lesions.

Epithelial Neoplasms

Use of this exposure enlarges the scope of sphincter preserving surgery for epithelial neoplasms of the rectum. It is customary to divide these into two groups, benign and malignant, and accordingly to prescribe different surgery for each group. However it is important to appreciate that there is a sequence of events in the change from normal mucosa, through a benign adenomatous stage to invasive cancer, progressing predictably at first by direct invasion across the rectal wall and then, less preditably, going on to involve local pararectal tissues and finally to disseminated disease. These are all stages in a neoplastic process, which, from his examination of a radically resected specimen, a histopathologist can recognise with accuracy and can predict five-year survival. But this is knowledge after the event.

Pre-Treatment Clinical Staging

This is the real challenge to clinicians, to achieve a system of pre-operative clinical staging sufficiently accurate to justify its use as a basis for planning selective management of the individual patient, and this is particularly important if the lesion is sited in the lower rectum. A transsphincteric approach is one of several alternative techniques for sphincter preservation; crucial for the success of any technique is accurate recognition of the stage of the neoplastic process before embarking on treatment.

RECTAL DIGITAL EXAMINATION

Fortunately, all lower sited lesions are within easy reach of the index finger, and also, forunately, this happens to be the most readily available instrument. An inquisitive, well-trained index finger is capable of deciding whether:
(a) the lesion is still a benign adenoma or an invasive cancer;
(b) if invasive cancer, it is still confined to rectal wall or has breached the barrier of fascia propria;
(c) if through rectum, the extent of local extra-rectal spread, slight, moderate, or extensive.

This examination needs to be carried out methodically, observing a defined protocol and recording the facts required from the finger on an agreed proforma. The most important ingredient for success is 'motivation'. This was understandably lacking during the many years when orthodox teaching was that the best treatment for all rectal cancers was abdominoperineal resection, and even when restorative resection became accepted for upper third cancers, the role of the index finger in assessment was a minor one. We now know that restorative surgery can be extended, without prejudice, to cancer cure in carefully selected patients, and that lesions still confined to rectal wall are potentially capable by local excision or destruction. The need to recognise the clinical stage of the local lesion should provide the necessary motivation, and increasing use of digital assessment will confirm the value of 'touch'.

Having made these necessary preliminary explanations about the difficulty of drawing a clear line of demarcation between benign and malignant neoplasms, and the value of rectal digital examination in the pre-treatment clinical assessment and staging of epithelial neoplasms, I can continue discussion of technique.

TRANSSPHINCTERIC SURGERY FOR VILLOUS TUMOURS

There are many factors which influence the decision about whether resection can be completed from below, or whether a combined approach is advisable or indeed necessary. I will illustrate a few examples.

Transluminal Resection

Fig. 4. This was a large, rather coarsely lobulated villous tumour which seemed to fill the rectum. It was felt to be soft throughout, a protuberant type of growth and broad-based, but because of its bulk it was difficult to determine exactly the size and location of the base. It could not be prolapsed through the anal canal. When the rectum was opened up the tumour prolapsed to fill the transsphincteric wound. However, by wrapping the growth in moist towels, (not shown in this drawing) it was possible to identify the base as being about 10 cm from the anal verge and about 5 cm in diameter. The growth was resected by full-thickness elliptical excision between paired guide sutures. Fig. 5 illustrates transverse closure of the defect using a single layer of interrupted catgut sutures (and I would recommend a vertical mattress, mucosa-inverting type of stitch).

Fig. 6 illustrates a smaller sessile type villous growth, being lifted out of the wound, suspended on the inner circle of guide sutures. This lesion had been assessed as a villous growth with invasive change still confined to rectal wall. The patient, an old man in poor health, had refused a permanent colostomy. Care was taken to include perirectal fat, cleaning the back of the prostate and the left seminal vesicle.

These two examples of transsphincteric, transluminal, full-thickness, local excision represent both ends of the spectrum. Between them lie a large variety of growths, differing in morphology, size and site, treated basically in similar

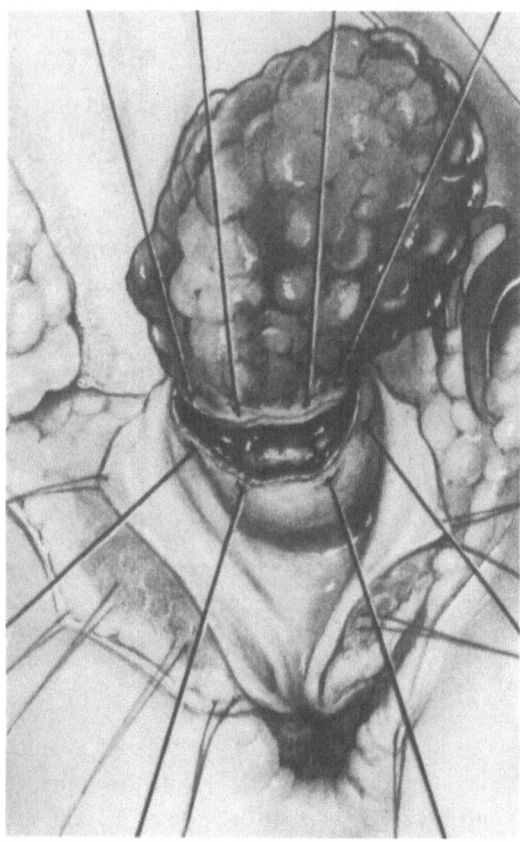

Fig. 4. Transluminal full-thickness elliptical excision of a protuberant type villous tumour.

manner, but with variations appropriate to individual circumstances. For example, for posterior quadrant growths, the anal canal and rectum are opened up to just below the lower edge of the growth. The posterior wall can now be mobilised from the front of the sacrum, via the para-rectal space, in order to prolapse the growth into the lumen of the rectum and it can now be dealt with 'en face'. For growths with a lower edge above the level of the internal sphincter, and with a diameter of less than about 8 cm full-thickness excision is the treatment of choice, and for higher sited anterior wall growths, an ellipse of peritoneum may be safely included. It may facilitate closure of the defect if this is extended to 'tube resection'.

For patients treated by simple full-thickness local excision there is usually no need for a temporary protective colostomy, but this advice must be qualified by the general condition of the patient and the smoothness or otherwise of the resection. If in doubt, establish a protective colostomy. For pre-operative bowel preparation I abandoned, some years ago, the antibiotic

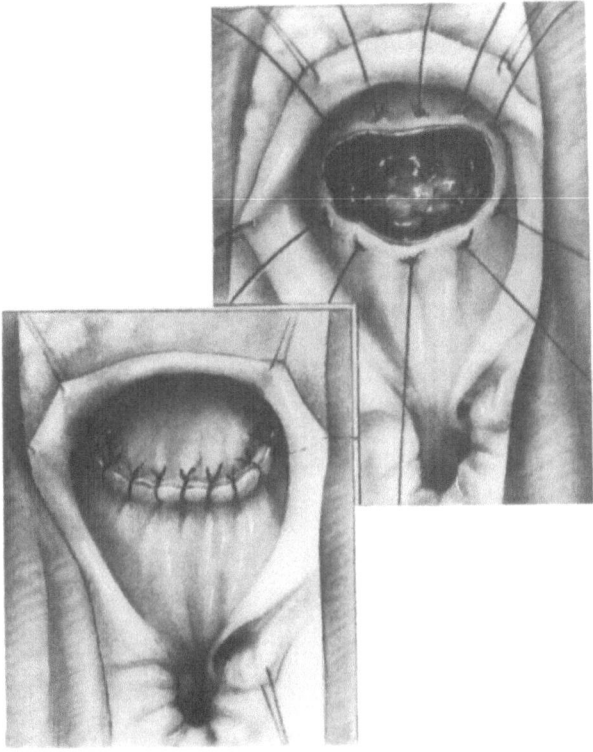

Fig. 5. Transverse closure of the defect by means of a single layer of interrupted catgut sutures.

regime prescribed by mouth for several days before surgery. Instead I now use a wide spectrum antibiotic given by injection at the time of operation and, more recently, have added metronidazole. However, mechanical cleansing of the bowel would seem to be the main factor in avoidance of wound infection. Gentle handling of tissues is also important. I was concerned about the danger of cell implantation when I first used the transluminal resection and washed out the wound with oxychlorosene. The value of specific cytoxic chemical solutions is not proven, and a good wash-out of the wound before closure, using ordinary sterile water, is probably sufficient. Apart from any other consideration, this lavage removes blood clot and other debris.

The patients illustrated both healed cleanly by first intention and defaeca-tion, on or about the third post-operative day, was normal with full anal control. This has been the usual sequence of events in patients treated by full-thickness local excision.

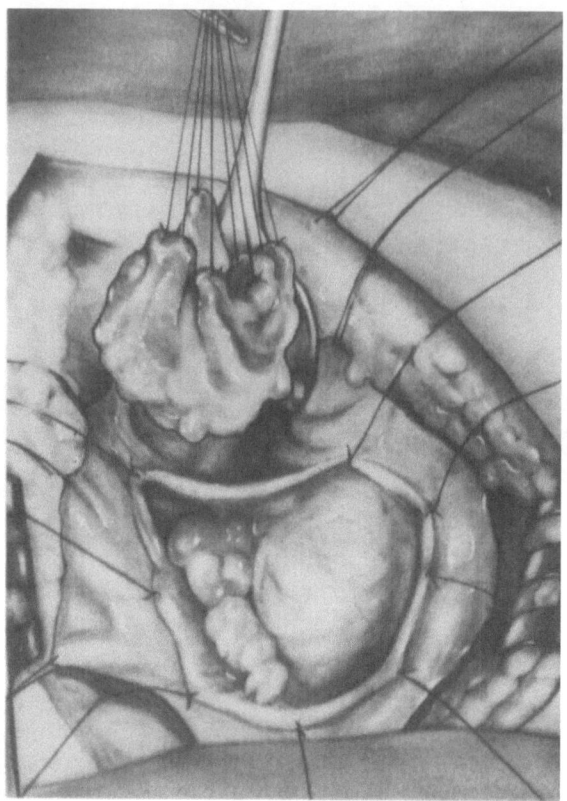

Fig. 6. Full-thickness elliptical excision of a flat type villous growth, assessed to have early invasive change.

SUB-MUCOSAL RESECTION

Fig. 7 illustrates submucosal resection of a circumferential benign flat carpet type growth, with a lower edge extending virtually down to the dentate line.

Blood vessels passing across this plane can be visualised clearly during the course of dissection, and can be diathermied before scissor division. It is important to maintain a clean field in order to be able to recognise any transgression by growth of this clean submucosal plane. Submucosal dissection should be limited strictly to those carpets assessed with confidence to be still benign, and, over the past 15 years, I have tended more and more to reserve its use to the kind of lesion illustrated in fig. 7, circumferential lesions with a lower edge down or near to the dentate line. It is necessary to open up the lower end of the mucosal tube, as illustrated, in order to visualise the lower edge of the growth clearly. Upward dissection from this lower edge may be tedious because mucosa of anal canal is attached to underlying internal sphincter by strands of muscle; above the ano-rectal junction submucosal

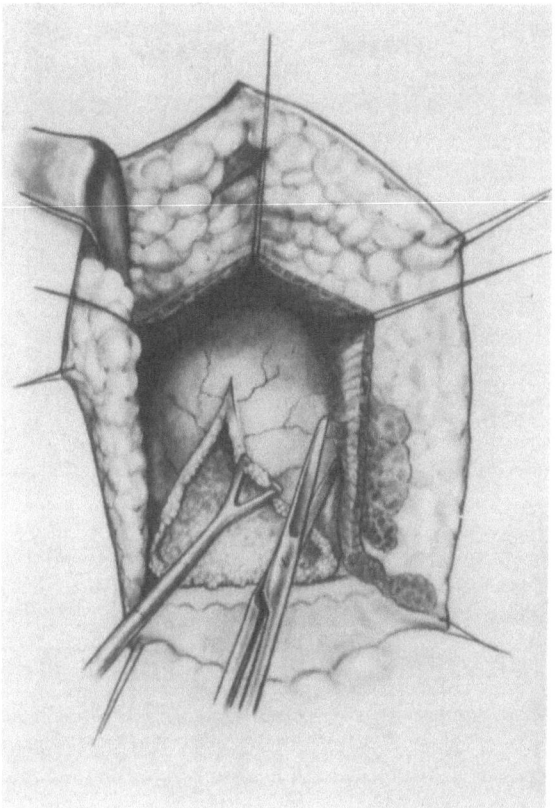

Fig. 7. Submucosal resection of an extensive flat type benign villous growth.

dissection is easy and proceeds quickly, and the growth can be dessected out as a 'closed tube'.

Fig. 8, an operation photograph, shows this long mucosal tube held out of the wound. Dissection had continued to above the level of the rectosigmoid junction and an opening made through the tube in order to visualise the upper margin of the villous carpet. These tumours are so soft that it is difficult to determine the upper limit by palpation.

Fig. 9 shows the resected specimen. Multiple sections confirmed that this was a benign carpet throughout.

CIRCUMFERENTIAL MUCOSAL DEFECTS

Up to about 10 cm lengths of raw muscle, left after extensive submucosal resection, can be covered by drawing the upper mucosal cuff down over the muscle and stitching it loosely to the mucosa left at the anal end. This is possible

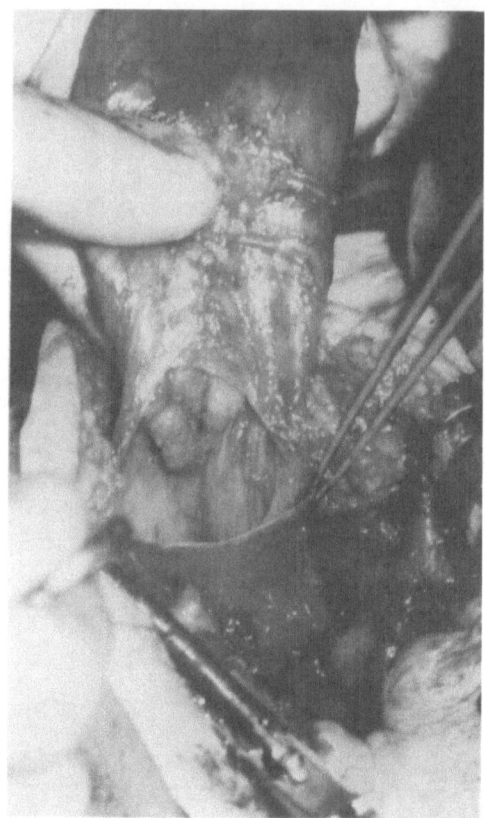

Fig. 8. Submucosal tube resection of a benign villous growth which carpeted the entire rectum, and an opening made to identify the upper limit.

because the muscularis propria of the rectum is mobile and can be 'telescoped' down, also there is a certain 'give' in the loose connective tissue of the sub-mucosa.

For defects longer than 10 cm complete mucosal covering is not possible. The upper mucosal cuff is drawn down as far as possible and tacked to underlying muscle, leaving some raw muscle to granulate and then to be re-epithelialised by growth of mucosa from the upper and lower edges. This is a slow process, from 3-4 months, depending upon the length of defect to be covered. *During this period regular daily dilatation is essential to prevent stricture formation.* A temporary protective colostomy is advisable. This can be closed as soon as the transsphincteric wound is soundly healed and before epithelialisation is complete.

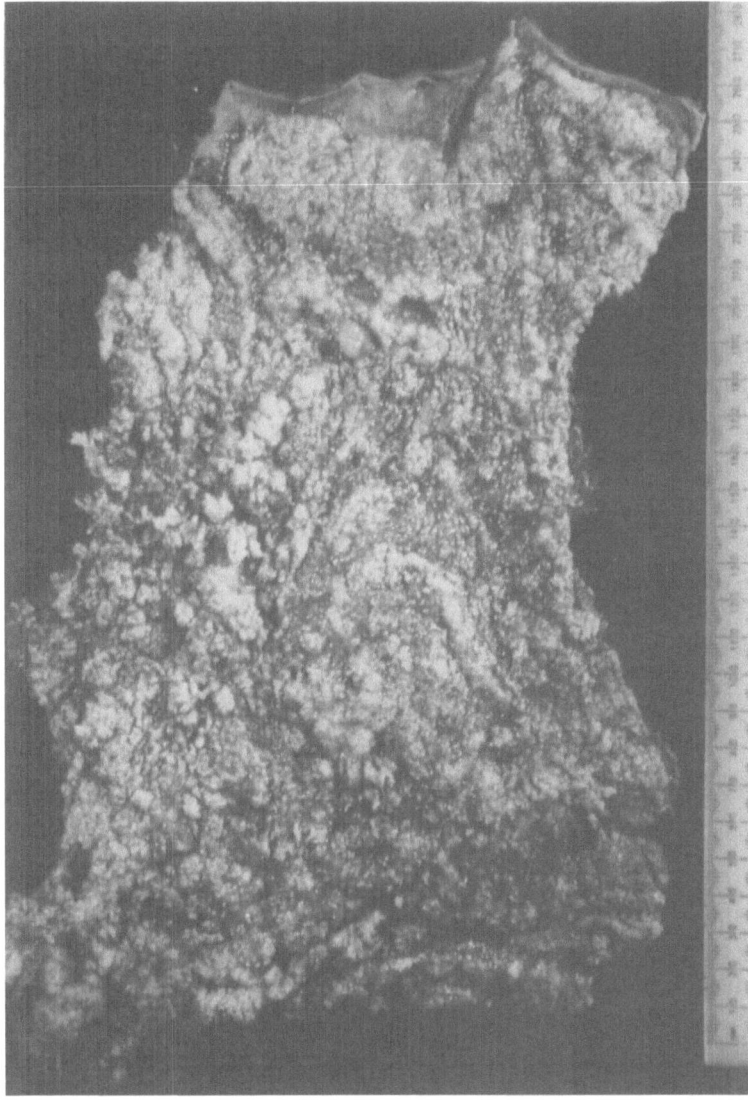

Fig. 9. The resected tube, opened and set out flat, correctly orientated for detailed histopathological examination.

COMBINED PROCEDURES

Villous tumours with a lower edge more than about 10 cm above the anal verge are best treated by trans-abdominal restorative resection, and when conditions are favourable, this can be extended to include growths with a distal edge at a lower level. The technical difficulty of carring out a really low anastomosis can be overcome by transsphincteric exposure.

A conventional trans-abdominal approach is used to mobilise the rectum down to the pelvic floor. In order to obtain an adequate length of healthy colon, it is good practice to mobilise the splenic flexure, and high ligation of inferior mesenteric artery and vein ensures a good blood supply. A temporary protective right transverse colostomy is recommended. The abdominal wound is now closed and the patient repositioned prone. The sphincters are divided, opening up the anal canal to visualise clearly the lower edge of the growth. If this is down to the dentate line, dissection upwards for the first 1-2 cm is carried out through the submucosal plane, then at full-thickness, to meet up with the pelvic dissection. The growth, and the previously mobilised, rectum and lower colon, are drawn down through the widely opened sphincters. The colon is transected at a chosen site, and continuity restored by colo-anal anastomosis. Repositioning does not seem to upset patients if this is carried out correctly and carefully. Alternatively, the need can be obviated by carrying out the combined procedure with the patient lying in the right lateral position.

These combined procedures do carry a higher morbidity than submucosal resection. This is, however, counterbalanced by the real advantage of complete removal of foci of microscopic invasion. For old, poor risk patients the danger of residual microscopic foci of invasive cancer in an extensive carpet, assessed clinically to be benign, is an acceptable risk and submucosal resection is justifiable. In fit patients, and certainly if there is any suspicion of invasive change, then I would certainly advise combined resection.

RESULTS

Over the past fifteen years I have used a transsphincteric approach in the treatment of 58 patients referred as having benign villous tumours. By rectal digital examination these were divisible into three groups:
1. invasive cancers (12 patients),
2. doubtful (6 patients),
3. benign (40 patients).
In the time available I can only describe briefly the outcome in each of these groups and try to convey the lessions I have learnt.

1. In 12 patients I made a confident diagnosis of invasive cancer. Two patients with comparatively small villous growths had easily palpable hard extra-rectal growth. Both were treated by palliative restorative resection and both died from pre-existing disseminated disease. Three patients had large villous growths with areas of hardness and diminished mobility. All were treated by radical combined restorative resection; examination of the resected specimens showed no invasive change in two; the hardness and fixity were due

to fibrosis from previous surgery. They were fit patients and came to no harm from radical surgery, and I have no regrets about my overassessment. The third specimen confirmed invasive cancer with slight extra-rectal spread and involvement of an immediately adjacent node. Seven patients with sessile villous cancers about 5 cm in diameter were treated by full-thickness local resection, 'disc' or 'tube'; histopathology confirmed that the invasive cancer was still confined to rectal wall. Followup, admittedly less than five years in some, nevertheless, seems to indicate that this has been adequate curative surgery.

2. There were 6 patients in the doubtful group, 'doubtful' because of previous deep biopsies or partial diathermy snare. In two patients, and this was in my early and overoptimistic period, I began by attempting submucosal resection, became confused by scar tissue? invasive cancer, and proceeded to a compromise deeper resection. My pathologist colleague found definite invasive cancer in scar tissue, but it was difficult for him to say whether excision in depth had been adequate. I adopted. wrongly as I now know, a 'wait and see' policy, and waited too long. Both manifested extra-rectal cancer, and, despite abdomino-perineal resection at this late stage, both died from disseminated disease. The right management policy, adopted subsequently, would seem to be to treat doubtful cases as cancers, to make sure that dissection is well clear of doubtful scar tissue, and this makes it much easier for a pathologist to give a difinite answer. One patient in this doubtful group has had a radical combined resection for a benign lesion. He has come to no harm from this major surgery, and all his potentially unstable rectal mucosa has been removed.

3. Forty patients were assessed by me pre-operatively as having benign villous tumours. The only two operative deaths were in this benign group, one due to coronary thrombosis and he had a past history of cardiac failure and the picture had been obscured by hypokalaemia. The other death was thought to be due to pulmonary embolism in a patient who had presented with dehydration and profound electrolyte disturbance. In the surviving patients, the real difficulty in assessment of results is in those patients with very extensive villous carpets treated by submucosal resection, and two of these were old, poor risk patients who died from natural causes less than five years after resection. Meticulous histopathology found microscopic foci of invasive cancer in 5 patients. In 4 of these a policy of 'wait and see' seems to have been justified. In one it was wrong because he manifested extra-rectal growth and it is doubtful whether this has now been cleared by abdomino-perineal resection. More disturbing, is a similar manifestation of extra-rectal growth, four years after resection of a very large villous carpet in which a pathologist had not found any foci of invasive cancer.

The main conclusion must be that, while it is possible to carry out submucosal resection of very extensive villous carpets, this should be limited to old, poor risk patients, those who are fit enough, should have complete rectal excision, because in the majority it is still possible to restore continuity by colo-anal anastomosis and to leave the patient with an acceptable pattern of defaecation.

In the preceding section, while concentrating mainly on a peculiar variant, I have discussed most aspects common to the 'neoplastic sequence'. I will try, therefore, to avoid repetition.

In order to resolve the dilemma of how best to manage the individual patient presenting with a low-sited rectal cancer, we need a system of pre-treatment clinical staging. There are, of course, many factors to be taken into consideration, but I have come to rely mainly on digital assessment, and I have found that the study of macro-sections has been of the greatest help in checking and improving the accuracy of my index finger. On this basis I evolved a numerical staging (3).

Fig. 10 is a good example of an early invasive carcinoma. Before removal, an index finger should have had no difficulty in recognising that this was a protuberant lesion with an area of superficial ulceration, that the hardness of the central area, contrasting with the soft periphery, was a sign of invasive change in a previously benign polyp. It would have appreciated the free mobility over the underlying muscle coat because invasion is still confined to submucosa. I classify this as a clinical stage 1 cancer. Errors of staging have been due to fibrosis due to previous biopsy and the lesson is that clinical evaluation should be recorded before histological diagnosis.

Cancers at this stage are curable by local excision or destruction; this can be done via the dilated anal canal, but I find that opening up the lower bowel provides clearer vision, and I prefer excision rather than destruction because I need a specimen!

Fig. 11 is an example of invasion reaching muscularis propria. Note the muscular hypertrophy which precedes invasion. Cancers at this stage feel mobile, but less freely so than those at the preceding stage. They cannot be moved independently of the underlying true muscle coat. I would classify this as a stage 2 cancer, and curable by adequate local resection. Although there is only a poor correlation between surface area and depth of invasion, for technical reasons a tube resection rather than disc excision is appropriate. Sphincter division facilitates this, and there are variations of the basic technique to suit individual circumstances. I have already stressed the importance of close surgeon-pathologist collaboration in deciding whether local resection

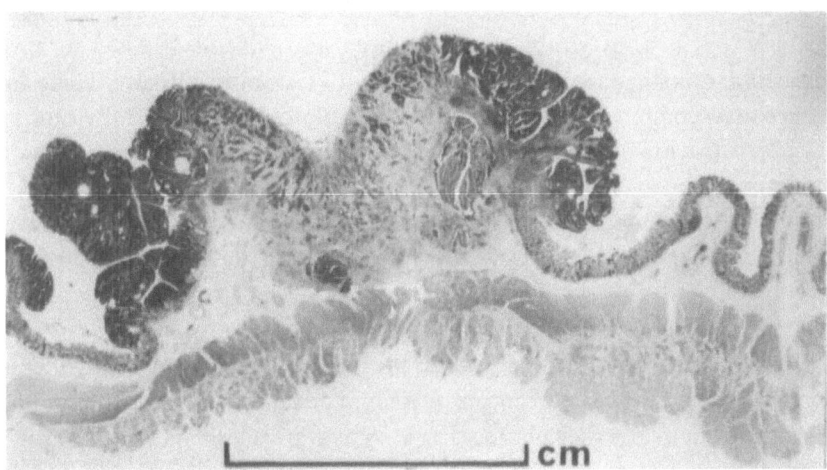

Fig. 10. Early invasive cancer. CSI.

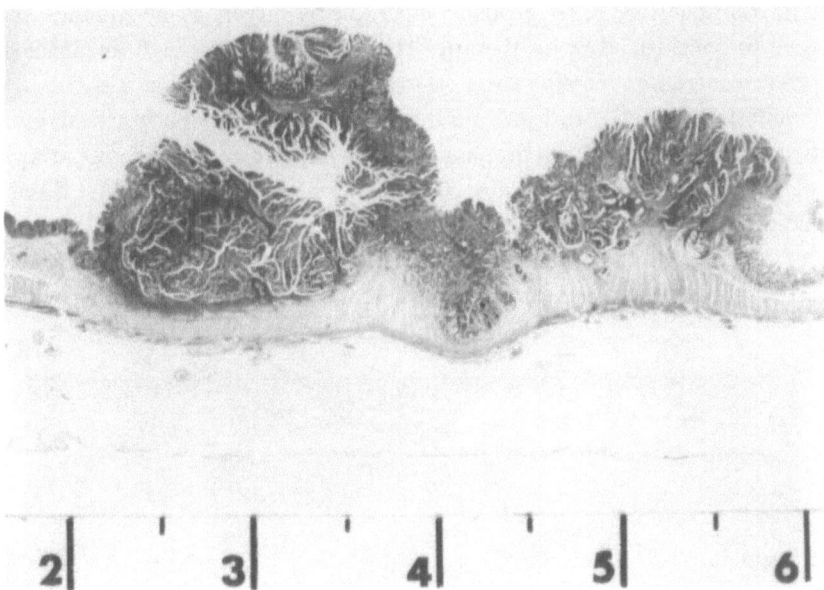

Fig. 11. Invasive cancer confined to rectal wall. CSII.

has been adequate treatment.

Fig. 12 exemplifies a cancer correctly assessed pre-operatively as having invaded full thickness rectal wall but with only slight extra-rectal spread. Looking at this photograph of a longitudinal slice through the centre of the growth one can understand why this lesion coveyed to the finger a sense of 'tethered' mobility and by palpation of its deep aspect through adjacent rectal wall, the finger could only just detect an impression of extra-rectal growth. I classify this as a favourable stage 3 cancer, and patients assessed to have cancers at this stage are all good candidates for restorative surgery. There are alternative combined techniques; I have exploited sphincteric division to facilitate the low anastomosis, but I appreciate the advantages of Parks' endo-anal anastomosis (4).

It would seem that a definite dividing line can be drawn at this stage, and it is of interest that by grouping cancers confined to rectal wall with those through rectum but with only slight extra-rectal spread, finger assessment approaches 90% accuracy.

Fig. 13 exemplifies the really major problem of how best to treat patients presenting with low-sited cancers at a more advanced stage. Although the lesion shown in this slice photograph is comparatively small, it is rather flat and deeply ulcerated. Extra-rectal growth is definitively palpable and in addition to this spread in continuity there is palpable node involvement. Although resectable, the majority of cancers at this stage, which I classify as unfavourable stage 3, are probably incurable by surgery alone and there is a need to consider adjuvant therapy. There is, however, a high incidence of pelvic recurrence even after the most radical clearance possible; it is clinically manifest sooner after restorative surgery than after abdominoperineal resection. Unfortunately, from past and ongoing trials of adjuvant radiotherapy, we have not as yet received any clear answer as to when or in what dosage radiotherapy should be added to surgery, but I remain hopeful.

I come now to the problem of how best to manage patients presenting with 'fixed' growths, which I classify as stage 4 cancers. Certainly, there is no place

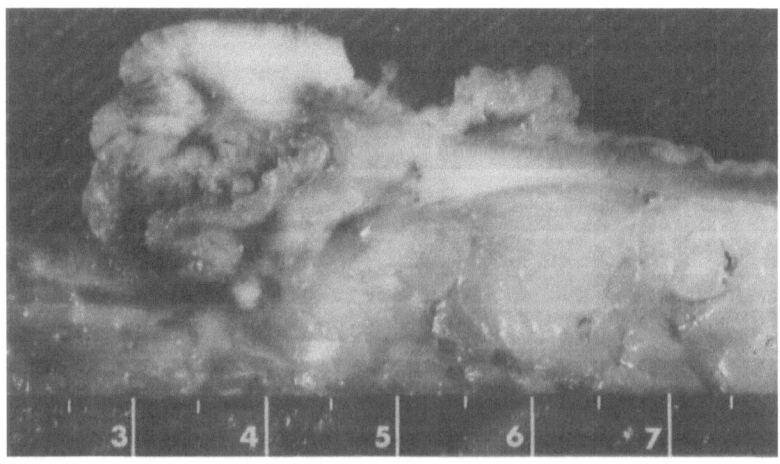

Fig. 12. Invasive cancer with slight local extra-rectal spread. A favourable CSIII.

233

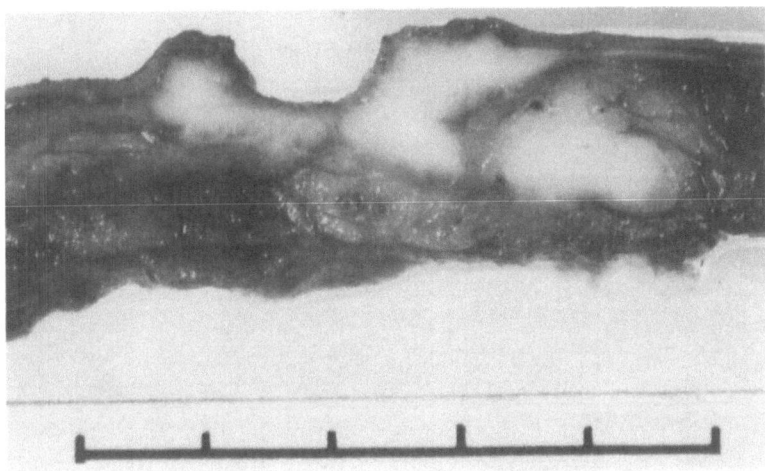

Fig. 13. A small deeply ulcerated cancer with palpable local extra-rectal spread and palpable node involvement.

here for local excision hoping the palliate troublesome symptoms. Some large fixed growths have responded remarkably well to radiotherapy, and, some years ago, I tried transsphincteric resection of the small residual lesion. There was no difficulty with excision, but wound healing was very long delayed, and because of post-radiation fibrosis, it seemed unlikely that these patients would regain satisfactory sphincter function. Fortunately, by this time they had come to accept their 'temporary' colostomy, and did not press for its closure.

However, the possibility remains that some of these problems could be overcome by a combination of alternative radiotherapy and surgical techniques. Also, although the results to date have been disappointing, we need to remember that there are other potentially valuable adjuvant therapies.

ACKNOWLEDGEMENTS

Figures 1-7 reproduced by courtesy, the Editor Proceedings of the Royal Society of Medicine.

REFERENCES

1. Mason A York: Surgical access to the rectum – a transsphinctive exposure. Proc Roy Soc Med, Suppl to Vol 63, 1970, p 91-94. (International Conference on Proctology, June 23-26, 1969.)
2. Mason A York: The place of local Resection in the treatment of rectal carcinoma. Proc Roy Soc Med 63, No 12, 1970, p 1259-1262.

3. Mason A York: Local excision. Malignant tumours of the rectum. Clin Gastroen 4: 582-593, 1975. (W.B. Saunders Company Ltd.)
4. Parks AG: Endoanal technique of low colonic anastomosis. In: *Surgical techniques illustrated* Vol 2, No 2, 1977 (Little Brown and Company).

25. SURGICAL TREATMENT OF LIVER METASTASES FROM COLORECTAL CANCER

L.H. BLUMGART AND C.B. WOOD

INTRODUCTION

Liver metastases are found in 15-25% of patients with colorectal cancer at initial presentation (2, 17, 29) and the incidence is even higher in post mortem studies (11). The presence of liver metastases has more effect on prognosis than any other factor known to influence survival. Although there are occasional reports of long-term survivors, most patients with untreated metastases die within 2 years of diagnosis and average survival rates of approximately 6 months are usually reported (12, 20, 28).

The dismal prognosis is influenced by the extent of secondary spread within the liver and this has an important bearing on the subject of hepatic resection for metastatic spread. Thus, Jaffe et al. (12) reported a study of patients with liver metastases from primary tumours of pancreas, biliary tract, stomach, colon and rectum. They found a median survival time of 72 days for patients with widespread liver metastases, 93 days for patients with metastases localised to a single lobe of the liver, whereas patients with solitary liver metastases had a median survival time of 136 days. Similar results were reported by Nielsen et al. (18). They showed that patients with 'few' liver metastases had a mean survival rate of 18 months, whereas patients with 'several' metastases survived on average 9 months, compared to 5 months for patients with multiple metastases. Wood et al. (28), in a retrospective study of 113 patients with colon cancer and hepatic metastases, showed the one year survival rate to be 5.7% for patients with widespread liver metastases, 27% for those with metastases localised to a segment or lobe of liver and 60% for patients with solitary metastases. They also noted that the mean survival time was 25 months for patients in whom solitary liver metastases were the sole evidence of metastatic spread. Thus, survival is related very much to the extent of metastatic spread within the liver. This is an important factor in the natural history of patients with liver metastases and in assessing results of various forms of treatment for secondary liver deposits. However, it should be noted that despite this more favourable prognosis for patients with solitary metastases, there remain few, if any, 5-year survivors if the metastases are left untreated. For this reason, patients with solitary metastases or metastases confined to a single lobe of liver should be considered for liver resection. The results of surgical removal of secondary liver tumours are far from conclusive, but such data as are available are encouraging.

A greater understanding of the detailed anatomy of the liver (10, 16), has led to technical developments in liver surgery and more widespread use of hepatic resection in a variety of conditions. In 1970, Foster (8) reviewed the world literature and found 83 patients who had undergone liver resection for metastases. Of these patients, 47% survived 2 years and 21% were alive 5 years after resection. Wilson and Adson (27) reported the Mayo Clinic experience with 60 patients who had undergone resection of hepatic metastases from colorectal cancer. Solitary deposits were removed from 40 patients, while the remaining 20 had multiple deposits excised. Their results of surgical resection of apparent solitary metastases showed 5- and 10-year survival rates of 42% and 28% respectively. No patient who had resection of multiple secondary deposits survived 5 years. Wanebo et al. (25) found that of 25 patients with resected solitary liver metastases, 9 (36%) survived 4 years after resection, compared to only 3 (17%) of 18 patients with unresected solitary metastases. The 4-year survival rate was only 1% for the 149 patients with unresected multiple liver metastases in the study. Somewhat less optimistic results were reported by Fortner et al. (7). Of the 17 patients in their study who had resection of liver metastases from colorectal cancer, only 2 survived beyond 3 years. We have performed resection of secondary hepatic deposits in 11 patients, most of whom had primary tumours in the colon or rectum. Of these, 7 died between 1 month and $4\frac{1}{2}$ years after surgery. The remaining patients are alive and apparently free of tumour between 3 months and $6\frac{1}{2}$ years. Thus, the presence of a solitary metastasis in the liver arising from a primary tumour site in the colon or rectum need not be viewed with undue pessimism. Indeed, an aggressive approach in selected patients may be rewarded by good long-term results.

In the routine surgical practice of any one surgeon, the number of patients that would be suitable for hepatic resection is small, since only approximately 10% of those with liver metastases have solitary or localised lesions. Thus, it would be difficult to obtain sufficient experience in the complex operative and postoperative management of these patients unless such surgery was being performed in specialist centres and by surgeons with the necessary expertise.

Before embarking on hepatic resectional surgery, it is essential to exclude the presence of multiple deposits in both lobes of the liver and of extra-hepatic metastases. A chest X-ray, isotope or ultrasound liver scan and bone scan should be performed. Local tumour recurrence should be excluded by performing a Barium enema and/or colonoscopy. It is our policy to perform selective hepatic arteriography in all potential candidates for liver resection. This not only outlines a large number of secondary deposits in the liver, but also demonstrates the arterial anatomy. Splenoportography and inferior vena cavography are also performed, particularly in cases with large metastatic deposits, since these investigations can give valuable information regarding operability (26). Thus, a tumour may still be resectable even if it is involving one branch, but not both branches, of the portal vein. Similarly, resection may be possible even though a tumour is compressing the inferior vena cava, provided there is no actual tumour involvement of the vein. We would consider liver resectional surgery to be contra-indicated if there are tumour deposits in both anatomical lobes of the liver, proven extra-hepatic disease, involvement of both main branches of the portal vein, or tumour invasion of the inferior vena cava. In our experience, liver resection would be ill-advised in patients with extensive local invasion of the primary tumour, since this has been shown to carry a poor prognosis (see chapter on 'Prognostic Factors in Staging of Colorectal Cancer, this volume).

The standard techniques for liver resection have been described in detail elsewhere (1, 4, 6, 7, 21, 23). Up to 80% of the human liver can be excised with relative safety due to the amazing capacity of the liver to undergo regenerative hyperplasia. This phenomenon occurs with predictable and remarkable rapidity and results in restoration of liver mass, micro-anatomy and function of the liver (3). The precise mechanism controlling the process of liver regeneration is unknown, but an adequate portal flow to the remaining liver is essential (5, 23).

During the period of active regenerative hyperplasia, much of the cellular energy is diverted towards this process with the result that metabolic functions of the liver are depressed and a degree of liver failure exists. This state of affairs usually lasts for 2-3 weeks after surgery and fairly rapid recovery occurs thereafter. During this period of depressed function, certain metabolic and haematological sequelae can have serious, and even fatal, consequences. Hepatic ischaemia, or a decrease in liver blood flow, which may occur as a result of intra-operative haemorrhage, may increase the effect of these metabolic defects (9, 15).

Hypoalbuminaemia is frequently seen after major hepatic resection and may not be averted by the administration of albumin supplement. Hypoglycaemia is a serious risk, since glycogen stores within the liver are rapidly used up after liver resection. The main danger period is within the first 48 hours and infusion of Dextrose is almost always necessary.

A small rise in serum bilirubin level is frequently seen after partial hepatectomy. Deepening jaundice is a worrying feature, since this may be due to centri-lobular damage as a result of hypoperfusion of the liver, or alternatively, may be the result of extra-hepatic obstruction. There has been considerable debate regarding the use of T-tube drainage of the biliary tree after liver resection. It has been argued that the insertion of a T-tube offers no advantage and even increases morbidity after liver resection for trauma (14).

Certainly it has been shown that there is no reduction of intra-hepatic pressure by external biliary drainage (13). However, the distinct advantage of having a T-tube in the biliary system is that it allows measurement of the bile output and also allows cholangiography to be performed and thereby demonstrate any extra-hepatic cause for increasing jaundice.

The liver is the only site of fibrinogen synthesis and the main site of synthesis of Factors II, V, VII, IX and X. Thus, decreased synthesis of these Factors, particularly Factors V and IX because of their relatively short half-life, can lead to haemorrhagic problems (24). Specific therapy for the complex coagulation defects encountered can be difficult. In our experience, the mainstay of treatment has been fresh blood, since this provides platelets and coagulation factors. Fresh frozen plasma, triple strength plasma, platelet concentrates and Vitamin K have also been useful.

An important consideration is the optimal timing of liver resection, in relation to resection of the primary colonic tumour. Because of the risk of infection, the two resections should only be performed rarely at the same time. On the other hand, there is no need to wait for a prolonged period before proceeding to hepatic resection. Furthermore, there is no particular advantage in only selecting cases for resection who present with secondary tumours some years after removal of the primary.

In experienced hands, the mortality for liver resection is acceptable (19). The long-term results for patients undergoing hepatic resection offer at best the prospect of cure and at the very least, significant prolongation of life for many patients. In addition, hepatic resection can provide excellent palliation in some patients, particularly those presenting with symptoms referrable to the metastatic tumour.

REFERENCES

1. Balasegaram M: Hepatic surgery: present and future. *Ann Roy College Surg England* 47: 139 158, 1970.
2. Bengmark S and Hafstrom L: The natural history of primary and secondary malignant tumours of the liver. *Cancer* 23: 198-202, 1969.
3. Blumgart LH, Leach KG and Karran SJ: Observations on liver regeneration after right hepatic lobectomy. *Gut* 12: 922-928, 1971.
4. Blumgart LH: Biliary tract obstruction – New approaches to old problems *Amer J Surg* 135: 19-31, 1978a.
5. Blumgart LH: Liver atrophy, hypertrophy and regenerative hyperplasia in the rat: The relevance of blood flow. In: 'Hepatotrophic Factors': *Ciba Foundation Symp* 55, Porter, Ruth and Whelan, Julie (eds.), p 181-205, North-Holland, Elsevier/Excerpta Medica.
6. Blumgart LH, Drury JK and Wood CB: Hepatic resection for trauma, tumour and biliary obstruction *Br J Surg* 66: 762-769, 1979.
7. Fortner JG, Kim DK, Maclean BJ, Barrett MK, Iwatsuki S, Turnbull AD, Hawland WS and Beattie EJ: Major hepatic resection for neoplasia. Personal experience in 108 patients *Ann Surg* 188: 363-371, 1978.

8. Foster JH: Survival after liver resection. *Cancer* 26: 493-502, 1970.

9. Furnival CM, Mackenzie RJ, MacDonald GA and Blumgart LH: The mechanism of impaired coagulation after partial hepatectomy in the dog. *Surg Gynecol Obstet* 143: 81-86, 1976.

10. Goldsmith NA and Woodburne RT: The surgical anatomy pertaining to liver resection. *Surg Gynecol obstet* 105: 310-318, 1957.

11. Goligher JC: *Surgery of the anus, rectum and colon.* 3rd edition p. 505, London: Bailliere Tindall, 1975.

12. Jaffe BM, Donegan WL, Watson F and Spratt JS Jr: Factors influencing survival in patients with untreated heptic metastases. *Surg Gynecol Obstet* 127: 1-11, 1968.

13. Lucas CE and Walt AJ: Critical decisions in liver trauma. *Arch Surg* 101: 277-281, 1970.

14. Lucas CE and Walt AJ: Analysis of randomised biliary drainage for liver trauma in 189 patients. *J Trauma* 12: 925-930, 1972.

15. Mackenzie RJ Furnival CM, Wood CB, O'Keane Maureen A and Blumgart LH: The effects of prolonged hepatic ischaemia before 70% partial hepatectomy in the dog. *Br J Surg* 64: 66-69, 1977.

16. McIndoe AH and Counsellor VS: The bilaterality of the liver. *Arch Surg* 15: 589-594, 1927.

17. Morris MJ, Newland RC, Marks JE, Levin B, Platz CE and Skinner DB: Factors influencing local recurrence after abdomino-perineal section for cancer of the rectum and rectosigmoid. *Br J Surg* 62: 727-730, 1975.

18. Nielsen J, Balslev I and Jensen HE: Carcinoma of the colon with liver metastases: Operative indications and prognosis. *Acta Chir Scand* 137: 463-465, 1971.

19. Ong GB and Lee NW: Hepatic resection. *Br J Surg* 62: 421-430, 1975.

20. Oxley EM and Ellis H: Prognosis of carcinoma of the large bowel in the presence of liver metastases. *Br J Surg* 59: 149-152, 1969.

21. Smith R: Carcinoma of the gall bladder and extrahepatic bile ducts. Operative procedures. In: *Abdominal Operations.* Maingot R (ed.), Ch. 50, Appleton Century Crofts, New York 1974.

22. Starzl TE, Putnam CW, Porter KA, Halgrimson CG, Corman J Brown BI, Gotlin RW, Rodgerson DO and Greene HL: Portal diversion for the treatment of glycogen storage disease in humans. *Ann Surg* 178: 525-539, 1973.

23. Starzl TE, Bell RH, Beart RW and Putnam CW: Hepatic trisegmentectomy and other liver resections. *Surg Gynecol Obstet* 141: 429-437, 1975.

24. Vajrabukka T, Bloom AL, Sussman M, Wood CB and Blumgart LH: Post-operative problems and management after hepatic resection for blunt injury to the liver. *Br J Surg* 62: 189-200, 1975.

25. Wanebo HJ, Stearns M and Schwartz MK: Use of CEA as an indicator of early recurrence and as a guide to a selected second-look procedure in patients with colorectal cancer. *Ann Surg* 188: 481-493, 1978.

26. Williamson BWA, Blumgart LH and McKellar NJ: Management and tumors of the liver. Combined use of arteriography and venography in the assessment of resectability, especially in hilar tumors. *Amer J Surg* 139: 210-215, 1980.

27. Wilson S and Adson MA: Surgical treatment of hepatic metastases from colorectal cancer. *Arch Surg* 3: 330-334, 1976.

28. Wood CB, Gillis CR and Blumgart LH: A retrospective study of the natural history of patients with liver metastases from colorectal cancer. *Clin Oncol* 2: 285-288, 1976.

29. Wood CB and Blumgart LH: Unpublished data, 1980.

26. MAGNETIC COLOSTOMY

W. SCHELLERER

A simple method to establish a continent ostomy, using magnetic material, was described by Feustel and Henning (1). This device is commercially available and used all over Europe. Our years of experience with the magnetic closure system for colostomies and ileostomies are summarized briefly here.

GENERAL DESCRIPTION

The Erlanger Magnetic Continent Ostomy system consists of a samarium cobalt ring, encased in palacos, a PMMA plastic, which is implanted in the abdominal wall during ostomy construction, and a corresponding magnetic cap which is composed of the external magnet, and a core magnet and a washer.

INDICATIONS

The system can be used in colostomy patients. As a secondary operation, a magnetic ring can be placed around a preexisting ostomy (except a loop ostomy).

The magnetic ostomy system is not recommended under certain conditions:

1. Obesity: In the obese patient with a subcutaneous fat tissue of more than 3.5 cm, a magnetic closure system should be strenuously avoided, since the magnetic power will be diminished and the distance between ring and cap will be too great.
2. Thinness: In a thin patient with subcutaneous fat tissue of less than 1 cm, the magnetic power is too strong and may lead to pain when the cap is in situ. The patient with fat tissue of more than 1 cm and less than 3.5 cm seems to be the ideal candidate.
3. Advanced disease: If palliative surgery results in a clear survival period of only a few months, it is of questionable worth to implant the magnetic ostomy system. However, if longer survival is contemplated, the device may be advantageous.

K. Welvaart et al. (eds.), Colorectal Cancer, 241-247. All rights reserved.
Copyright © 1980 by Martinus Nijhoff Publishers, The Hague/Boston/London.

4. Contamination: If the rectum was lacerated during mobilization and the peritoneal cavity soiled by feces, implantation of a magnetic ring should be performed at a second stage.

5. Impaired cerebral function: Patients must be mentally allert in order to cope with using the magnetic colostomy system. Cerebral deterioration, which renders the patient incapable of self-care, contraindicates the use of the magnetic device.

6. Scarring: Abdominal scars in the choice areas for ostomy siting can prevent secure fitting of the magnetic cap. Unless a flat, smooth, abdominal surface can be provided, the device should not be used.

7. Crohn's disease: implantation of a magnetic ring should not be considered in patients with granulomatous colitis.

THE PREOPERATIVE CARE

Informing the Patient

Prior to surgery, the patient should be thoroughly advised concerning the magnetic device. The purpose of the cap and ring should be discussed, and the patient must be made aware of the results of implanting this device.

Bowel Preparation

Preparation is the same as for traditional large bowel surgery. Physical bowel preparation should be thorough to minimize fecal content.

Stoma Siting

Colostomy placement. 'We must take as much care in constructing our 'magnetic' colostomies as we are accustomed to taking with our ileostomies. 'This statement by Goligher (6) has to be kept in mind.

The maintenance of continence depends on the ability of the magnetic cap to fit flat to the abdominal wall. This necessitates a flat, smooth skin surface, free of folds, away from bone prominences, and away from the waistline. The colostomy and laparotomy wounds have to be kept separate. Septic complications of the laparotomy wound are frequent after rectal excision. To prevent spreading of the infection from the laparotomy wound to the magnetic ring, an entirely separate colostomy incision should be established. Using a median incision, the colostomy should be sited lateral to the left rectus muscle above the external oblique muscle. It should not be placed too close to the costal margin, not on top of a vault, and not too far laterally. Once the stoma site has been selected, it has to be observed with the thighs reflexed, in the sitting position, standing upright, bending forward, walking, and dressed in order to observe the formation of a fold of skin. The skin around the colostomy has to remain flat. In general the selected site is situated higher than is customary for an ileal colostomy.

Preparation of the Magnetic Ring

The ring should not be autoclaved but gas-sterilized with ethylene. (It is delivered by the manufacturer gas-sterilized.) The PMMA plastic of the ring will become porous if the system is heated to over 90°C. When inside the body, the magnetic material would then be oxidized.

At the beginning of the operation, the magnetic ring has to be soaked in an antibiotic solution (kanamycin). In primary implantation, two separate tables should be prepared by the assisting nurse: one for the intraabdominal part of the colonic recession and the other with the instruments and the magnetic ring. The surgeon should change gloves before putting the ring in place.

Antibiotic Preparation

Antibiotics should be parenterally administered just before the operation and continued for six days postoperatively. We prefer a combination of ampicillin and oxacillin.

OPERATIVE TECHNIQUE

Principles

The final decision to implant the magnetic ring is made after the abdomen is opened. In constructing the stoma the surgeon must be aware of the shape and size of the standard plug. If the stoma embraces the plug perfectly and evenly, the result will be good. Pressure points may lead to ulceration or secondary infection.

Listed below are some principles which will help avoid potential problems that may lead to postsurgical difficulty in providing a continent system.
1. Excise a disk of skin, for colostomies 2.5 cm in diameter. Too tight a fit will lead to pressure necrosis, too loose a fit to incontinence.
2. The bowel must lead through the abdominal wall at a right angle.
3. The ring must be fixed in order to avoid migration in the subcutaneous tissue. The sheath of the muscle must be sutured to Scarpa's fascia inside

the buried ring so as to avoid drawing in the skin (thus distorting the stoma). The sutures must not, therefore, include any fat superficial to Scarpa's fascia.

4. The skin-to-mucosa stitch must not be placed so as to evert a flange of mucosa. Nonabsorbable sutures should be used.

General Guidelines

Creation of a pocket for the ring. At the chosen stoma site a disk of skin with underlying subcutaneous fat is excised. The deeper fibrous portion of the subcutaneous tissue, the fascia of Scarpa, is incised. The fascia is separated by sharp and blunt dissection from the underlying muscle sheath. Between the subcutaneous tissue and the muscle aponeurosis a space for the ring is created by finger dissection. Now a cruciate incision is made through the muscle aponeurosis, and the muscle fibers are cut by means of diathermy. The cruciate incisions of the aponeurosis are 2.5 cm long.

Route of insertion. After removal of the rectum in colostomy construction, the left-lateral peritoneum is incised at its deepest point. An extra-peritoneal tunnel is created by blunt finger dissection up to the ostomy site. The magnetic ring is brought to its position through this tunnel. Care has to be taken that the flange of the magnetic ring (south pole) points toward the outside. The magnetic ring is positioned in the prepared space. Although most surgeons prefer to insert the ring through the excised skin opening of the ostomy, some prefer to open a pocket anterior to the muscle sheath via the laparotomy incision and to close the pocket with a few stitches after insertion.

Suturing of the magnetic ring. The cruciate incised muscle fascia is stitched to the edges of the dense plane of subcutaneous tissue (Scarpa's fascia). It is essential for good function of the magnetic closure that the ring be placed strictly parallel to the skin above. The stitches, therefore, must not include undue parts of fat lying superficial to Scarpa's fascia. Four stay sutures, one at each quadrant, are placed first and remain untied, held by a clamp. A circumferential series of eight to ten sutures is done next. The sutures are of absorbable material (Vicryl 3-0 or Dexon 2-0) and are tied immediately. The stay sutures are tied last. The placing of the sutures requires some skill, since the magnetic power of the ring attracts the forceps, the needleholder, and the needle. The ring must be covered totally with tissue, so that inspection from the front shows the ring completely concealed from view. Then the ring remains in place and cannot migrate in the subcutaneous tissue. However, one must take care not to narrow the lumen of the ring too much by taking too large a-bite with the needle. It is advisable to remove a too large bite and replace it. Occasionally, in this people, a stitch is made through the corium of the skin above, producing unevenness of the surrounding of the stoma. The skin must be separated with plastic surgery scissors or a small scalpel. The surroundings of the stoma have to remain even, otherwise skin shrinkage and scar formation, which lead to minor leakage afterward, will occur.

Drawing through the terminal bowel. The next step is to put the terminal bowel in place. After division with the aid of an autosuture machine, the bowel is covered with a latex contraceptive sheath firmly tied by a ligature. the bowel stump is guided through the retroperitoneal channel by pulling on a hemostat, which was inserted from the outside, and gentle pulling of the bowel with the other hand. Now, further attention is brought to reconstruction of the peritoneum and closing of the laparotomy incision. The laparotomy wound is covered with sterile dressing, and the bowel is shortened to its definitive length at the skin level.

Appositional sutures of bowel to skin should not go through the mucosa. We prefer reverse stitches with nonabsorbable material. Four to six stitches are sufficient to achieve a good adaption of the bowel to the skin.

Ostomy dressing. An adhesive appliance should not be placed around the colostomy in the operation room. This might create a moist chamber and lead to infection of the ring. We prefer to dress wound with gauze pads. The area surrounding the ileostomy is covered with Stomahesive, and an adherent bag is applied immediately.

In secondary implantation it is best, provided the stoma is in a correct position, to make a circular incision around the stoma, by means of a circular knife, through the skin down to the fascia. Then the magnetic ring is buried just above the fascia and it is fixed, somewhat differently from a primary implantation technique, by suturing the Scarpa's fascia to the dense fibrous tissue along the bowel going through the subcutaneous tissue. Then a Redovac drain is inserted and the skin stitches are tied. This is a simple method that can be performed under local anesthesia.

If the stoma has to be resited, a laparotomy should be performed. If the stoma is too large, it should be made smaller.

Temporary Care of Magnetic Ostomy

Colostomy. In the postoperative period the management of the EMCO is not different from that of a colostomy without a magnetic ring. The gauze should be renewed daily until the bowel starts to work again and produces stools or gas. The onset of stool production is unsually somewhat delayed, as compared to the conventional colostomy. There is some swelling of the colon, as it is held by the ring, and the lumen is narrowed. By the fifth day an adhesive appliance is attached.

The area surrounding the stoma must be watched carefully every day. Infection during the first 10 days postoperatively indicates a poor prognosis for the healing of the ring. If there is pus escaping at the mucocutaneous junction, or if a part of the inner circle of the ring can be seen, one should not hesitate to remove the ring as soon as possible. Reinforcing sutures will not suffice to keep the ring. It inevitably will be rejected.

Diet. A special diet is not necessary after implantation of a magnetic ostomy system.

Evacuation methods. When the patient begins to wear the cap it is possible to effect bowel evacuation in several ways. The surgeon, nurse, or stomal therapist, together with the patient, will have to determine the best method for each individual. Here are two of the recommended methods for easy bowel evacuation:

1. The cap may simply be removed when the need to evacuate occurs and the bowel contents allowed to pass directly into the toilet.
2. The cap may be removed and a temporary adhesive bag placed over the stoma; the bowel contents then pass into the bag. The appliance is then removed and discarded, and the cap with the washer is reapplied. This can be done at bedtime or upon rising and may work well with those ostomates with fairly regular bowel evacuation patterns. The bag may be worn through the night if it is convenient for the patient.

Following bowel evacuation, the peristomal area should be cleansed and the cap reapplied, always being sure that the washer is clean. Tissues or toilet paper are natural materials for this procedure. Small amounts of mucous secretions can be wiped off the filter washer with a moistened tissue, but a soiled washer should be changed to prevent leakage.

Now what are our results? These are our latest figures: 219 magnetic colostomies: There are 138 primary and 81 secondary operations. 26% of the patients died in the follow-up period. 20% of the rings had to be removed and there was no significant difference whether they were primary or secondary operations. The 'continence' – which is a debatable word, I could better call it 'success rate' – is 68 to 66%.

As you may see in our first series, when we were not aware of all the technical details necessary for good function, we had poor results. We had to remove more rings than in the second series where we had 80% good results and 10 to 20% rings to remove.

In the last few years we have not made as many magnetic rings, as we did before. The reason for this is that we had a nurse trained in the Cleveland

Clinic as a stoma therapist and we started to use the irrigation technique routinely. It is our policy now to tell the patient first to try the irrigation technique and, only if it fails, to have the magnetic colostomy inserted.

Another reason for implanting fewer magnetic rings in recent years is that we realized that a lot of patients with a perfectly fitted cap do not use it and use an adhesive bag instead of the cap. This is not a very encouraging result.

The next problem is the price of the ring. A magnetic system costs DM 900 now. However, these expenses can be repeated, as the cap is easily destroyed if it falls onto stony ground. Then the question of who must pay for the cap arises. The hospital cannot provide the patient with more and more new caps, to be paid for by the hospital.

I want, at least, to present a newly developed closure system for colostomies that is called STOMAVENT. This is an inexpensive, simple thing that avoids the disadvantages of a magnetic ring. It costs about as much as a month's supply of adhesive bags. It is fixed by a girdle and may be used in combination with the irrigation technique.

REFERENCES

1. Feustel H, Hennig G: Kontinente Kolostomie durch Magnetverschluß. *Dtsch Med Wochenschr* 100: 1063, 1975.
2. Feustel H: Kontinente Kolostomie durch Magnetverschluß. Erlangen, Habilitationsschrift, 1975.
3. Goligher JC: MACLET Symposium, London, Dec 10-11, 1976.
4. Heald: MACLET Symposium, London, Dec 10-11, 1976.
5. Hansen HH, Stelzner F: Zur chirurgischen Anatomie der Arterienversorgung der Dickdarmwand. *Langenbecks Arch Chir* 340: 63, 1975.
6. Goligher JC: Extraperitoneal colostomy or ileostomy. *Br J Surg* 46: 97, 1958.
7. Schellerer W.: The magnetic ring and the ostomy. In: *Surgery Annual* 10: 152-173, 1978. Herausgeber: Lloyd M. Nyphus. Appleton-Century-Crofts, New York (angeforderte Arbeit) Springer-Verlag, Berlin-Heidelberg-New York.
8. Schellerer W.: Erlanger Continent Magnetic Colostomy. In: *Intestinal Stomas*, 36-50, 1978. Herausgeber: Iann B. Todd, William Heinemann Medical Books, Ltd., London (angeforderte Arbeit). ISBN 0433325011.

27. COLOSTOMY CARE

ANNE EARDLEY

Colostomy care is associated in most people's minds with teaching patients
how to change their bags. Although that is obviously a necessary skill, I am
not going to discuss such specific aspects of caring for the patient with a
stoma. I prefer to treat colostomy care in a much wider sense. The dictionary
defines caring for someone as 'giving them serious attention or feeling concerned for them'. If we are to care for patients in the fullest sense of the word,
then it helps to have something more than an impressionistic understanding
of the impact of stoma surgery on the lives of patients and their families. As
Sutherland et al. (1) in a celebrated study published in 1952, wrote:

> 'Effective management of the colostomy patient cannot be achieved
> unless the widespread impact [of the operation] is clearly recognised.'

There is another reason for finding out how patients manage with their
colostomy: the problem of getting patients to come for treatment when the
cancer was at an early stage has been raised by more than one of the speakers
at this conference. Could it be that some potential patients (particularly those
of an older generation) delay because they are frightened of the possible cure?

Consider this statement from one of the people I interviewed:

> 'It was a shock when I heard I'd got to have a colostomy. I'd heard
> about people who had to wear a bag at the side – I'd always had a
> dread of it, because a friend had told me once about someone who had
> had it, and she said she could hardly bear to go into the same room.'

There have been a number of investigations over the years into this topic of
life with a stoma. It seems paradoxical that the more recent studies have
presented more pessimistic views than the earlier ones did, as the last two
decades have shown a marked improvement in the quality and variety of
stoma appliances and related products.

In 1934 Lockhart-Mummery (2) wrote the following:

> 'Many patients who have colostomy openings live very active lives –
> hunt, play golf, shoot, dance, dine out, travel and perform all the
> other activities of a normal person. A little patience and practice are
> required to learn how best to manage themselves, but once this is

acquired, they should experience little, if any, inconvenience and no-one but themselves and their family need know that they are in any way abnormal.'

Contrast this with the sober words of Devlin et al. (3) who drew our attention to

'The immense price paid by the patient for his cure from cancer, a price paid in physical discomfort, and in psychological and social trauma.'

and Dudley (4), writing in the *British Medical Journal* in 1978 on the salutary subject of 'If I had carcinoma of the middle third of the rectum', stated

'However managed, however much we delude ourselves, a permanent, potentially incontinent abdominal anus is an affront difficult to bear, so that I marvel that we and our patients have put up with it so long. It says much for the social indifference of the one and the social fortitude of the other.'

Most clinicians will be able to recall patients of theirs who have, to all intents and purposes, made a successful adjustment to living with a stoma, and if they are honest, may also recall others who have never been able to come to terms with it. The aim of my study was to attempt to explain these differences, by seeking to identify factors in the patient's experience of living with a stoma which affected his or her current adjustment.

As the first step in my research, I reviewed the literature on the social and psychological effects of colostomy. As the above quotations indicate, conclusions were varied, but this in itself suggested that the experience of living with a stoma was not easily predictable; on the other hand, few studies could explain such differences in psychological terms, that is, no pre-existing personality factors have been consistently identified as likely to produce problems after surgery.

METHOD

The names of 101 patients who had had their operation within the last five years were drawn from the operations registers of the four hospitals participating in the study. All were sent a letter explaining the purpose of the survey and requesting an interview. Ninety-four replied – a response rate of 93%. Eighteen of these patients had an ileostomy. Men and women were represented in equal proportions; the social class distribution was as shown in table 1. Seventy-two patients had had their operation for cancer, 14 for ulcerative colitis, 3 for diverticular disease and 5 for Crohn's disease. One-third had had

Table 1. Social class.[a]

Class	Percentage
Non-manual	34
Skilled manual	36
Unskilled	30
Total	100

[a] Based on Registrar-General's *Classification of Occupations.*

Table 2. Information about the operation.

Did not understand operation	—	16%
Not satisfied with information	—	30%

Table 3. Information given on management

Satisfied	Number	Percent
Yes	61	65
No	33	35
Total	94	100

their stoma for less than a year, 45% for between 1 and 3 years, and 25% for between 3 and 5 years.

I will divide the presentation of the data into three parts relating to the three sections of the interview schedule, namely, the hospital experience, experiences in the first few weeks after discharge, and the current position.

The hospital experience. The majority of those interviewed said that they understood what sort of operation they were going to have, but 16% had not understood, and over a third said that they had not been told where the stoma would be sited. Most felt that they had been given enough information about the operation beforehand, but 30% said they would have liked more information (table 2).

Although most patients were proficient in the use of their appliance by the time they left hospital, taking all aspects of *managing* the stoma together, with regard to appliance, diet, obtaining further supplies or further advice, 35% felt they could have been given more practical information before leaving hospital (table 3). To quote one of those interviewed,

'It was a bit worrying trying to use these bags at home. I thought that's where they were a little bit lax. Perhaps they thought I could cope. There could have been someone who dealt just with this. You saw different nurses and not one individual who knew enough about it.'

Early problems. Patients were asked what they thought had been their biggest problem in the early days after discharge from hospital. Only 10% said they could not recall having any problems. The largest category of problems mentioned by 44% were those related to managing the stoma:

'Equipment was the biggest problem. The appliance they sent me home with wasn't odourproof, so I was confined to the house. Life came to a standstill.'

Almost a fifth mentioned more general problems of adjustment:

'The only problem I was having to face was "would I be able to do what I'd done before?"'

and 60% said that they had felt depressed at first:

'I couldn't pull myself together; I'm not used to feeling defeated.'

What impact did the *follow-up care* provided by the hospital have upon the resolution of these early problems? A rather limited one on the evidence of these interviews. Thirty-seven per cent of patients expressed dissatisfaction with some aspect of aftercare: this patient's comment was typical:

'It's all very brief – they just ask me if I've any pain, that's all – I know time is a factor, but I feel – well, why do they ask me to go?'

Current problems. By the time patients were interviewed, some of these early problems had been resolved, in some cases through trial and error, in others with the help and support of relatives, friends, community nurses, occasionally general practitioners or the self-help organisations, but the picture was far from ideal.

When asked whether they felt their appliance could be improved in any way, almost half expressed some dissatisfaction with the appliance they were currently using. Problems with sore skin, leakage and odour were far from uncommon. As far as diet was concerned, for almost half eating habits had not changed substantially since the operation, but a quarter of colostomy patients reported several restrictions and a similar proportion found control over bowel movements a problem because of their frequency or unpredictability. Taking all these problems together, 63% of all patients had some current problem related to managing the stoma (table 4).

Table 4. Current management problems.

Some dissatisfaction with appliance	—	48%
Several dietary restrictions	—	25%
Problems of 'control' over bowel movements	—	25%
Some current management problem	—	63%

Coming on to the wider effects of the colostomy, of those who were working, one-third had either changed their job because of the stoma or were working fewer hours because of it, although only one person felt markedly restricted in his current work. As far as social and leisure activities were concerned, 24% of colostomy patients said that their social life had been curtailed because of the stoma and 17% reported some restriction in leisure and household activities. Sixteen per cent found travelling a problem and 15% had not been on holiday for reasons connected with the stoma. All in all, 40% of those interviewed were experiencing some form of restriction attributable to the stoma.

Thirty per cent said that the operation had had some effect on their sex life: two-thirds of these patients were men. Although it is likely that some of the difficulties experienced were organic in origin, psychological factors and problems of managing the stoma were undoubtedly responsible for some restrictions:

> 'I wouldn't approach my wife – not with this at the front.'

How did people feel about having a colosomy once they had got over the initial shock? As already mentioned, 60% experienced early feelings of depression. At the time of the interview, two-thirds of patients said that they either never felt depressed about having a colostomy, or only occasionally did so:

> 'I sometimes feel it's a nuisance – I wish I'd had gallstones or something that wasn't permanent.'

Only 4 people experienced a continuing depression or resentment:

> 'It's like waking up and the nightmare's real.'

But 19% had occasional feelings of depression which were not easily dismissed:

> 'Sometimes I think "I wish I could cut this thing off – why should it happen to me?"'

However, when asked whether they were now used to living with a stoma, 94% replied that they were:

'Yes, I forget I've got it.'

'Once I got into a routine I was all right.'

And in answer to the question 'Do you ever regret having it done?' only 8 patients expressed unqualified regret. When asked to say what they felt was the biggest drawback to having a colostomy, 41% could not think of any (table 5). Of those who could think of some, the largest category related to some aspect of managing the stoma. As one patient put it:

'The inconvenience of the bag.'

Before going on to discuss the implications of these findings, it is relevant to present three correlations. First, present depression was more prevalent among those experiencing current problems of managing the stoma (table 6). Secondly, those who reported some restriction due to having a stoma were more likely to be experiencing current problems of management (table 7). And finally, patients with current management problems were more likely to have expressed dissatisfaction with the amount of practical information they had received before leaving the hospital (table 8). I would argue that it is these correlations which provide us with new insights into the experience of the patient with a stoma, and suggest ways of improving current practice.

Although I have concentrated on the negative side of patients' experiences after stoma surgery, my intention has not been to paint a gloomy picture, or to imply that having a colostomy invariably leads to a decline in the quality of life. What I hope to have shown is that restrictions are not inevitable. Hospital staff have three main opportunities for affecting the course of the patient's rehabilitation: before the operation, after the operation but before the patient is discharged, and in the follow-up clinic. But at each of these stages it is vital that the information conveyed should go both ways. Good practice on the part of hospital staff does not consist solely of dispensing a standard 'pre-scription of information' to every patient. Although it is important that certain concrete aspects related to having a stoma should be conveyed rou-tinely, it is equally important to recognise the variation among patients. Such

Table 5. Biggest drawback to having a stoma (n = 76).

Drawback	Percent
None	41
Management	34
Psychological/social factors	12
Physical factors	13
Total	100

Table 6. Problems of management/ present depression (percentages).

Problems	Present depression	
	Yes	No
Problems of management	91	56
No problems of management	9	44
Total	100	100

Table 7. Problems of management/restricted activities (percentages).

Problems	Restriction	
	Yes	No
Problems of management	84	38
No problems of management	16	62
Total	100	100

Table 8. Problems of management/satisfaction with information on management.

Problems	Satisfaction with information on management	
	Yes	No
Problems of management	59	70
No problems of management	41	30
Total	100	100

variation in attitudes and experiences can be detected only by carefully listening to the patient.

BEFORE THE OPERATION

I would not presume to recommend that every prospective stoma patient be given a standard lecture on surgical technique. A far more satisfactory service can be provided if doctors and nurses are receptive to the patient's reaction to the operation: what does he or she know already about colostomies? Are their fears warranted, or are they based on out-of-date information? How far does the patient understand what is being done to him or her?

Orbach and Tallent's study (5) shows that stoma patients who were confused about the nature of the surgery could be left with a sense of having been assaulted and with a conception of one's body as fragile. If this sense of weakness did not lessen with time, it led to a curtailment of activity not warranted by the operation.

Conversely, a recent study by Johnson et al. (6) indicates that where patients are provided with what they term 'sensory information' – on what the patient can expect to feel about the results of surgery, post-operative stress is reduced.

AFTER THE OPERATION

After the operation it is self-evident that every patient should be proficient in the use of an appliance before leaving hospital. The consequences of difficulties over managing the stoma have been clearly illustrated in the data already presented. What is less commonly realised is the danger of supplying dogmatic advice to patients – whether it be dispensing the same type of appliance, the same rigid dietary strictures, or the same timetable for a return to normal activities to all patients.

AFTER CARE

The visit to the follow-up clinic is the clinician's only chance to ascertain whether the patient is achieving an optimum level of rehabilitation. Ironically, the barriers to communication between staff and patient which pervade the hospital system are often most apparent in the out-patient setting. Few of the problems experienced by the patients in my study had been resolved by a visit to the out-patient department, although there was evidence that some had received helpful advice by paying an informal visit to the ward on which they had been a patient.

It is beyond the scope of this paper to discuss the nature of these barriers to communication. But where such barriers can be lowered, the benefits to doctors and patients alike are potentially very great indeed. For example, a sensitive interview by the doctor who provides the after-care service can ascertain whether or not the individual patient is sustaining any unwarranted restrictions and appropriate intervention can follow. If, on the other hand, such restrictions go undetected, then as Druss et al. (7) have pointed out, there is a risk that for the elderly person in particular, whose operation comes at a time of 'declining social, vocational and sexual prowess', the creation of a stoma could lead to what they term 'an early retirement from life'.

Is it the doctor's responsibility to ensure that the patient is not incapacitated by the treatment he provides? Devlin (8) has written

'There is no doubt that in the final analysis any surgeon who in any way mutilates a patient must make himself aware of, and responsible for, the necessity of rehabilitating that patient. But he cannot do this unaided.'

The author was referring here to the role of the stoma therapist. I would suggest that he cannot do it without the help of the patient, either. Although some problems after colostomy can be solved by technical expertise, others – typically those affecting interpersonal relationships in the areas of sex, social life and leisure – do not have a strictly medical solution. The answers to these problems can only be gained from patients who have experienced them, and overcome them. If patients are treated as active participants in rehabilitation, with a valuable contribution to make in building up an effective advisory service, this would go some way towards minimising the present social costs of this type of surgery.

REFERENCES

1. Sutherland AM, Orbach CE, Dyk RB and Bard M: The psychological impact of cancer and cancer surgery. Adaptation to the dry colostomy: preliminary report and summary of findings. *Cancer* 5: 857-72, 1952.
2. Lockhart-Mummery JP: *Diseases of the rectum and colon and their surgical treatment*, Baillière, Tindall and Co., London, 1934 (2nd edition).
3. Devlin HB, Plant JH and Griffin M: Aftermath of surgery for anorectal cancer *Br Med J* 3: 413-18, 1971.
4. Dudley HAF: If I had carcinoma of the middle third of the rectum. *Br Med J* 1: 1035-1037, 1978.
5. Orbach CE and Tallent N: Modification of perceived body and of body concepts following the construction of a colostomy. *Arch General Psych* 12: 126-35, 1965.
6. Johnson JE, Fuller SS, Endress MP, Rice VH: Altering patients' responses to surgery: an extension and replication. *Res Nursing Health* 1: 3, 111-121, 1978.
7. Druss RG, O'Connor JF, Stern LO: Psychologic adjustment to colectomy. Part II. Adjustment to a permanent colostomy. *Arch General Psych* 20: 419-27, 1969.
8. Devlin HB: Colostomy care. *Nursing Mirror* 70: 16, 576-577, 1974.

PART VI

POSTOPERATIVE MANAGEMENT

28. CHEMOTHERAPY IN METASTATIC DISEASE

M.G. HERBEN

The results of the medical management of patients with metastatic colorectal cancer are still very disappointing. Large bowel cancer has been one of the most extensively evaluated solid tumors with regard to drug treatment. However, at the present time, little progress has been made in the effective treatment of symptoms due to metastatic spread of the disease.

Since its introduction into clinical trial over 20 years ago, 5-fluorouracil (5FU) remains the most effective palliative agent.

In contrast with other solid tumor treatment trials, combination chemotherapy has failed to improve the response rates reported with the use of 5FU alone.

SINGLE AGENT CHEMOTHERAPY

Although there has been vast experience with the use of 5FU, the literature devoted to this drug is replete with confusing and contradictary data. There exists a lack of uniformity in criteria for selecting patients and for evaluating therapeutic response.

The lesions of colorectal cancer can frequently be very difficult to measure; this phenomenon is well illustrated by the results of a comparable method of administration of 5FU therapy in large bowel cancer. The percentage of objective regressions, as reported in the literature, ranges from 8 to 85% (table 1).

Moertel (1) has reviewed the relationship between the site of metastatic disease and therapeutic results with systemic 5FU and found that objective response rates varied from 6.4% (lungs) and 24% (liver) to 32% (abdomen) and 41% (skin and nodes) (table 2).

Many trials have been conducted to determine the optimum dose, schedule and systemic route of administration of 5FU. These studies have included comparisons of i.v. and oral loading courses, prolonged i.v. infusions versus i.v. push schedules, and weekly i.v. or oral schedules. All of the trials suffered from an intrinsically low response rate with 5FU. This makes it difficult to show definite superiority for any particular regimen. Table 3 shows the results of different systemic methods of administration of 5FU in colorectal

Table 1. Reported results of 5-fluorouracil therapy of large bowel cancer.

	Patients treated	Objective response %
Sharp and Benefiel	13	85
Hall and Good	19	63
Rochlin et al.	47	55
Allaire et al.	17	47
Cornell et al.	13	46
Everly	12	42
Field	37	41
Bell	22	36
Weiss and Jackson	37	35
Ferguson and Humphrey	12	33
Hurley	150	31
Eastern Cooperative group	48	27
Hyman et al.	30	20
Asnfield	141	17
Ellison	87	12
Kennedy	22	9
Knoepp et al	11	9
Olson and Green	12	8

from Moertel (1).

Table 2. The relationship of the site of primary (most clearly measureable) indicator lesion to therapeutic results of fluorinated pyrimidines.

Site of indicator lesion	No. of patients treated	Objective regressions (%)
Liver	118	24[1]
Lungs	78	6.4[1]
Abdomen	34	32[1]
Cutaneous and subcut.	31	16
Peripheral nodes	8	25
Other	8	25

1. $P < 0.01$ from Moertel (1).

Table 3. Systemic 5FU treatment of metastatic colon cancer.

	No. of patients	Response rate %
– Loading courses by i.v. push followed by either monthly reinduction or weekly maintenancy	277	22
– Oral loading courses	86	16
– Weekly i.v.	231	19
– Weekly oral	103	15
– Nontoxic loading	54	13
– Prolonged infusion	154	25

carcinoma. Data have been collected from randomized Mayo Clinic, COG, ECOG, WCSG series (table 3).

The use of *oral* 5FU has been based in part on the premise that the drug might be more efficacious by this route, especially in the treatment of hepatic metastases. The results obtained by randomized double blind studies by the Mayo Clinic and the Western Cancer Study Group failed to show any advantage of the oral route with respect to the effect of treatment upon liver metastases.

The *prolonged* infusion method reduces hematologic toxicity, but with an increased incidence of severe stomatitis. This method may allow more effective use of the drug in combination with other myelosuppressive agents. There seems to be no therapeutic advantage to prolonged infusion of 5FU.

In summary, *Systemic 5FU* treatment has given the most consistent response rates by loading courses or aggressive weekly maintenance with or without loading. It is now generally agreed that an objective response rate of 20% in advanced colorectal cancer is a realistic one. The remissions with 5FU are only of a short duration (2-3 months) with no significant increase in survival time for the responders compared to nonresponders. A large number of additional chemotherapeutic agents have undergone evaluation of activity in advanced large bowel cancer. The available information has been well summarized by Carter and Friedman (2) (table 4).

The overall remission rates with single agents are low and the duration of response has been quite short, varying from 1 to 3 months. However, most of the patients had prior 5FU therapy. The minimal drug activity found in 5FU refractory patients showed that second line single agent chemotherapy after 5FU failure is usually unsuccessful or of only marginal clinical value.

Table 4. Single agents with some degree of activity in large bowel cancer.

Drugs	Response		% Response
	No. obj. resp.	No. evaluable patients	
5FU	454	2107	21
MTX	19	111	17
Mitomycin C	35	218	26
Adriamycin	8	92	9
BCNU	15	104	14.5
MeCCNU	7	75	10
CCNU	12	77	15
DTIC	8	71	11
Hexamethylmelamine	10	86	11.5
Cyclophosphamide	24	89	27
Hydroxyurea	16	151	10
Melphalan	19	110	17

from Carter and Friedman (2).

Until now, there are no new developed agents which could be added to the already five year old list of (only minimally) active drugs in colorectal cancer.

COMBINATION CHEMOTHERAPY

Most combination chemotherapy regimens which have been evaluated over the past 10 years included *5FU with MethylCCNU*, the most favorable nitrosurea for colorectal cancer.

Using a combination of 5FU, MethylCCNU and Vincristine, Moertel (3) and Co-workers in 1975 reported a response rate of 43%, compared to 19% with 5FU alone.

Macdonald et al. (4) were able to confirm these results using the same drug combination and weekly 5FU instead of the 5-day loading schedule used by Moertel et al. (3). Falkson et al. (5) in 1976 have reported a 37% response with the combination regimen, versus a 22% response rate for 5FU alone.

On the basis of these data various clinical trials have been conducted with slight alteration in dosage schedules or routes of administration. However, more recent reports indicate that these favorable results have not been duplicated by other investigators.

Kemeny et al. (6) obtained only a 11% response rate with the combination. A possible explanation for this low response rate could be that the most common sites of metastatic desease in Kemeny's study were liver (66%) and lung (43%). The predominant site of metastatic disease may be an important factor in the evaluation of the therapeutic results of chemotherapy regimens.

The differences in response rates obtained in studies using the same drug combination and comparable criteria in the evaluation of response may partly be due to unequal distribution of patients according to the predominant site of metastatic disease. (table 5).

Determination of response is difficult to quantify especially in abdominal sites of metastatic desease. This may be another possible explanation for the contrasting experience with combined drug therapy in colorectal cancer.

The study by Baker et al. (7) failed to show a difference in response rate for liver metastasis (31.7%), compared to other sites of metastatic disease (31.5%). Buroker et al. (8) reported a 18% response rate in 93 patients with liver metastasis treated with MethylCCNU and 5FU administered as a 5-day continuous intravenous infusion.

Survival data in those studies indicating a higher response for the combination have failed to demonstrate a statistically significant difference between the 5FU alone and the 5FU plus MeCCNU treated groups of patients. This lack of effectiveness with regard to survival and the (hematologic) toxicity of the combination does not make the 5FU, MeCCNU regimen suitable for

Table 5. Comparison of studies using MeCCNU and 5FU in advanced colon cancer.

Study	No. of patients	Obj. resp	Site of *metastatic* disease		
			Liver	Lung	Abdominal, skin and nodes
Moertel (3)	39	43.5%	56%	38%	38%
Falkson and Falkson (4)	91	37 %	50%	26%	43%
Macdonald et al. (5)	25	40 %	64%	12%	48%
Kemeny et al. (6)	67	11 %	60%	43%	16%
Baker et al. (7)	151	31.8%	59%	25%	52%

Table 6. Drug combinations with only minimally activity in advanced colorectal cancer.

Study	Drug treatment	No. of pat.	Obj. resp.
Buroker et al. (8)	5FU inf. + Mitomycin	136	18%
Haller et al. (9)	5FU, Adria, Mitomycin	53	17%
Davis and Park (10)	5FU, Mitomycin, Adria., cytosine arabinoside	54	17%
Presant et al. (11)	Mitomycin, Cyclophosph. Methorexate	14	29%
Bedikion et al. (12)	5FU, Cycloph., CCNU	37	25%
White et al. (13)	5FU, MeCCNU, Daunorubicin	38	16%
Seligman et al. (14)	5FU + Streptozotocin	51	21%

standard clinical use in advanced colorectal carcinoma.

Many *other drug combinations* have been investigated. However, there is no regimen at this moment showing more effectiveness than could be expected from 5FU alone. (table 6).

In *summary* progress in systemic chemotherapy of metastatic colorectal cancer remains discouragingly slow. The most effective regimens produce only transient and incomplete tumor regression with considerable side effects.

It is evident that there is no chemotherapeutic regimen available at this moment of sufficient value to the patient with clinically established metastatic disease to justify its consideration as standard treatment.

REFERENCES

1. Moertel CG: Alimentary tract cancer: Large Bowel In: *Cancer Medicine*, Holland JF and Frei E III (eds.), Lea & Febiger, Philadelphia, 1974, p. 1597-1627.
2. Carter SK and Friedman M: Integration of chemotherapy into combined modality therapy of solid tumors. II. Large bowel carcinoma. *Cancer Treat Rev* 1: 114-128, 1974.
3. Moertel CG, Schutt AJ, Hahn RG et al.: Therapy of advanced colorectal cancer with a

combination of 5-fluorouracil, methyl-1,3-cis(2-chlorethyl)-1-nitrosourea and vincristine. *J Natl Cancer Inst* 54: 69, 1975.

4. Macdonald JS, Kisner DF, Smythe T et al.: 5-Fluorouracil (5-FU), Methyl-CCNU, and Vincristine in the treatment of advanced colorectal cancer: Phase II study utilizing weekly 5-FU. *Cancer Treat Rep* 60: 1597-1600, 1976.

5. Faldson G and Falkson HC: Fluorouracil, Methyl-CCNU and Vincristine in cancer of the colon. *Cancer* 38: 1468-1470, 1976.

6. Kemeny N, Yagoda A, Braun Jr. et al.: a randomized study of two different schedules of methyl CCNU, 5-FU and vincristine for metastatic colorectal carcinoma. *Cancer* 43: 78-82, 1979.

7. Baker LH, Vaitkevicius VK and Gehan E: Randomized prospective trial comparing 5-Fluorouracil (NSC-19893) to 5-Fluorouracil and Methyl.CCNU (NSC-95441) in advanced gastrointestinal cancer. *Cancer Treat Rep* 60: 733-737, 1976.

8. Buroker T, Kim PN, Groppe C, et al.: 5FU infusion with mitomycin-C versus 5FU infusion with Methyl-CCNU in the treatment of advanced colon cancer. *Cancer* 42: 1228-1233, 1978.

9. Haller DG, Woolley PV, Macdonald JS, et al.: Phase II trial of 5-Fluorouracil, Adriamycin, and Mitomycin C in advanced colorectal cancer. *Cancer Treat Rep* 62: 563-565, 1978.

10. Davis S, Park YK: Chemotherapy for colorectal cancer with a combination of 5-fluorouracil, miomycin C, adriamycim, and cytosine arabinoside; a pilot study. *Cancer Treat Rep* 62: 1557-1559, 1978.

11. Presant CA, Ratkin G, Klahr C: Phase II study of mitomycin C, Cyclophosphamide, and Methotrexate in drug-resistant colorectal carcinoma. *Cancer Treat Rep* 62: 549-550, 1978.

12. Bedikian AY, Staab R, Livingston R, et al.: Chemotherapy for colorectal cancer with 5-fluorouracil, cyclophosphamide, and CCNU; comparison of oral and continuous in administration of 5-fluorouracil. *Cancer Treat Rep* 62: 1603-1605, 1978.

13. White Jr. LA, Perry MC, Kardinal CG et al.: Phase II study of 5-fluorouracil, methyl-CCNU, and daunorubicin in colorectal cancer; a Cancer and Leukemia Group B study. *Cancer Treat Rep* 63: 215-217, 1979.

14. Seligman M, Bukowski RM, Groppe CW et al.: Chemotherapy of metastatic gastrointestinal neoplasms with 5-fluorouracil and streptozotocin. *Cancer treat Rep* 61: 1375-1377, 1977.

29. THE MANAGEMENT OF PAIN IN COLORECTAL CANCER

JOH. SPIERDIJK

In this paper I shall not deal with either the temporary postoperative pain which is expected to follow surgery or the treatment of intractable pain by palliative methods (surgery, radiotherapy and chemotherapy).

In contrast to the many patients with intractable pain, the cancer patient shows a direct relationship between the pain stimulus and the pain itself.

Although a specific disease can cause pain or intensify it, other factors can play a role. These factors are mainly affectional and emotional in nature and include the following.

Fear: of the diagnosis, the effectiveness of the therapy, the future (both their own and that of their family), the pain still to come, or a combination of these.

Experience: past experience with pain similar to that which made surgery or irradiation necessary.

Reactions of those around the patient: how do they react, what do they want to know about what the patient is experiencing, are they afraid of developing the same disease, do they show exaggerated concern or cheerfulness?

Personality: the patient's personality of course plays an important role in how they react to the pain. All of these points must be taken into account when pain control is attempted.

For these reasons the cancer patient with pain needs the good support of his family doctor and the surgeon who performed the operation. For these patients, drugs prescribed in a precise way by the doctor can often control the pain. These drugs are mostly analgesics, tranquilizers and anti-emetics.

I shall in the first part of this paper deal with drugs to be used in cancer patients. In the second part I shall discuss the use of neurolytic drugs in colorectal cancer, as well as the possibilities of percutaneous cordotomy.

In the first place, if after his surgical, chemical or X-ray treatment, a cancer patient starts to complain about pain you must be sure that you are not dealing with a recurrence of the tumor or a metastasis, which can still be treated by the original therapy. This means that sometimes a second operation or a new course of chemotherapy will be necessary. What I am saying is that before we start with treatment of pain we must be sure that we can no longer use any therapy directly related to the tumor.

ANALGESICS

It is preferable to start with oral drugs. Many patients have a favorite home remedy, usually a combined preparation with a pleasing name, which is taken irregularly and in uncontrolled amounts. In our opinion, the patient is benefited by strict regulation. Simple preparations or even combinations are often more helpful than the original one. The important thing is that the patient be given strict rules for taking his analgesic preparation. In this respect it is important to stay ahead of the pain. Analgesics must be given at fixed times, regularly and prophylactically. In some cases the patient will require a schedule including a dose to be taken during the night. A brief awakening to take the tablet can prevent hours of sleeplessness during the early morning hours. The patient must also know whether he is allowed to take an extra dosage and when it is allowed. An ideal analgesic has not yet been found.

The so-called 'as required' medications are both irrational and inhuman, according to Twycross (1). The use of a good schedule often means that the patient will respond well to simple analgesics. In our schedule we make a choice between:

acetosal	250-500 mg	4-6 daily	1 tablet
paracetamol	500 mg	4-6 daily	1 tablet
codeine	10- 30 mg	4-6 daily	1 tablet

These preparations can also be used in combination. In some cases glafenine (Glifanan®) in a dosage of 1 tablet 3-6 times daily is effective when these drugs do not give satisfactory results. If all four prove ineffective or are known to have been tried before and we are not ready to use opium derivatives, we make use of pentazocine (Fortral®). Pentazocine is available in 50 mg tablets, 50 mg suppositories and 30 mg/ml ampoules for injection. These dosages can be given 4-6 times daily. Fortral can lead to habituation. A higher dose must then be given, which is not objectionable if there are no side-effects (sweating, dizziness, nightmares or hallucinations). It should be mentioned that Fortral⁽ᵇ⁾ can be combined with the four medications mentioned above.

If painkilling is not achieved with any of these combinations we must resort to morphine preparations or other methods. Morphine preparations have the following characteristics:

a. Effects on the central nervous system:

    the patient becomes soporous,

    the pain threshold rises,

    the respiration frequency drops,

    the depth of respiration increases,

    coughing is depressed,

    the emetic chemoreceptor center is stimulated,

pupil contraction is induced via the oculomotor nerve;
b. Effects on the digestive tract:

the secretion of digestive fluid decreases,

the tones of the gut increases (mainly that of the sphincters).
c. Effect on metabolism:

the rate of metabolism decreases, leading

to a decrease in oxygen consumption.

All morphine preparations have the same side-effects. In addition it must be kept in mind that habituation is rapid, which means that the dose must be steadily increased to achieve the same analgesic effect. In the final stage of the disease there is no reason to withold high doses of morphine. Morphine can be given subcutaneously or intramuscularly in a dosage of 5-10 mg every 4-6 hours. Metadone (Symoron®) and nicomorphine (Vilan®) have the same side-effects as morphine.

When we prescribe analgesics it is good to know the equi-analgesic dosages i.e. the dosages which have approximately the same effect. For example, 100 mg pethidine is as effective as 10 mg morphine.

Equi-analgesic doses.

	mg
Morphine	10
Heroin	±5
Methadone	10
Idemerol	
= Pethidine	100
Nicomorphine	
= Vilan	10

The oral route of morphinomimetic drugs is still under discussion. In a liquid form the use of diamorphine and morphine is possible. The use of diamorphine was very popular in the United Kingdom, and is advocated by Saunders and Twycross (2). During the past few years it has been proven that if used in equi-analgesic dosages, there is no difference in the pain relief produced by these two drugs. Diamorphine makes the patient more euphoric. Drug addiction arises sooner with heroin than with morphine; this is not a problem for the patient but for those surround the patient.

Heroin is a very dangerous drug and must be avoided in medical practice. It has been proven that morphine in water is as effective as the 'Brompton Cocktail'. As an antidote for the respiratory side-effects of morphinomimetic drugs we recommend the use of 0.4-0.8 mg Nalloxone®. Because of the possibility of acute withdrawal effects, it is recommended that these drugs be given in small dosages until the desired effect is obtained.

Janssen Pharmaceutica has placed Burgodin or Bezitramide on the market in the Benelux (3). A tablet contains 5 mg. It is a strong analgesic with heavy side-effects. In experienced hands and with knowledge of the side-effects the drug is of great value.

If the patient cannot take a drug orally, injections have to be given. In my opinion morphine is the drug-of-choice in these cases. Nearly all patients treated with morphinomimetic drugs need a laxative. When vomiting exists because a trigger in the cerebrum is stimulated by drugs, an anti-emetic drug can help. If this vomiting arises from stimuli in the abdomen anti-emetic drugs will not help.

As already mentioned, pain and fear are inseparable. The abolition of fear must be carried out mainly by the people around the patient, but a good supportive effect can often be obtained by psychopharmaceutics. It must be kept in mind, however, that some of these drugs induce 'depression'.

NEUROLYTIC DRUGS

Cancer pain of colorectal origin, especially in the perineum and the sacral region, can be treated by the injection of neurolytic drugs intrathecally. Phenol (3-5% in water or glycerin) and absolute alcohol are the most commonly used neurolytic agents. In his book *Intractable pain*, Mehta (4) states that the intrathecal administration of 5% phenol in glycerin is the standard method for controlling pain in the cancer patient. When the dose is chosen precisely and the patient is placed in exactly the right position for the injection, the sensory fibers are eliminated and the motoric fibers are unaffected. This is particularly important for the maintenance of adequate bladder and bowel control. This treatment can give a dramatic reduction of pain.

Special Areas

Perineum. This is a common area of cancer pain, usually the first indication of secondary spread after pelvic operations, such as abdominoperineal resection. Good results are obtained if chemical neurectomy is performed early, as soon as the pain is 'fixed' and appears to be unresponsive to mild oral analgesics. It is unwise to wait for clinical or X-ray confirmation or neoplastic invasion when relief is much more difficult to attain.

The initial punture is made between L_5 and the sacrum, where withdrawal of C.S.F. may be difficult because the dural sac begins to taper at this point and the needle must be placed accurately in the mid-line. The main problem is to get the phenol from this level to the painful segments in the perineum ($S_{4,5}$ and L_4) which lie in between.

After the puncture at L_5-S_1 in the sitting position, the patient is tilted backwards at an angle of 15-30° with respect to the edge of the table, and 0.5 ml of 5% phenol in glycerin is injected slowly, taking at least a minute for the procedure. The needle is then withdrawn and the position maintained for 30 min. This maneuver also encourages slow gravitation of the hyperbaric phenol in glycerin along the posterior aspect of the subarachnoid space, away from the important sacral nerve roots, until it settles in the perineal hollow, where it exerts its destructive action on the pain fibers. Some authors advise doing this procedure first on one side and then, a few days later, on the other side. In our clinic, we normally give a local analgesic drug intrathecally as a prognostic block.

Sacral region. In the sacral region, the lumbar puncture is located at L_{4-5} or L_5-S_1 and the patient is turned onto the painful side with a slight cephalad inclination (10-15°). The position is maintained for 30 min after the injection of 0.5 ml of 5% phenol in glycerin, which drifts slowly downwards onto the painful segments. Complications of the bladder and rectum do not occur if control is normal before injection and phenol is administered on one side only. Pain in the outer regions of the buttock is notoriously difficult to relieve.

GENITO-URINARY COMPLICATIONS

Bladder and Bowel Dysfunction

This is the most common complication of this technique and is possible when sacral roots are involved or when there is a pre-existing disturbance of normal control. A common presentation is retention with overflow, and catheter drainage must be instituted at once. The nerves which innervate the urinary bladder are the following:
1. Nervus hypogastricus (sympathetic) arising at L_{2-5} with preganglionic fibers to the inferior mesenteric ganglion and the vesical plexus.
2. Nervus pelvicus (parasympathetic) arising at S_1-S_2-S_3.
3. Nervus pudendus (somatic) arising at S_3-S_4.
The pudendal nerve also innervates the external sphincter muscle of the anus. After resection of only the pudendal nerve incontinence occurs but micturition is still possible. If after resection of the pelvic nerves the pudendal nerves are also cut, micturition is abolished and replaced by continuous dribbling and a large residual volume of urine; however, eventually an automatic bladder appears.

Fortunately, as incontinence or retention is rare, permanent and normal conditions should return within six weeks. With meticulous attention to detail, the incidence of bladder complications can be kept below 5%. According to Maher the common sites where serious damage can be produced by phenol are:

1. At the sacral cord and the origin of the cauda equina, dysfunction follows injection between D_{12} and L_1. This is probably caused by the needle going too deeply into the theca.
2. Crossing the cauda equina at the level of L_3-L_4, retention is less serious and is due to involvement of the cauda equina.

Recommendations for Avoiding Bladder Dysfunction

1. Withdraw the point of the needle to the edge of the subarachnoid space, just within the theca.
2. Rotate the patient backwards before injection of phenol, because this also keeps the neurolytic solution away from the center of the subarachnoid space.
3. Injections should be stopped immediately if, after the test dose, symptoms and signs are noted at locations neurologically remote from the injection site.
4. When treating upper lumbar sites, it is safer to introduce the needle at L_{2-3} or L_{3-4} and tilt the table in a slight Trendelenburg position. Phenol drifts away from the vulnerable sacral roots and gravitates onto the upper lumbar nerves.

In the higher parts of the colon innervation is supplied via the celiac ganglion. This ganglion can play an important role in the conduction of pain, directly from the colon or from liver metastases.

In some patients nerve fibers from the lower part of the colon can pass the celiac ganglion, as well as the superior mesenteric ganglion. The introduction of alcohol into the celiac ganglion can give dramatic pain relief. Our method is to do so under direct X-ray control. Before the alcohol, we inject on each side 5 cc 1% Lignocaine (lidocaine). Five minutes later we introduce 25 cc 50% alcohol on each side.

Other Methods of Pain Relief

1. Intrathecal saline E.S.O.
2. Percutaneous cordotomy
3. Electrostimulation
4. Introduction of alcohol into the sella turcica and hyperthermia

1. Intrathecal Saline E.S.O. The reluctance of some physicians to accept the irreversible consequences of the intrathecal infection of phenol or alcohol has led to the development of a number of variants of this technique. One of these is the intrathecal injection of a hypertonic saline solution. For this purpose NaCl (8-14%), either at normal body temperature or cooled to 4°C, is recommended. This treatment is said to selectively affect the pain-conducting C fibers. Large series have not been reported yet. The alleviation sometimes persists for more than three months.

Another method currently under development is that of the barbotage of cerebrospinal fluid, 20 ml of lumbar fluid being withdrawn and re-injected at the level of L3/L4. This is repeated 15-20 times in one session. The procedure is thought to lead to demyelinization of the nerve fibers. The results range from nil to good. Alleviation lasting longer than six months is sometimes obtained.

2. Percutaneous cordotomy. Surgical cordotomy provides the most certain method of relieving intractable pain of organic origin. On logical grounds it might be thought that surgical cordotomy would be in considerable vogue for the treatment of the intractable pain of inoperable carcinoma but such is not the case. Most neurosurgical units did, and do, relatively few such operations and it is not difficult to understand the reasons for this if one bears in mind the heavy surgical and nursing burdens involved in treating this group of patients.

Furthermore, many patients suffering from intractable pain due to malignant disease have already undergone one or more major operations. They are often in poor health and are unwilling to submit to further surgery, and their medical advisors are reluctant to insist on such a course.

In recent years, the introduction of percutaneous cervical cordotomy has changed some of these attitudes. Percutaneous cordotomy is performed by inserting an intrathecal spinal needle laterally below the mastoid process. An electrode is passed down this needle into the spinothalamic tract which is subsequently destroyed by an electromagnetic current (diathermy). Thus there is no incision, no removal of bone, no opening of the dural sheath and, therefore, no waiting for healing of wound and skin. The stay in the hospital is short: five or six days suffices for the uncomplicated unilateral case. Rarely is a patient so ill that a percutaneous cervical cordotomy cannot be carried out.

Lipton (5) from the Center for Pain Relief at Liverpool wrote the following:

Value of cordotomy

It must be stated that the Centre for Pain Relief uses all commonly accepted techniques for relieving pain but in the malignant group of patients has found that there is no other method that can approach the high percentage of total freedom of pain attained by the percutaneous cervical cordotomy. It must be emphasised that although freedom from pain is produced, the patient still has all the other concomitants of malignant disease – the anorexia, debility, weakness, general discomfort, and the like, which are unaltered. Relief of their constant pain removes an intolerable burden from these patients but life may still be somewhat miserable and therefore it is suggested that the use of the percutaneous cervical cordotomy should be encouraged at an early stage of the disease.

3. Electrostimulation. Electrostimulation, either transcutaneous or dorsal column, can be used for pain relief in cancer patients. It is known that in some cases the patients develop tolerance to electrical stimulation but, as with opiates, in the case of cancer patients this is of no importance.

4. Injection of the pituirary with alcohol. This method is used mainly in patients with hormone-dependent tumors. But some reports mention the choice of this method for severe pain due to generalized metastases of all kind of tumors (6).

5. Hyperthermia. There is a revived interest in this method, which has been known for over a hundred years. Tumor cells, especially of mesodermal origin, are more vulnerable to temperatures over $40\,°C$, which do not affect normal tissues, and regression of tumors has occurred in patients who have had attacks of erysipelas. Technical problems have been encountered in raising the body temperature, perhaps several times, without endangering an already precarious hold on life. Toxins are debilitating, pyrogenic solutions are unreliable, a mechanical heat-exchanger using an arteriovenous shunt involves surgery, and the surface application of heat, as in a hot bath sufficient to raise the body temperature $4\,°C$, carries a high risk of thermal damage to the skin.

It appears that a $4\,°C$ rise in temperature is optimum and this requires a quarter of a million calories of energy. Hyperthermia should be induced rapidly, and special measures for insulation must be instituted because the body loses heat to the outside atmosphere at a prodigious rate.

The results of this small series are encouraging, but much more work is needed to confirm this promise. It appears that a malignancy of mesodermal origin, like bone metastasis, is particularly susceptible to hyperthermia and it remains to be seen whether other tumors will also respond well to this treatment. In the meantime, improved methods of heating inhaled gases, and more efficient circuits are being investigated.

REFERENCES

1. Twycross RG: Diseases of the central nervous system. Relief of terminal pain. *Br Med J* 4: 212-214, 1975.
2. Saunders C: The need in patient care for the patient with terminal cancer. *Middlesex, Hospital Journal* 72: no. 3, 1973.
3. Spierdijk J and Kweekel-De Vries WJ: Experiences with bezitramide (an oral morphinomime-

tic) and Aspegic (a parenteral acetylsalicylate). Multidisciplinary approach to pain patients in Leyden University Hospital. *Anaesthesiology, Proceedings of the Fifth World Congress of Anaesthesiologists, Kyoto, September 19-23, 1972.*

4. Mehta M: *Major problems in anaesthesia: intractable pain.* W.B. Saunders, 1973.

5. Lipton S: Percutaneous cervical cordotomy and the injection of the pituitary with alcohol. *Anaesthesia* 33: 953-957, 1978.

6. Morica G: Chemical Hypophysectomy for cancer pain. *Adv Neurol* 4, 1974, Raven Press.

30. FOLLOW-UP: FREQUENCY AND METHODS

RENÉ C.J. VERSCHUEREN

Numerous reports in the literature confirm the fact that salvage of patients with colorectal cancer treated by surgical resection has reached a plateau in the past decades. There is no doubt that early detection, screening of the population-at-risk and awareness of the need to perform 'good' cancer surgery are possible means of increasing the survival rate. The duration of survival and the cure rate are neat statistical data that everybody tries to improve. However, for those patients for whom surgery was not curative, the quality of life during the remaining years is equally important as the duration of survival.

There is a general acceptance of defeat and hopelessness among surgeons when facing tumor recurrence, and patients are condemned to linger miserably without a sound attempt to evaluate their condition. During a careful follow-up a recurrent tumor may be detected at an early stage when curative treatment is still possible or at least good palliation can be provided. Should the recurrent cancer not be eligible for surgery or radiotherapy, the surgeon is in the best position to prescribe the appropriate pain medication when needed. Being aware of the spread of the disease and the origin of the pain, the surgeon should be able to tailor the medication to the individual needs of the patient.

Today's patients are aware of scientific progress and of exotic treatments that are spreading like wildfire. If we want the patients to keep believing in traditional surgery we should offer them a sound follow-up after resection for colorectal cancer, thus providing them with the support of knowing that their surgeon cares and is honestly trying to keep them out of trouble or is at least attempting to limit the problems should cancer recur.

The follow-up should be done by the surgeon. It is very bad practice to rely on the general practitioner to refer the patient back to the surgeon when problems arise. The family doctor cannot be expected to be aware of the early signs of recurrent disease, and if he does refer the patient he is likely to do so after considerable delay.

Since the vast majority of the Dutch population is satisfactorily covered by health insurance, frequent follow-up visits do not put a financial burden on the patient. However, the surgeons ought to be aware of the fact that over-consumption of diagnostic procedures during follow-up contributes towards making our health system tremendously expensive. Knowledge of when and where recurrent disease is likely to develop in the individual case and awareness of the indications and limitations of available diagnostic procedures are the essential prerequisites for providing appropriate follow-up.

1. GOALS OF THE POST-OPERATIVE FOLLOW-UP

1.1. Early Post-Operative Control

During the first weeks after surgery most patients are still in the process of recovering from the mental stress of surgery, the knowledge of their diagnosis and eventually the mutilating effect of an abdomino-perineal excision or a temporary colostomy. During this period of decreased psychological balance the slightest abdominal discomfort is likely to make the patient fear that something is seriously wrong. The family doctor is often unable to convince the patient that he is unduly concerned, and only the surgeon will succeed in making the patient believe that the small aches are the normal consequences of surgery. Moreover the patients derive an enormous emotional reassurance from repeated 'negative' examinations.

Bladder dysfunction, often arising after pelvic surgery, can successfully be taken care of if early warning signs, such as urinary tract infection, are recognized.

The presence of a temporary or permanent stoma can be the origin of discomforting practical problems. Very often the patient is taught how to manage his stoma while recovering from surgery, but once at home he has to face minor unforeseen problems. Lack of adequate follow-up in stomal care and leaking appliances may have a very detrimental influence on the quality of life and put an additional burden on both the patient and his family. Regular visits in the early post-operative period will allow the patients to reveal their problems and receive appropriate advice from the surgeon or the enterostomal therapist.

1.2. Detection of the Metachronous Second Primary in the Colon

After surgery for colorectal cancer 3 to 5% of the patients will develop a second primary in the colon (1, 2). We should bear in mind that some of these metachronous tumors may be synchronous tumors that were overlooked at the time of surgery for the first primary. Therefore it is very important early in the follow-up to thoroughly examine the remaining colon whenever this was not done before emergency resection had to be carried out.

It is generally accepted that the majority of the colonic cancers arise in a pre-existing polyp (3). Detection and removal of newly formed polyps which become obvious during follow-up are a warranted means of staying ahead of the polyp-cancer sequence. This is confirmed by the results of the 25-year study of periodic proctosigmoidoscopy carried out among an asymptomatic population at the University of Minnesota Cancer Detection Center (4). All the polyps detected at the yearly proctosigmoidoscopy were removed. As a result 85% of the statistically anticipated cancers of the rectosigmoid colon did not develop. In all but one of the cancers that developed between examinations, invasion did not penetrate deeper than the submucosal layer. Extrapolating these results to the population-at-risk after surgery for colorectal cancer, removal of all neoplastic polyps appearing during the follow-up should considerably decrease the likelihood of second cancers elsewhere in the colon. The widespread use of colonoscopy allows for safe removal of the vast majority of the polyps by the endoscopic route (5). This technique being safe in experienced hands, an aggressive attitude towards asymptomatic polyps is warranted.

1.3. Detection of Recurrent Cancer

Although follow-up examinations are time-consuming and expensive, they should be scheduled to permit timely discovery of recurrent cancer with the intent of allowing control of the disease or at least extending the period of comfortable life. Two-thirds of the recurrences are apparent within two years of the initial operation (6, 7). If recurrent disease does not develop within the first five years of surgery, it is highly likely that it will not develop at all.

1.3.1. Local recurrences. Recurrence of rectal carcinoma within the confines of the pelvis after complete excision of the primary tumor is considered to be the cause of more than half of the surgical failures of these operations (8, 9). Ten to twenty-five percent of the patients with an anterior resection subsequently develop a suture line recurrence (10). Pelvic recurrences usually involve the posterior vaginal wall and the cul-de-sac in females. In males recurrent pelvic disease often becomes obvious in the presacral space, the perineum, the bladder and the prostate gland (11).

1.3.2. Pulmonary metastases. In the joint postmortem study carried out by several Japanese Institutes, 35.2% of the patients proved to have pulmonary metastases (12). Sixty-four percent of the lung metastases occur within the first five years of follow-up and their excision may yield a five-year survival of 35% (13).

1.3.3. Liver metastases. In Shindo's series (12) 66.4% of the patients who died due to recurrent tumor had hepatic metastases. These hepatic metastases are solitary and thus resectable in only 5% of the cases. After hepatic lobectomy a five-year survival of 42% has been obtained (14).

1.3.4. Miscellaneous locations of recurrent disease. Hematogenic dissemination can give rise to a variety of localizations of metastasis, such as bone and brain, but the relative frequency is too small to warrant the inclusion of investigations such as bone scans or brain scans in the routine follow-up.

2. DIAGNOSTIC TECHNIQUES FOR THE DETECTION OF RECURRENT OR SECOND PRIMARY CANCER

During the past decade new diagnostic tools have become available. Some of these techniques are relatively inexpensive; for others, such as axial computer tomography, a vast investment is required. Cheap routine laboratory tests can make the total expense of the follow-up very high when performed too frequently. When setting up the follow-up schedule and deciding which investigations should be carried out, the surgeons should consider patients factors, expenses, yield and local technical factors. For elderly debilitated patients, who have to travel a long distance to reach the hospital, some compromise with respect to the frequency of the follow-up visits is justified. For every investigation the cost-effectiveness ratio and the degree of expertise available at the individual institute should be taken into consideration. The surgeon should select those diagnostic techniques that give an acceptable yield without causing too much discomfort to the patients or imposing an undue financial burden on the public health system or the individual.

2.1. History

The initial symptoms of recurrent colorectal cancer are often so unspecific that they contribute to the delay in diagnosis in may patients. Moreover, the average patient will tend to repress and deny alarming symptoms like weakness, vague abdominal pain or perineal discomfort. Dull, aching perineal discomfort aggravated by sitting often precedes detectable perineal recurrence by several months (6). The surgeon should actively elicit such a history instead of deferring pursuit of these symptoms until more obvious signs of recurrence are present.

2.2. Physical Examination

A palpable mass, often nodular, in the perineal scar, the abdominal incision, the cul-de-sac, the liver or the orginal bed of the primary neoplasm may be the

early sign of recurrence in asymptomatic patients. Careful digital examination may disclose a recurrence in the suture line or in the soft tissue of the
pelvis after sphincter-preserving operations. In a retrospective review of the
material from the Ellis Fischel State Cancer Hospital the diagnostic yield of
physical examination was investigated (6). In 121 patients with recurrent
disease, examination of the perineum and digital examination disclosed the
tumor in 15% of the cases. Palpation of the liver and vaginal examination
were positive in 7% of the patients. Palpation of the site of resection of the
primary cancer disclosed tumor recurrence in 10% of these 121 patients.

2.3. Proctosigmoidoscopy

This easy and highly reliable examination should be used every six months
during the first three years after a sphincter-preserving type of resection, and
on a yearly basis in all the cases after surgery for colorectal cancer. The goal of
this examination is to detect suture line recurrences or second primaries. The
effectiveness of this technique has been proven by the prospective study at the
Cancer Detection Center of the University of Minnesota (4). With the recent
developments in the field of flexible colonoscopy, flexible sigmoidoscopes
with a working length of about 50 cm have become available. These sigmoidoscopes have a large-bore suction channel and obviate the need of thorough
bowel cleansing before the examination. As a consequence flexible sigmoidoscopy can be carried out as an office procedure. With some experience the
descending colon can be reached in about ten minutes, thus considerably
increasing the extent and the yield of the examination when compared with
conventional rigid proctosigmoidoscopy (15). Some experts even use the
flexible sigmoidoscope instead of the rigid scope for all their diagnostic
procedures.

2.4. Colonoscopy

During the past decade colonoscopy has developed and spread to such an
extent that endoscopists claim that they achieve better results than the radiologist and can complete a total colonoscopy in about 15 min. An experienced
radiologist can perform a complete double-contrast examination of the colon
in about the same time. The major advantage of radiology is the fact that a
permanent document is available for further study and even for a second
opinion. After a colonoscopy the only document left is a written report, and I
sincerely believe that the colonoscopist too is likely to miss smaller tumors,
especially around the hepatic and splenic flexure. Therefore I do not think
that total colonoscopy should be included as a routine procedure in the
follow-up of patients after surgery for colorectal cancer. However, when the

air-contrast barium enema is equivocal, colonoscopy will help to clarify the situation and may lead to the detection of metachronous cancers or polyps (16).

2.5. Chest X-Ray

In the Study of Sloan Kettering, 42% of the patients who developed a solitary lung shadow during follow-up of colorectal cancer proved to be asymptomatic; the opacities were discovered on routine chest films (13). Therefore it is justified to repeat the chest X-rays every 6 months during the first three years of follow-up. Subsequently one X-ray a year is enough. The solitary lung shadow eventually seen on the X-ray has a equal chance of being a primary lung tumor or a metastasis. This ambiguity requires clarification without delay in order to allow for early institution of the proper treatment.

2.6. Barium Enema

The double contrast enema is a very reliable technique for the detection of a second primary tumor and, if properly performed, does not cause more discomfort than colonoscopy. By repeating this examination every two years, one is being very careful to detect metachronous tumors at a early stage.

2.7. Intravenous Urography

This examination should only be used when symptoms require examination of the urinary tract. Routine use of the I.V.P. gives a very low yield.

2.8. Axial Computer Tomography

The C.T. scan is still too new to have a place in the routine follow-up, but it may be useful for localization of suspected local recurrences after an A.P. resection. When the liver scans are equivocal, computer tomography may help clarify the situation.

2.9. Liver Function Tests

Alkaline phosphatase, 5 nucleotidase and LDH have such a poor sensitivity that they can only be used for screening purposes.

2.10. Liver Scan

The accuracy of liver scans in detecting hepatic metastasis is very poor and therefore they have no place in the routine follow-up schedule. However, when liver metastases are suspected on clinical or biochemical grounds, the liver scan can be useful if followed by hepatic angiography. The combination of these two techniques is a highly accurate tool.

2.11. Carcino-Embryonic Antigen

One of the major practical applications of the carcino-embryonic antigen (CEA) assay is the post-operative monitoring of patients with colorectal carcinoma. However, it is absolutely necessary to have preoperative CEA levels available in order to determine whether the malignancy is producing CEA. Some cancers of the colon do not produce significant CEA elevations even before surgery so that the CEA level may be an unreliable marker in the postoperative period (17). In the retrospective study of Sloan Kettering (18) 92% of the patients with liver metastases had an elevated CEA level, whereas the CEA level was increased in only 50% of the patients with local recurrences. The CEA assay nevertheless may predict tumor recurrence several months in advance of the clinical diagnosis and thus permit surgical intervention in selected patients and earlier initiation of palliation in others. Herrera even advises contemplating a second-look procedure if three successive elevations of CEA are found within a two-week interval (19.) Ultimately only randomized clinical studies will determine whether second-look surgery motivated by elevated CEA levels can improve the quality and length of survival for patients with colorectal carcinoma.

CONCLUSIONS

The goal of the follow-up of patients with colorectal carcinoma is to detect local recurrences, metastases and metachronous lesions as soon as possible in order to allow prompt institution of the appropriate therapy. This follow-up schedule should be adapted to the risk factors and the therapeutic consequences while taking the age of the patient into consideration. For patients over the age of 70 the detection of distant metastases to lungs or liver in the postoperatieve period has very few therapeutic consequences, and the follow-up schedule should be drawn up accordingly. However for younger patients the early detection of recurrent disease may lead to cure or at least effective palliation. If the first operation was a proper standard cancer operation, the chances of cure by re-resection are very small. Some authors obtain a good cure rate after re-resection (7, 20) but do not comment on the adequacy of the primary resection. In this respect Polk and Spratt state that they have yet to 'cure' a patient of his local perineal recurrence after a standard primary operation (21). There is no doubt that every patient should have a chance of repeat surgery, but we have to wonder whether the individual case in going to benefit from it and to what extent survival and the quality of life will be influenced. In the majority of the cases the treatment of recurrent disease will not be curative, but the palliative effect will be better if careful follow-up leads to early detection and hence early initiation of the appropriate treatment.

REFERENCES

1. Bussey H Jr, Wallace MH and Morson BC: Metachronous carcinoma of the large intestine and intestinal polyps. *Proc Roy Soc Med* 60: 208-210, 1967.
2. Ginzburg L and Dreiling PA: Successive independent (metachronous) carcinomas of the colon. *Ann Surg* 143: 117-119, 1956.
3. Muto T, Bussey HJR and Morson BC: The evolution of cancer of colon and rectum. *Cancer* 36: 2251-2270, 1975.
4. Gilbertsen VA: Proctosigmoidoscopy and polypectomy in reducing the incidence of rectal cancer. *Cancer* 34: 936-939, 1974.
5. Wolff WI and Shinya H: Earlier diagnosis of cancer of the colon through colonic endoscopy (colonoscopy) *Cancer* 34: 912-931, 1974.
6. Polk HC Jr and Spratt JS Jr: Recurrent colorectal carcinoma: detection, treatment and other considerations. *Surgery* 69: 9-23, 1971.
7. Berge T, Ekelund G, Mellner C, Pihl B and Wenckert A: Carcinoma of the colon and rectum in a defined population. *Acta Chirur Scand (Suppl)* 438, 1973.
8. Stearns MW Jr and Debbisch MR: Five-year results of abdominopelvic lymph node dissection for carcinoma of the rectum. *Dis Colon Rectum* 2: 169-172, 1959.
9. Gunderson LL and Sosin H: Areas of failure found at reoperation (second look or symptomatic look) following 'curative surgery' for adenocarcinoma of the rectum. *Cancer* 34: 1278-1292, 1974.
10. Wilson SM and Beahrs OH: The curative treatment of carcinoma of the sigmoid, rectosigmoid and rectum. *Ann Surg* 183: 556-565, 1976.
11. Gilbertsen VA: Adenocarcinoma of the rectum: Incidence and location of recurrent tumor following present-day operations performed for cure. *Ann Surg* 151: 340-348, 1960.
12. Shindo K: Recurrence of carcinoma of the large intestine. A statistical review *Amer J Proctol* 25: 80-90, 1974.
13. Cahan WG, Castro EB and Hajdu SI: The significance of a solitary lung shadow in patients with colon carcinoma. *Cancer* 33: 414-421, 1974.
14. Wilson SM and Adson MA: Surgical treatment of hepatic metastases from colorectal cancers *Arch Surg* 111: 330-334, 1976.
15. Marks G, Boggs HW, Castro AF, Gatright JB, Ray JE and Salvati E: Sigmoidoscopic examinations with rigid and flexible fiberoptic sigmoidoscopes in the surgeon's office: a comparative prospective study of effectiveness in 1.012 cases. *Dis Colon Rectum* 22: 162-168, 1979.
16. McKelvey STD: The management of suspected tumours of the colon: the role of colonoscopy in general surgery. *Br J Surg* 66: 306-308, 1979.
17. Martin EW, Kibbey WE, DiVechia L, Anderson G, Catalano P and Minton JP: Carcinoembryonic antigen, clinical and historical aspects *Cancer* 37: 62-81, 1976.
18. Wanebo HJ, Stearns M and Schwartz MK: Use of CEA as an indicator of early recurrence and as a guide to a selected second-look procedure in patients with colorectal carcinoma. *Ann Surg* 188: 481-492, 1978.
19. Herrera AM, Chu TM and Holyoke ED: Carcinoembryonic Antigen (CEA) as a prognostic and monitoring test in clinically complete resection of colorectal carcinoma. *Ann Surg* 183: 5-9, 1976.

20. Welch JP and Donaldsoo GA: Detection and treatment of recurrent cancer of the colon and rectum *Amer J Surg* 135: 505-511, 1978.
21. Polk HC Jr and Spratt JS Jr: The results of treatment of perineal recurrence of cancer of the rectum. *Cancer* 43: 952-955, 1979.